2024

全国医学博士英语统考

综合应试教程 第15版

环球卓越医学考博命题研究中心 / 组编

张秀峰 / 主编　梁莉娟 / 副主编

机械工业出版社

CHINA MACHINE PRESS

本书是卫健委组织的全国医学博士英语统一考试辅导丛书的一个分册。

　　本书共分为五章，第一章为听力理解，第二章为词汇，第三章为完形填空，第四章为阅读理解，第五章为写作。本书具有讲解内容全面、针对性强、编写质量过硬三大特点。全书紧密围绕大纲要求和历年真题这一主线进行编写，包含最新医学考博真题，详细讲解各种题型的命题特点和应试方法，是一本很有针对性的应试辅导用书。

图书在版编目（CIP）数据

全国医学博士英语统考综合应试教程／环球卓越医学考博命题研究中心组编；
张秀峰主编. —15版. —北京：机械工业出版社，2023.7
卓越医学考博英语应试教材
ISBN 978-7-111-73505-2

Ⅰ.①全…　Ⅱ.①环…②张…　Ⅲ.①医学－英语－博士生入学考试－教材　Ⅳ.①R

中国国家版本馆CIP数据核字（2023）第127860号

机械工业出版社（北京市百万庄大街22号　邮政编码100037）
策划编辑：孙铁军　　　责任编辑：孙铁军　苏筛琴
责任校对：张晓娟　　　责任印制：张　博
保定市中画美凯印刷有限公司印刷
2023年9月第15版第1次印刷
184mm×260mm・27.25印张・727千字
标准书号：ISBN 978-7-111-73505-2
定价：89.80元

电话服务　　　　　　　　　网络服务
客服电话：010-88361066　　机　工　官　网：www.cmpbook.com
　　　　　010-88379833　　机　工　官　博：weibo.com/cmp1952
　　　　　010-68326294　　金　书　网：www.golden-book.com
封底无防伪标均为盗版　机工教育服务网：www.cmpedu.com

丛书序
PREFACE

　　这是一套由全国知名医学博士英语统考培训机构"环球卓越"（优路教育旗下品牌）策划，联手医学博士英语资深辅导专家，为众多志在考取医学博士的考生量身定制的应试辅导用书。国家医学考试中心于2019年底修订了考试大纲，对全国医学博士外语统一考试的题型及各部分分值进行了局部调整。新大纲仍然设置了听力对话、听力短文、词语用法、完形填空、阅读理解和书面表达6种题型，但调整了具体命题形式，其中听力部分变化最大。"15个短对话＋1个长对话＋2个短文"的经典组合成为历史，从2020年开始，"5个短对话＋5个小短文"的搭配将在很长一段时间内成为考生要面对的题型。考试时间为3个小时（含播放录音及收发卷时间）。

　　考纲的变化并未改变对考生能力的考查方向，因此为了帮助广大考生在较短的时间内系统备考，在听、说、读、写4个方面得到强化训练，全面提高英语应用和交际能力，顺利通过考试，本套"卓越医学考博英语应试教材"仍然是广大考生朋友们很好的选择。本丛书紧密结合最近几年卫健委组织的医学博士英语统一考试命题情况，针对最新考试大纲进行了修订，并针对新题型编写了大量针对性练习。本丛书包含《全国医学博士英语统考词汇巧战通关》《全国医学博士英语统考综合应试教程》《全国医学博士英语统考实战演练》三本传统综合分册，《医学考博阅读理解高分全解》《医学考博英语听力28天训练计划》两本专项分册，以及《18天攻克医学考博英语核心词》的单词小分册。传统分册从基础到综合再到真题实战，从模块详解到全套试题，高屋建瓴，逐步推进。阅读专项分册对分支较大的阅读理解进行字、词、句、语篇的详解和训练，从技术（语言知识）到技巧（做题方法），精讲多练。听力专项分册则根据听力训练的规律和考试考查目标，按天设置训练内容，分解目标，逐步达成最终目标。

　　本丛书的特点如下：

一、紧贴考试，实用性强

　　策划编写本丛书的作者常年在教学一线授课，从基础英语到医博考前辅导，积累了大量的应试辅导实战经验。丛书内容是他们多年辅导经验的提炼和结晶，实用性非常强，专为医学考博考生定制，是目前市面上较全面、系统的医学考博英语应试教材。

二、紧扣大纲，直击真题

　　本丛书紧扣最新大纲，体例设置与大纲保持一致；各部分考点紧密结合最新历年真题，还原真实考场环境，命题思路分析透彻，重点突出，讲解精确；各部分内容严格控制在大纲规定的范围之内，让考生准确把握考试的重点、难点及命题趋势。

三、内容精练，讲练结合

传统分册《全国医学博士英语统考词汇巧战通关》《全国医学博士英语统考综合应试教程》和《全国医学博士英语统考实战演练》简单精练，通过突破词汇基础关、学习各个题型应试方法以及在高质量实战中历练，考生可在有限的时间内进行全面复习，把握重点，比较系统地完成考前准备。阅读分册《医学考博阅读理解高分全解》则是根据考生的具体情况，分模块予以详解，提升基础，总结技巧，各个击破。听力专项《医学考博英语听力28天训练计划》则专练听力，循序渐进，按天分配学习任务，力争高分。核心词汇专项《18天攻克医学考博英语核心词》在使用词频软件完整统计近十年全套真题的基础上，将该统计结果和大纲词汇进行比较，最后确定出记忆任务的内容和安排。按天设置，不断重复。

四、超值服务，锦上添花

本丛书附带赠送精品服务，由优路教育为每位购书读者提供专业的服务和强大的技术支持。具体为：

1. 《医学考博英语听力28天训练计划》附赠内容：优路教育"2024年医学考博（统考）《英语听力28天训练计划》图书赠课英语（20节）"网络视频课程。使用方法：刮开书籍封底的兑换码，扫描书籍封底二维码关注【优路医学考试】微信公众账号后，点击【兑换课程】-【点击这里兑换课程】的链接，输入兑换码，输入姓名手机号，将自动跳转至您的课程页，开始观看课程。后续看课路径：关注【优路医学考试】服务号，在底部菜单栏【我要学习】-【我的课程】查看课程。（可通过扫描文末二维码，关注后兑换课程）

2. 《18天攻克医学考博英语核心词》附赠内容：优路教育"2024年医学考博（统考）《18天攻克医学考博英语核心词》图书赠课英语（20节）"网络视频课程。使用方法：刮开书籍封底的兑换码，扫描书籍封底二维码关注【优路医学考试】微信公众账号后，点击【兑换课程】-【点击这里兑换课程】的链接，输入兑换码，输入姓名手机号，将自动跳转至您的课程页，开始观看课程。后续看课路径：关注【优路医学考试】服务号，在底部菜单栏【我要学习】-【我的课程】查看课程。（可通过扫描文末二维码，关注后兑换课程）

3. 《全国医学博士英语统考实战演练》附赠内容：优路教育"2024年医学考博（统考）《实战演练》图书赠课英语（10节）"网络视频课程。使用方法：刮开书籍封底的兑换码，扫描书籍封底二维码关注【优路医学考试】微信公众账号后，点击【兑换课程】-【点击这里兑换课程】的链接，输入兑换码，输入姓名手机号，将自动跳转至您的课程页，开始观看课程。后续看课路径：关注【优路医学考试】服务号，在底部菜单栏【我要学习】-【我的课程】查看课程。（可通过扫描文末二维码，关注后兑换课程）

4. 《全国医学博士英语统考综合应试教程》附赠内容：优路教育"2024年医学考博（统考）《综合应试教程》图书赠课英语（10节）"网络视频课程。使用方法：刮开书籍封底的兑换码，扫描书籍封底二维码关注【优路医学考试】微信公众账号后，点击【兑换课程】-【点击这里兑换课程】的链接，输入兑换码，输入姓名手机号，将自动跳转至您的课程页，开始观看课程。后续看课路径：关注【优路医学考试】服务号，在底部菜单栏【我要学习】-【我的课程】查看课程。（可通过扫描文末二维码，关注后兑换课程）

5.《全国医学博士英语统考综词汇巧战通关》附赠内容：优路教育"2024年医学考博（统考）《词汇巧战通关》图书赠课【学习卡】英语（10节）"网络视频课程。使用方法：刮开书籍封底的兑换码，扫描书籍封底二维码关注【优路医学考试】微信公众账号后，点击【兑换课程】-【点击这里兑换课程】的链接，输入兑换码，输入姓名手机号，将自动跳转至您的课程页，开始观看课程。后续看课路径：关注【优路医学考试】服务号，在底部菜单栏【我要学习】-【我的课程】查看课程。（可通过扫描文末二维码，关注后兑换课程）

6.《医学考博阅读理解高分全解》附赠内容：优路教育"2024年医学考博（统考）《阅读理解高分全解》图书赠课【学习卡】英语（8节）"网络视频课程。使用方法：刮开书籍封底的兑换码，扫描书籍封底二维码关注【优路医学考试】微信公众账号后，点击【兑换课程】-【点击这里兑换课程】的链接，输入兑换码，输入姓名手机号，将自动跳转至您的课程页，开始观看课程。后续看课路径：关注【优路医学考试】服务号，在底部菜单栏【我要学习】-【我的课程】查看课程。（可通过扫描文末二维码，关注后兑换课程）

优路教育技术支持及服务热线400-8835-981，可以帮您解决兑换及观看课程中的技术问题。您也可以登录优路教育网站www.youlu.com，在"医学博士英语"栏目下获取更多的学习资料和资讯。

编　者

2023 年 3 月于北京

扫码关注后兑换课程

前 言
FOREWORD

　　本书是卫健委组织的全国医学博士英语统一考试辅导丛书之一，编者在结合 2019 年出版的最新考试大纲和对最新真题进行分析的基础上进行了修订。

　　本书是为了帮助广大考生在较短的时间内系统备考，顺利通过考试而量身定制的。修订版增加了部分最新真题，以便考生掌握最新考试动向。

　　全书共分五章：

　　第一章为**听力理解**，通过新大纲样题和仿真模拟题讲解了听力理解部分的测试特点、应试技巧与方法以及听力常考用语，并配有专项练习和解析；修订版的听力部分结合最新大纲的要求全部更新了题型和讲解，解析部分更是精心制作，不仅含有听力原文和题目、选项对应的中文翻译，还针对不同题型的解题技巧做出了详细讲解，真正做到讲练结合，旨在帮助考生有效地运用应试技巧，具有极强的指导性。本次修订增加了 2020—2023 年部分真题，考生能更加真切地体会到新大纲指导下的命题思路。

　　第二章为**词汇**，通过真题演练讲解了词汇部分测试内容和应试方法，并详细介绍了几种词汇记忆方法和重点的词根和词缀；结合例句对常考词组进行讲解，并配有专项练习和详细解析。此外，修订版将近三年真题作为词汇测试部分中的真题演练，并根据不同题型重新编排。这样，考生在掌握了必要的解题技巧后，能够最直接地将不同的解题技巧运用到相应的真题中，可大大增加考生的应试能力。

　　第三章为**完形填空**，结合最新真题讲解了完形填空的命题特点和应试方法，通过专项练习进行训练，并给出详细解析。

　　第四章为**阅读理解**，通过真题分析了阅读理解必备的语法知识、长难句结构、阅读理解各类题型应试方法，以及阅读理解整体答题方法。通过专项练习进行训练，练习部分附有详细解析，并重新修订配套练习的解析，附上题目、选项的中文详解，将答案出处清楚标明，并给予详细中文解释。考生认真练习后，能从答案、解题技巧等多方面得到有益帮助。

　　第五章为**写作**，依据真题对评卷人掌握的评分原则、写作常见问题和对策、写作常用词语和句子、写作常用医学词汇进行一一讲解，同时配有大量练习，并根据解题要领和步骤给出详细的解析和参考范文，有助于考生解决"不知如何写、写什么"的难题，让考生真正掌握正确完成英文摘要写作的要领。"命题作文和翻译解析"简明扼要地对这两种题型进行了解读，让考生有备无患。本次修订增加了 2022—2023 年真题详解，让考生真正掌握作文和翻译题型的命题思路和应对技巧。

本书具备以下特点：

1. **讲解内容全面。**本书根据考试题型，分专项编写，各章详细讲解了各个专项复习的要点和方法，内容全面，重点突出。

2. **配套最新真题及详解。**修订版将最新真题作为各项题目的配套练习，这样考生能直接接触真题，并在真题训练中，重点演练各项解题技巧。

3. **针对性较强。**本书各个部分都是在分析历年医学博士考试的基础上编写的，紧紧围绕考试要求进行讲解，完全为医博考生定制，是一本专业的医学博士应试教材。

4. **编写质量过硬。**作者常年在医学院校任教，多年参与医学博士的阅卷工作，对医学博士英语考试的命题有比较深入的研究，对医学博士英语考试的材料来源有深入的追踪和分析。在这一背景下，作者进行了有效的选材，使本书非常适合医学博士英语考生的考前复习。

在编写过程中，本书始终围绕大纲要求和历年真题这一主线来讲解各个题型的命题特点和应试方法，提高了其作为应试教材的针对性。

由于编者水平有限，书中不妥之处在所难免，衷心希望广大读者批评指正！

编　者

2023 年 5 月于北京

目 录
CONTENTS

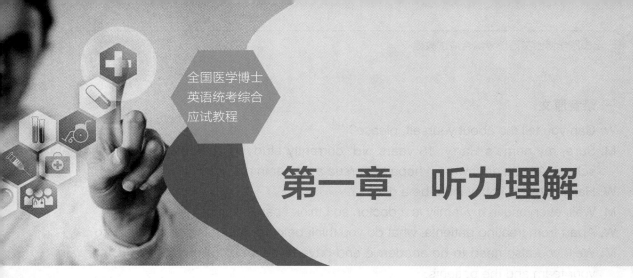

全国医学博士
英语统考综合
应试教程

第一章　听力理解

一、考试大纲要求、试卷结构与考试特点

（一）考试大纲要求及试卷结构

《全国医学博士外语统一考试英语考试大纲》于 2019 年 12 月进行了修订，并于 2020 年考试启用（以下简称新大纲）。与旧大纲相比，新大纲题型中对听力部分做出了重大修订。

根据 2019 年国家考试中心出版的最新大纲，全国统考听力理解分两部分：Section A 和 Section B，答题时间为 30 分钟。

Section A：对话

本部分共 5 个对话，每个对话分别由 100 个左右的单词组成，旨在测试考生对英语对话的听力理解能力，要求考生能理解对话的中心思想和主要内容，并能根据听到的内容进行逻辑推理、分析概括和归纳总结。题型包括大意概括题、具体细节题和判断推理题。每个对话附有 3 个小题，每个小题附有 4 个选项，要求考生在听完每个对话之后，根据所听内容于 12 秒内选出 1 个最佳答案。对话及问题只读 1 遍。

Section A 部分共 15 小题，序号 1~15，每题 1 分，共计 15 分。

我们先来看看新大纲 Section A 部分的例题。🎧

1. A. Switching to biology and chemistry.　B. Choosing to be a family physician.
   C. Going to college.　D. Being a doctor.
2. A. Because of his family's influence.
   B. Because of the fact that he's young.
   C. Because of the practical skills he has.
   D. Because of his love for biology and chemistry.
3. A. A strong sense of responsibility.　B. Good communicative skills.
   C. Excellent health.　D. Great patience.

▶ 录音原文

W: Can you tell me about yourself, please?

M: Sure, my name's Harry, 18 years old, currently studying biology and chemistry at school. As you are aware, I hope to pursue a career in medicine.

W: Harry, why do you want to be a doctor?

M: Well, everyone in my family is a doctor, so I think I can follow on nicely.

W: Apart from treating patients, what do you think being a doctor is going to require?

M: Well, you also need to be academic and have to be an excellent communicator with your team and the patients.

1. What are the two speakers talking about?

2. Why does Harry choose to be a doctor?

3. What is mentioned by Harry as one of the requirements for a doctor?

✓ 答案速记　DAB

🔍 题型分析

1. 从场景上看，本对话与医患场景无关，而是面试场合，对话中涉及与医学相关的极为基础简单的词汇，比如 doctor。

2. 从考点上看，第 1 题为大意概括题，第 2、3 题均为具体细节题。因此，把握细节仍是得分的重中之重。

3. 从对话轮次上看，该对话为多轮次（老大纲多为一个轮次），因此把握轮次间的语义走向是很重要的。

4. 从命题数量上来看，一个对话对应三道题（老大纲为一个对话对应一道题），即平均下来一个轮次对应一道题。因此，听懂每个轮次的问题和答案，往往都会有收获。

Section B：短文

本部分共由 5 篇短文组成，每篇短文由 150 个左右的单词组成。旨在测试考生对英语篇章的听力理解能力。要求考生能理解所听短文的中心思想和主要内容，并能根据所听到的内容进行逻辑推理、分析概括和归纳总结。题型包括大意概括题、具体细节题和判断推理题。每篇短文附有 3 个小题，每个小题附有 4 个选项，要求考生在听完每篇短文之后，根据所听内容于 12 秒内选出 1 个最佳答案。短文及问题只读 1 遍。

Section B 部分共 15 小题，序号 16~30，每题 1 分，共计 15 分。

下面我们来看看新大纲 Section B 部分的例题。

▶ 录音原文

16. A. The role of genetic factors.

　　B. The factors that affect health.

　　C. The impact of lifestyle on health.

D. The importance of working conditions.

17. A. People with jobs have less stress.

B. The more education, the less stress.

C. Many factors affect health via stress.

D. Stress is not related to genetic make-up.

18. A. More challenging research on workplace stress.

B. A better understanding of stress-health relationship.

C. A better connection between medical research and practice.

D. More research on the combined effects of health-related factors.

We commonly think that our health is affected by our age, gender, lifestyle and genetic factors that we inherit from our parents. However, these factors are only a small part of what affects our health. Other factors include our social relationships, income, education and working conditions. Let's look at stress for example. Unemployment or poor working conditions create unstable life situations and cause stress, which has negative effects on health. One major factor, education, determines income or employment. However, even if you are employed, some workplace conditions, such as lack of flexibility and control over your workday can cause stress. As you can see, many complex social processes and other factors are connected with one another to affect your health. Studying how these factors work together in large populations is a challenge for researchers and that is what we would like to look at next.

16. What is the passage mainly about?

17. What does the speaker intend to say by mentioning stress?

18. What does the speaker call for at the end of the passage?

✅ 答案速记 **BCD**

🔍 题型分析

1. 从选材上看，短文以医学研究、社会现象或者最新发现为主旨，逻辑清楚，层次分明。

2. 从考点上看，第16题为主旨大意题，第17、18题为简单推理题，短文不像对话那样有提问进行提示，因此，短文是有难度的。

3. 从长度上看，150词左右的文章对应3道题目，文中有的句子就是支撑性内容，并无实际对应考点出现。因此，听懂文章的结构，即"起承转合"的句与句关系，非常重要。

（二）听力理解考试特点

通过对历年考题的分析，可以看出听力理解考试有以下特点：

1. 听力材料内容兼顾日常交际与医学背景

在 Section A 里，多数题目围绕日常对话展开，涉及医学领域、日常生活、现象讨论等，有时对话材料里也会提到医学常用词汇，如常见病或症状。因而，考生应该储备一定量的医学常用词汇，但医学词汇不作为听力测试第一部分的主要考点。在 Section B 中，医学为听力材料的主要背景，涉及常见病症、医学常识等。

2. 题型较为常见且为客观选择题

无论是 Section A 还是 Section B，所有题目均为选择题，这样的题型是考生较为熟悉的形式。而且考试测试点与其他重大英语考试类似：Section A 的题目以测试习惯用语、特殊句式、词组含义、细节与推断题为主，详细的分析将在本章后面阐述；Section B 主要以测试细节和细节衍生为主。因而，从题型上看，考生不会有完全不适应的地方。

3. 口音较为固定、语速较快

对于考生来说，听力测试部分较为不适应的地方应该是听力材料的口音以及语速。每个考生可能对某一种英语口音较为熟悉，如英音或美音。医学博士英语统考听力测试中的发音常为标准的英音，因而，考生在平时应该多接触英音，这样才不至于在考试时觉得很陌生。另外，医学博士英语统考听力测试的语速也较快，连读处更是难点。因而，考生在平时听力训练时，应多加强发音规则和规律训练，以适应考试的语速和口音，这样在正式考试时，心理上就会占一定优势。

二、考查内容及相应的应试技巧

综观听力部分各类考题，考生要重视以下方面的问题：

1. 知识储备很必要

听力中经常会出现句式、词组、习语等，而这些表达往往是解题的关键，因而，考生应在考前注重积累与听力考试相关的语言知识点。

2. 语境信息是关键

无论是 Section A 还是 Section B，听力题目均在一定的语言环境下提出，无论听力材料的长或短，都会给考生足够的语言信息，因而抓住了关键信息或信号词（cue words）就等于找到了解题的密钥。

3. 预读选项有帮助

当听力录音在播放 Directions 或者例子的时候，考生可利用这段时间预读选项。有些题目选项很有特点，考生通过预读选项可以提前知道考点，或者可以通过突出某个选项关键词对选项进行分类，或者还能够提前知道听力对话或短文的话语情景。所以，考生要养成提前看选项的习惯，做到料敌在先。

4. 简单笔记是依靠

在听力考试过程中，由于极度紧张，人的记忆力在那时是有限的。考生经常会有这样的尴尬：在听对话或短文时，信息在脑海里清晰呈现，但是当问题提出后，即将解题时，却怎么也想不起来自己刚才所听到的信息了，结果无法正确解题，同时，紧张情绪增加，十分不利于考试。所以，考生在平时做听力训练的时候，就应养成记笔记的习惯，边听边记是训练听力的好办法。

三、提高听力的技巧

1. 加强短时记忆力

平时训练时，考生听完一段对话或文章后可以进行复述。通过复述可以知道自己是否听懂了，不但巩固了听的内容，而且加强了记忆。因此，考生会发现，只有在听的过程中，按意群捕捉讲述内容，才会有助于记忆。加强记忆力训练，不是一朝一夕的事情，坚持训练，才能循序渐进、不断提高。

2. 精听和泛听相结合

精听是指在有时间保障的情况下对一段内容反复听若干遍，尽量把所有内容都听明白，也可以通过听写把关键的信息（如重点词汇，与事件有关的任务、地点、原因、结果等）写下来检测自己是否听懂了。泛听是指在不特定的空间或时间里听各种材料，这种方法不要求把所有的内容听懂，而是通过听大量的不同材料来熟悉各种人的话语、口音及语速，积累经验，找到语感。因此，精听和泛听应该相结合。

3. 加强辨音能力

近音、同音异义给听力测试增加了难度，往往使考生误选答案。要解决这一问题，就要加强辨音及提高根据上下文正确辨义的能力。另外，还要注意速读、弱读、停顿、英音与美音之间的区别以及发音特点。所以我们平时应该多听读、跟读录音，纠正自己不正确的发音。

4. 听写

考生常常这样抱怨：听的过程中问题很多，跟不上、听不明白、走神、听懂了解不出题。不仅仅是因为听不懂单词导致听不懂句子，也因为耳朵磨得不够多、练习得不够多，导致大脑反应不出来，所以有充足备考时间的同学要花时间做精听练习，坚持三个星期，对解决以上问题有非常大的帮助。听写便是一个很好的练习精听的方式。

什么样的材料是好的听写素材呢？对考博学生来说，听写材料其实可以根据个人的喜好选择，但是需要注意的是：（1）听写的材料不宜过长。如果材料过长，听写的过程就会花费比较长的时间，容易疲倦，难以坚持下去；（2）听写的材料尽量挑选贴近考试水平的文章。

下面简单说一下听写练习的流程：

第一步：总听。了解文章主旨大意，同时把握文章的逻辑框架。

第二步：细听。分节点听写。所谓节点，就是短时记忆能承载的最长的意群，通常是一个短句、从句、较长的形容词、名词短语等。

第三步：精听。反复琢磨遗漏信息的地方。借用基本的语法、语义及语音知识，对即将进行确认的空缺处设定一个信息预期，然后再次听录音，填补信息。

第四步：核对。对照文本，进行最终的核对。

第五步：总结期间碰到的难点和疑点，包括陌生的单词、词组，没听明白的各种发音方式和语音现象等。

第六步：跟读。丢开文本，在短时记忆能承载的最长意群处暂停并进行跟读。

在听写练习中，切忌以下几种情况：

- 对无关紧要的细节过于纠结。切实抓准句子大意是根本，对语气词、名字、特殊名词等，用首字母或者符号代替。
- 把 80% 的精力花在 20% 的事情上。练习过程中听了 5 遍仍没听出所以然的，应该直接对照文本去研究症结在何处。
- 逐词听写。我们听写时按意群停顿，而非 word for word，听两三个词就暂停录音来记录，是绝对不可行的。
- 硬听。能听出来就写，听不出来就坐等第二遍，这与听写练习的初衷背道而驰。练习听写的核心本质其实是为了提高我们快速理解和记忆的能力。听写真正应该做的是记忆和总结的工作，而不是听和写的工作。
- 用对话来作为练习听写的材料。对话类型的材料是不适合拿来练习听写的。对话的难点往往来自于一些音变现象、俚语习惯表达或者对上下文语境的理解，而非句型的表达或内容本身。更合适的材料是某些长度为一分钟左右的话题型文章，最好是与医学相关的话题短文。

听写练习一（A New Blood Test for Cancer）

非考点难点词汇：

University of Swansea in Wales

Gareth Jenkins

esophagus

esophageal cancer

▶ 录音原文

Cancer is a leading cause of death around the world.

When it comes to cancer, the sooner you know you have it, the better your chances of surviving.

A new blood test could change the way doctors and researchers find cancer in patients. Researchers say the test could provide clues to the early forms of the disease.

Scientists at the University of Swansea in Wales came up with the idea.

Gareth Jenkins is a professor at the university. He says he and his team did not look for cancer. They instead looked for a by-product of cancer. They looked for, what Jenkins calls, the collateral damage of cancer — the damage left by the disease.

In this case, the by-product was mutated red blood cells.

The researchers tested blood from about 300 people, all of whom have cancer of the esophagus. Patients with esophageal cancer have high levels of mutated red blood cells. Jenkins says that at this point he is not sure if other cancers would produce similar results.

The hope is that the new test and other non-invasive methods could one day become part of commonly used medical methods. He says that using a battery, or series of tests will be the best way to find out if a person has cancer.

These new technologies could save millions of lives.

听写练习二（Electromagnetic Waves to Treat Depression）

▶ 录音原文

People suffering from depression are finding help when electromagnetic waves enter their brains.

Mental health experts estimate that depression affects more than 120 million people worldwide. It severely affects the person's quality of life and, in extreme cases, can lead to suicide.

Anti-depressant medicines have been shown as an effective treatment for many patients. But the drugs are unable to help some people with the disorder.

For such persons, doctors may suggest deep transcranial magnetic stimulation or DTMS for short.

In this treatment, patients wear a helmet — a large hard hat on their head. The helmet is connected to a machine.

An electric coil in the helmet sends out regular pulses of electromagnetic energy. These beating sounds produce changes in the brain area responsible for the disorder.

Electromagnetic brain stimulation is not new. It was first used to treat depression over 30 years ago. Now, a new generation of wiring can direct the energy to one part of the brain. DTMS starts with daily 20-minute-long treatments for 20 to 30 days. The patient then returns for treatment two to three times a week for several weeks.

The only side effect is sometimes minor head pain.

听写练习三（The Treatment of Alzheimer's）

非考点难点词汇：

Alzheimer's
menstrual pain
mefenamic acid

 录音原文

A surprising discovery has been made in the treatment of Alzheimer's, the brain disease that causes memory loss and other problems.

A drug used to treat women's menstrual pain made memory problems disappear in laboratory animals with Alzheimer's disease.

The researchers gave the medicine — mefenamic acid — to mice with Alzheimer's disease. The scientists say treatment reversed the animals' memory-loss problems.

Alzheimer's is a progressive disease. It worsens over time. It affects many parts of people's lives, including the ability to remember, think and make decisions.

The findings were published in the journal *Nature Communications*. David Brough of Britain's University of Manchester led the research.

听写练习四（The Treatment of Alzheimer's）

录音原文

The scientists did experiments with mice that were engineered to develop Alzheimer's symptoms. Like humans who get the disease, the laboratory mice developed memory problems over time.

Ten of the Alzheimer's mice were treated with mefenamic acid for one month. The drug was contained in very small pump devices placed under their skin. Ten other mice, also with memory problems, had devices placed under their skin too, but theirs did not contain medicine. Then the animals were placed in a maze — a complex group of connected paths. They had to learn how to move around the maze without problems.

Mike Daniels was a researcher on the study. In a Skype interview he said the mice who received the drug learned the maze easily. That was not true for the mice who did not get the medicine.

The researchers were excited by the results with the drug-treated mice.

The researchers say the drug is already approved by the U.S. government and is known to be safe. So, after more testing, mefenamic acid may be available quickly to treat Alzheimer's patients.

听写练习五（The Treatment of Alzheimer's）

非考点难点词汇：

amyloid

amyloid plaques

▶ 录音原文

In another recent study, researchers testing a drug on humans found it slowed the progress of Alzheimer's disease. People were given a drug that fights substances that build up in the brain of Alzheimer's patients.

The substances are called amyloid. They are sticky proteins that group together in the brain. Together, they form what are called amyloid plaques, and are thought to be a cause of Alzheimer's.

The researchers reported that in the brains of those given the treatment, there was an "almost complete clearance" of the amyloid plaques, according to the AFP news agency.

But researchers said that while the results are exciting, it is too early to know if this is an effective treatment for the disease. More tests are planned.

The study results were published in the journal *Nature*.

The World Health Organization says more than 47 million people worldwide are affected by dementia. Nearly eight million new cases are diagnosed each year.

听写练习六（Possible Genetic Causes of Autism）

非考点难点词汇：

autism

Princeton University in New Jersey

Princeton's Lewis-Sigler Institute for Integrative Genomics

▶ 录音原文

The human body has about 25,000 genes. Researchers already know of 65 genes they believe carry a risk for autism. Now, researchers at Princeton University in New Jersey have identified 2,500 more that could help create the conditions for autism.

The discovery is important because the genes could lead scientists toward finding a cause and, possibly, a treatment.

Autism is a condition that makes it difficult for some people to communicate, learn and socialize.

Arjun Krishnan is a researcher at Princeton's Lewis-Sigler Institute for Integrative Genomics. He says researchers used what they called a machine-learning computer program to identify autism-related genes.

Krishnan explains that the program identified similarities between brain-related genes and the 65 autism-risk genes.

Then, the program looked for other genes that are "friends" of both sets.

The findings can also help researchers understand why one person may be only mildly affected with autism, while another is severely affected.

Researchers still have not found a way to diagnose autism, beyond just observing the children. But they hope this new research into gene patterns will lead to a way to diagnose very young children. Then they can be helped as soon as possible.

听写练习七（Sleep Well in Childhood to Prevent Obesity）

▶ 录音原文

Getting a good night's sleep tonight could guard children against weight gain in the future. According to a new study, putting preschoolers in bed by 8 pm could reduce their chances of becoming overweight or obese later in life by half. Preschoolers are children around the age of 4 or 5.

The term "obese" refers to calculations of your Body Mass Index, what doctors call BMI. They use a person's height, weight and age to assess their amount of body fat. BMIS help tell whether a person is underweight, normal, overweight or obese.

The World Health Organization says obesity can lead to serious long-term health problems like diabetes, heart disease and stroke.

听写练习八（Sleep Well in Childhood to Prevent Obesity）

非考点难点词汇：

Ohio State University's College of Public Health
The Journal of Pediatrics
Sarah Anderson

▶ 录音原文

Researchers from the Ohio State University's College of Public Health have found that young children who go to bed after 9 pm are twice as likely to be obese later in life. The researchers wrote their findings in *The Journal of Pediatrics*.

The lead author of the study is Sarah Anderson. She is an associate professor of epidemiology. She studies how diseases spread and how they can be controlled. Anderson says that, for parents, the results of the study support the importance of creating a bedtime routine. She says that having a usual bedtime routine is something "families can do to lower their children's risk" of becoming overweight.

"A usual, early bedtime," Anderson adds, "is also likely to have positive benefits on behavior and on social, emotional and cognitive development."

听写练习九（Sleep Well in Childhood to Prevent Obesity）

非考点难点词汇：
Centers for Disease Control and Prevention

▶ 录音原文

Anderson said putting children in bed early does not mean they will immediately fall asleep. But, she adds, it makes it "more likely that children will get the amount of sleep they need to be at their best".

But Anderson says it is important to understand that having early bedtime may be harder for some families than others. She says that "families have many competing demands and there are trade-offs that get made". For example, she says, if some parents work late, that can push the children's bedtime to later in the evening.

Obesity among children in the United States is a major health concern. About 17 percent of children and teenagers in the U.S. are considered obese. That is according to the Centers for Disease Control and Prevention.

The World Health Organization reported in 2014 that the number of overweight babies and young children worldwide had increased from 31 million in 1990 to 44 million in 2012. If that trend continues, the WHO warns, there will be 70 million obese children in the world by 2025.

听写练习十（Pioneer Worked Hard to Gain Public Acceptance of IVF）

非考点难点词汇：
Huang Guoning
IVF in vitro fertilization

▶ 录音原文

Despite initial rejection, doctor still soldiered on after seeing many couples struggle to conceive. For thousands of infertile couples in China and abroad, Doctor Huang Guoning is the savior of their family dream.

Huang, 60, is considered one of the pioneers in reproductive medicine in the country. Through an in vitro fertilization procedure done by Huang, a baby boy — the first successful IVF baby in Southwest China — was born in Chongqing in 1997.

IVF is a process in which an egg is combined with sperm outside the body, or in vitro. The first human was born through this technology in 1978.

He was the first one in China to point out that the air quality in laboratories will affect the growth of embryos and even increase the health risks of fetuses. To address the problem, he took the lead in the design and development of a smart lab project which had been implemented in many reproductive centers in China.

听写练习十一（Pressured Speech）

非考点难点词汇：

mania

hypomania

insomnia

schizophrenia

dementia

cocaine

methamphetamine

phencyclidine

▶ 录音原文

Everyone occasionally experiences a pressing desire to talk—whether to share good news or an exciting or unusual experience. If you have bipolar disorder, however, a compulsive urge to talk might represent a symptom called pressured speech. This symptom occurs commonly in adults, adolescents, and children with bipolar disorder experiencing mania or hypomania.

A rapid-fire speech pattern is one of the most frequent initial signs of bipolar disorder. It usually occurs with other common signs and symptoms, such as increased energy and activity; reduced need for sleep or insomnia; elevated mood; irritability, agitation, or jumpiness; and racing thoughts. Pressured speech alone does not necessarily indicate bipolar disorder. This symptom can occur with other mental and nervous system conditions—such as schizophrenia, dementia, and stroke — and the use of certain drugs, like cocaine, methamphetamine, and phencyclidine (PCP).

听写练习十二（Science Has Proven that Fast Walkers Live 15 Years Longer than Slow Walkers）

非考点难点词汇：

Leicester University

the United Kingdom

▶ 录音原文

There are two types of people in this world — fast walkers and slow walkers. And they are practically mortal enemies. The most frustrating thing for a fast walker is to be stuck behind someone taking their sweet time. Maybe they're busy texting on their phone or they just have no sense of urgency. Either way, they're taking too darn long.

Science has shown that you're in the right, and slow walkers are in the wrong — at least when it comes to your health. Now, you have a reason to speed on by them.

Fast walkers have been proven to live fifteen years longer than slow walkers. The study was conducted by a team, at Leicester University in the United Kingdom.

The team analyzed date from 474,919 people within the United Kingdom. The age range varied and has an average age of 52. The numbers were gathered over a ten year period from 2006 to 2016, which means this data set is rock solid.

听写练习十三（Drinking Green Tea Is Good for You）

非考点难点词汇：

catechins

flavonoid

oxidative stress

▶ 录音原文

A lot of little lifestyle decisions can have a big impact on overall health. Taking the stairs for two minutes, choosing to grill rather than fry your food or refusing that extra glass of wine can all add up to a longer life.

Given the importance of these small choices, some are wondering whether they should give up their morning cup of coffee in favor of green tea. The evidence on green tea's benefits is still developing, and we don't know if it's the healthier choice. But if you're looking to make the switch, there is some information that might push you over the bean-leaf divide.

Green and black teas come from the same plant, but green tea is less processed. Because of this, it has a relatively high concentration of something called catechins. Catechins are part of a bioactive compound known as a flavonoid, which is thought to reduce oxidative stress.

听写练习十四（Princess Carry at the Cost of Fractured Arms）

非考点难点词汇：

Chinese Valentine's Day

录音原文

A man in central China fractured his arm after trying to please his girlfriend with a surprise "princess carry".

The incident in Wuhan, Hubei Province occurred while the couple celebrated the unofficial Chinese Valentine's Day on May 20.

In his apparent excitement, the man, age 20, carried this 65-kilogram (143.3 pound) girlfriend out of the blue, hearing a loud crack in the process.

His right arm suffered from severe pain shortly after, prompting them to rush to a nearby hospital.

A CT scan revealed that the romantic gesture left the young man with a fractured arm and a dislocated elbow.

The man's doctor explained that his injury may be caused by a lack of strength and faulty squatting — his girlfriend was heavier than himself.

听写练习十五（Students Join Efforts Against Sue of Tobacco）

 录音原文

More than 670,000 students in China have joined a national union to become tobacco control volunteers tasked with helping to curtail use among the young, the Chinese Association on Tobacco Control said on Wednesday.

The students, from 343 schools across China ranging from universities to primary schools, will help launch a national campaign on tobacco control aimed at the young, together with other organizations, said Zhang Xiaopeng, director for the association's adolescent tobacco control committee.

The bodies and minds of young children and adolescents are not fully developed, so they suffer more serious damage from smoking and exposure to second-hand smoke.

Promoting tobacco-free schools is essential to protecting students from the harmful effects of tobacco, and it's an important part of the overall tobacco control effort.

下面将针对听力理解考试的不同部分，结合部分真题，对考点和应试技巧进行有针对性的讲解。

（一）Section A 的主要考点及应试技巧

大纲未修订之前，该部分对话一般为一个轮次，解题相对容易，但在新大纲的命题设置中，对话变成了多个（3个以上）轮次，我们解题的难度和负担就加大了。我们可以采取以下行之有效的解题步骤。

第一步：充分利用录音中阅读题目指令和题与题之间的 12 秒间隙，提前阅读选项（这是录音开始前我们唯一能看到的提示），勾画出选项中重复的关键词和结构，预测该题的命题类型及对话的中心内容；

第二步：录音开始播放时，集中精力听懂第一个轮次的对话（记住：不仅仅是听，而是听懂），并将该轮次中的关键词记录下来，往往此处和第一题的选项会有所重叠，大多数时候第一题的答案会出自对话第一个轮次的细节；

第三步：在听的过程中，对关键细节信息进行记录。关键信息，往往对应的是该部分命题处：细节题、逻辑关系题、推断题、主旨题。

下面一一阐述这些考点和应试技巧。

细节题 此类题目是根据男女双方的对话细节提出问题，如时间、地点、事实等。细节题往往在选项上有特点，解题可以根据选项预先做出判断，如果选项都是表示时间或者数字的，就可以根据选项的指引，重点关注与数字或时间有关的信息，必要时要做简单的笔记。这种类型的考题重点较为单一，就是听力材料中的细节，解题切入点就是选项。

逻辑关系题 逻辑关系包含句内逻辑关系、句间逻辑关系、段间逻辑关系。比如 dedicated doctor（修饰与被修饰的逻辑关系），because 代表因果逻辑关系，but 则代表转折逻辑关系。

推理题 题干中往往有 learn，infer 等词，证明不是"所听即所得"，需要对细节进一步转换才是正确答案。

主旨题 虽说是主旨大意题，但更多是各种细节的重复和概括，比如对话谈论三种治疗高血压的方案的利弊，那么主旨便是"高血压治疗方案"；对话谈论毕业后干了些什么工作，主旨就是"从业经历"；对话谈论如何在新社区登记医疗保健，主旨就是"新社区的医保服务"等。对话往往比较细节，稍加总结即可。

在开始讲解前必须提示一点：我们在练习时应尽可能多地按照新的考试命题题型来储备应试技能。虽然借用老题型分析考点会更加清晰明了，但在实际考试时，因为语料多，会导致在记忆储存时长、输入输出转换时间、上下文逻辑关系复杂度等方面的难度有很大差别。

真题回顾

No.1

🎧 2020 年真题

Conversation One

1. A. The right medication for the woman.
   B. The advantage of regular medication.
   C. The popular medication on the Internet.
   D. The best medication for high blood pressure.

2. A. To teach her how to properly use drugs.
   B. To prescribe her newly-developed drugs.
   C. To add a drug to the medication she is on.
   D. To increase the dosage of her medication.

> 3. A. To prescribe two medications for her.
>   B. To allow her to buy medicine on the Internet.
>   C. To advise on the medicine her friend is using.
>   D. To provide some medical advice to her friend.

▶ **听力原文**

Conversation One

M: Your blood pressure is still too high. Are you sure you're taking your medication as directed?

W: Well, the truth is that medication makes me feel dizzy. I'm not sure it's the right one for me.

M: It's one of the best and I use it for almost all my patients with high blood pressure. And I want to add another drug to relieve your symptom.

W: You want me to take two medications every day? I don't want to do that. What about this medication? A friend of mine is just taking it and she says it's really good. I checked it out on the Internet.

Questions number 1–3 are based on the conversation you've just heard.

1. What are the speakers talking about?
2. What does the man intend to do to deal with the woman's complaint?
3. What does the woman want the man to do?

第一题解析：

分析选项：核心词为 medication，具体是什么样的 medication，是考生需要解决的问题。可判定本题为细节题。且根据命题顺序，应该是在第一轮次对话里。

分析问题：对话在谈论什么？看上去是主旨题，按照第一个轮次对话精听的原则，可知对话中男士首先说了女士的血压仍然很高，询问女士是否按照医嘱在服用 medication。女士抱怨并质疑 medication，因为男士开的药让她感觉晕乎乎的（dizzy）。

选择答案：对话讲的是如何调整女士的治疗方案，即 right medication for the woman。D 选项是最具干扰力的混淆项。medication 有可能是治疗 high blood pressure 的，但这只是个引子，重点是在讨论这个 medication 是否适合女士。

答案：A

第二题解析：

分析选项：选项为 to do 结构，可推测问题问的是目的或者未来要做的事情。四个选项各自表达的内容没有混淆性，对应细节题的命题方式。A 选项"教她如何正确用药"，B 选项"开新药"，C 选项"在现行药方上加药"，D 选项"增加药的剂量"。

分析问题：男士打算如何处理女士的主诉？很明显，这是细节题。在对话第二个轮次里男士就说了自己想做的事情：want to add another drug to relieve your symptom。

选择答案：原文中的 want to 和题干中的 intend to 同义。

答案： C

第三题解析：

分析选项：选项也是 to do 结构，可推测问题问的是目的或者未来要做的事情。四个选项各自表达的内容没有混淆性，对应细节题命题方式。A 选项"给她开两种药"，B 选项"允许她网购药品"，C 选项"给她推荐她朋友正在服用的药品"，D 选项"给她的朋友提供一些医疗建议"。

分析问题：女士想让男士做什么？细节题。对应的答案肯定在对话第二个轮次女士所说的内容里。

选择答案：女士不同意男士增加药品的建议，而是开始询问（what about）药方，并且称自己在网上进行了查询（check out）。to advise on 和 what about 的语义功能近似，都是询问意见。

答案： C

解题小结

该对话为二个轮次，第一个轮次点明主题（用药），明确场景（医院），讲清关系（医患）。两道细节题，一道主旨题。没有高难度的词汇和表达方式，简单常见的医学词汇完全没有造成考试的障碍。

No.2

2020 年真题

Conversation Four

10. A. Their positive effects.
    B. Their constant mutation.
    C. Difficulty in identifying them.
    D. Possibility of inheriting them.

11. A. You may suffer from mental illnesses.
    B. You may be alone without feeling bad.
    C. You may have high levels of blood pressure.
    D. You may develop great ability to tolerate failure.

12. A. Because he is always cheerful.
    B. Because he likes outdoor activities.
    C. Because he felt bad at the weekend.
    D. Because he was not at home last week.

▶ 听力原文

Conversation Four

W: It's interesting that some people are more likely to feel lonely than others, because our genes play a role.

M: I wonder if I inherited loneliness genes.

W: I don't know. But the professor says they do not only have negative effects. In some situations, it is an advantage to be able to tolerate high levels of loneliness.

M: So, inheriting genes for loneliness might not be a bad thing. But why is that?

W: Because it means you can tolerate being alone for a long time without feeling bad. Well, you probably don't have those genes, because you did feel bad at the weekend.

Questions number 10–12 are based on the conversation you've just heard.

10. What are the speakers mainly talking about with regard to loneliness genes?

11. According to the conversation, what does inheriting loneliness genes mean?

12. Why does the woman say the man may not have loneliness genes?

第一题解析：

分析选项：选项为名词＋名扩的结构。注意：当第一题出现一个名词词组时，出现主旨题的可能性非常大，往往对应的问题就是：他们谈论的核心内容是什么？需要考生定位"什么"？

A 选项"它们积极的效果"，B 选项"它们持续的变异"，C 选项"确定它们的困难"，D 选项"遗传它们的可能性"。

分析问题：关于孤独基因，文中主要谈论了什么？主旨题。精听第一轮次对话，女士说"因为基因原因，有的人更容易感到孤独"，男士回答"我在想是否遗传了孤独基因"。这里有个特殊的提示，即 I wonder，这实际在提问："Did I inherit loneliness genes?"因此要想完整理解第一轮次对话的含义，必须知道这个问题的答案。女士紧接着回答："我不知道，但教授说孤独基因不仅仅只有 negative effects。在某些情况下，这还会成为忍受强烈孤独的一种优势。"因此解题原则不变，仍是第一个轮次对话能解决主旨问题。

选择答案：not only have negative effects，答案则为反面的 positive effects。

答案：A

第二题解析：

分析选项：四个选项都为"You may ＋ 动词"，可推断本题问的是功效和效果。A 选项"会遭受精神疾病的折磨"，B 选项"独处时心情并不坏"，C 选项"血压升高"，D 选项"具备很强的失败承受能力"。

分析问题：遗传孤独基因意味着什么？即问孤独基因的作用。细节题。由第二个轮次对话中男士所说的 an advantage to be able to tolerate high levels of loneliness 可知，有这些基因的人，就能承受更高程度的孤独。

选择答案：不难对应，本题应该选择 You may be alone without feeling bad。A 和 C 选项原文根本没有提及；D 选项张冠李戴，tolerate 的对象是 loneliness，而不是 failure。

答案：B

第三题解析：

分析选项：四个选项均以 because 开始，证明这是针对原文因果关系的内容命题。A 选项"因为他一直很高兴"，B 选项"因为他喜欢户外活动"，C 选项"因为他周末不开心"，D 选项"因为他上周不在家"。

分析问题：女士为什么说男士没有孤独基因？因果关系题。根据最后一个轮次的对话，女士说"you probably don't have those genes, because you did feel bad at the weekend"，可知答案。

选择答案：A，B，D 在原文没有提及，没有任何干扰力。

答案：C

解题小结

本对话为 3 个轮次，一道主旨题，一道细节题，一道逻辑题。本对话有一个特殊的地方：第一个轮次的对话结束时，变相地提出了一个问题，此时就需要扩展范围，将该问题的答案纳入考查主旨的范围中去。除了带有问题的情况外，如果第二轮次对话是以 but 等转折逻辑关系词开始，也需要将转折后的语义囊括进去。

我们一起来看看最新真题对话中的命题点。

No.3

2022 年真题

Conversation One

1. A. In Aisle 2.
   B. In Aisle 4.
   C. In Aisle 6.
   D. In Aisle 8.

2. A. They are less effective.
   B. They are less expensive.
   C. They are more effective.
   D. They are more expensive.

3. A. Confirming drug ingredients.
   B. Comparing drug brands.
   C. Purchasing drugs.
   D. Comparing drug prices.

▶ **听力原文**

Conversation One

W: I have a really bad headache. What do you recommend?

M: You can purchase some over-the-counter pain relievers in Aisle 6.

W: Do I need a prescription for those?

M: No. You just pick whichever brand you prefer and pay for it at the register.

W: Is there a difference between the name-brand pills and store-brand pills?

M: Usually there isn't. Just compare the labels and look for the active ingredients.

W: The store-brand is less expensive.

M: Usually it is just as effective.

W: I surely hope so because I want to save money and not have a headache.

Questions number 1–3 are based on the conversation you've just heard.

1. Where would the woman find the pain reliever?

2. What do we know about the store-brand pills?

3. What are the two speakers mainly talking about?

命题点分析：

1 细节题：What's wrong with the woman?

W: I have a really bad headache. What do you recommend?

M: You can purchase some over-the-counter pain relievers in Aisle 6.

2 细节题：Where/What can the woman buy (it)?

W: Do I need a prescription for those?

M: No. You just pick whichever brand you prefer and pay for it at the register.

3 细节题：How can she buy the medicine?

W: Is there a difference between the name-brand pills and store-brand pills?

M: Usually there isn't. Just compare the labels and look for the active ingredients.

W: The store-brand is less expensive.

4 细节题：Which is TRUE/NOT TRUE about the store-brand pills?

M: Usually it is just as effective.

W: I surely hope so because I want to save money and not have a headache.

5 推理题：What will the woman probably buy?

第一题解析：

分析选项：选项为表示位置的介宾短语，且含有数字，但要有合理预期，听力原文中可能会有其他数字，对应其他药物所在的位置。

分析问题：下文命题点分析中有讲到，问题问的是 pain reliever 对应的位置。

选择答案：不难对应，本题选择 Aisle 6.

答案：C

第二题解析：

分析选项：四个选项均为 They are... 完整句子，有区别的部分是由 more /less+effective/expensive 两两搭配而来的。描述的药物是同一个，但该药物是效果更好还是更差，价格是更贵还是更便宜，需要我们对应题干中的药物。

分析问题：问题中问的是 store-brand pills 的情况，按照命题规律，对话中往往会有另一个 brand 来迷惑考生。

选择答案：原文中说到了 The store-brand is less expensive。

答案：B

第三题解析：

分析选项：四个选项均为动名词短语，证明回答的是"在干什么"，A 选项"确认药物成分"，B 选项"比较药物品牌"，C 选项"买药"，D 选项"对比药价"。

分析问题：主旨题，题干问的是两个人在谈论什么。

选择答案：最佳选项为"买药"，买药过程中既包含药效对比，还包含价格对比，是综合的。

答案：C

解题小结　　本对话为 3.5 个轮次，一个主旨题，两个细节题。从选项不难看出，往往听到即得到，本题相对简单，需要考生注意的是，需要将所问与所答对应。

No.4

 2022 年真题

Conversation Five

13. A. To keep the favored trees unified.
    B. To prevent trees from getting diseases.
    C. To trigger competition in the chosen trees.
    D. To ensure better growth of the favored trees.

14. A. Thrival of the favored trees.
    B. Thrival of the removed trees.
    C. Extinction of the remaining trees.
    D. Damage of underground fungal networks.

15. A. Restoration of forests.
    B. Species competition.
    C. Healthy forest ecology.
    D. Prevention of trees extinction.

▶ 听力原文

Conversation Five

W: Did you know that trees can communicate with each other?

M: Interesting! But how?

W: A professor of forest ecology at University of British Columbia observed how logging companies would cut down diverse forests and replace them with the single tree species. They believe that by removing competition, the favored trees would thrive as they would receive more space, water, and sun light.

M: Is that so?

W: However, the favored trees were actually more prone to diseases. 10% of them would die if the surrounding trees were removed. Trees communicate through underground network of fungi. The fungi help connect trees of different species across the forests.

Questions number 13–15 are based on the conversation you've just heard.

13. Why would logging companies remove some trees?

14. What can be inferred about the result of tree removal?

15. What is the subject of the conversation?

命题点分析：

W: Did you know that trees can communicate with each other?

M: Interesting! But how? —— 1 细节题：How do trees communicate with each other?

W: A professor of forest ecology at University of British Columbia observed how logging companies would cut down diverse forests and replace them with the single tree species.

2 细节题：What does the professor find out?

They believe that by removing competition, the favored trees would thrive as they would receive more space, water, and sun light.

M: Is that so? —— 3 因果关系题：Why do the favored trees thrive?

W: However, the favored trees were actually more prone to diseases. 10% of them would die if the surrounding trees were removed. Trees communicate through underground network of fungi. The fungi help connect trees of different species across the forests.

4 细节题：What is the function of fungi?

5 结构题：What is the result of cutting down diverse forests and replacing them with the same species?

第一题解析：

分析选项：四个选项都为 To do sth., 表示目的。A 选项"为了让所选树木成片生长"，B 选项"为了阻止树木生病"，C 选项"为了激发相邻树木的竞争"，D 选项"为了保证所选树木的生长"。这应该对应一个表示目的或者原因的考题。

分析问题：题干问"为什么伐木公司会移走一些树"，那就是因果关系。

选择答案：原文第二个轮次里讲到，logging companies 移走不同种类的树，只剩下单一树种，是为了让 favored trees 生长得更好（thrive）。因此本题正确答案为 D。

答案：D

第二题解析：

分析选项：四个选项都是"名词 + 后置定语"的形式：所选树木的繁荣 / 被移走的树木的繁荣（互为相反答案）、剩下树木的灭绝（与 B 选项相反）、地下菌群的伤害。从选项可以判断，心理预期应该对听力内容的 removed trees，favored trees，fungi 要敏感。

听力原文：根据最后一个轮次的对话可以得到正确答案，此处有一个 however，答案往往在转折后。男士问："为什么 favored trees 会长得好（在移除其他树种后）？"女士一个 however 暗示，并非如此，favored trees 更容易生病，因为地下帮助树木交流的菌群被破坏了。

选择答案：favored trees 长得并不好，被挪走的树种后况未被提及，只能选择"菌群的破坏"。

答案： D

第三题解析：

分析选项：四个选项均为名词词组。A 选项"森林修复"，B 选项"物种竞争"，C 选项"健康的森林生态"，D 选项"阻止树木灭绝"。合理的心理预期为：what 类问题或者主旨题。

分析问题：主旨题。根据对话和前两道题的选项，结合频繁出现的森林、竞争、菌群等，这讲述的是如何维持一个健康的森林生态。

选择答案：健康的森林生态是正确答案，其他选项都是片面之谈。

答案： C

解题
小结

本对话通过伐木公司移除树木的行为，开始谈论这种行为的影响和效果，命题为一个主旨题，一个细节题，一个推理题。要注意推理题中的命题点在转折后。

No.5

 2023 年真题

Conversation One

M: Take a seat, please, Mrs. Smith.

W: Thank you.

M: What seems to be the problem?

W: I've been getting a very bad headache lately.

M: You say, lately. When exactly did it start?

W: About two months ago?

M: Did anything happen to you at that time? Did you have a fall, or a hit on the head or something like that?

W: Nothing that I can remember. The headache just started.

M: Have you ever had headaches like this before?

W: Yes, but it was years ago, just after I got married. I was still trying to work, and we were living with my husband's parents.

Questions number 1–3 are based on the conversation you've just heard.

1. What is the woman's problem?

2. When did the problem start?

3. What did the man want to learn later on in the talk?

问题分析：

1. What is the woman's problem?

细节题。解题点在第 1 标注处。

2. When did the problem start?

细节题。解题点在第 2 标注处，要注意答案在该轮次的答语处。

3. What did the man want to learn later on in the talk?

归纳题。这是根据对话末尾设置的一道推理题，要求考生界定"Have you ever had headaches like this before？"的问题类型。

下面我们再来看看新大纲听力 Section A 的命题解析。这是介于 short conversation 和 long conversation 之间的一种考题。根据考试大纲的要求和规定，这部分由五段对话组成，目的在于测试考生的对话听力理解能力，要求考生能够理解所听材料的中心思想和主要内容，并能根据所听到的内容进行逻辑推理、分析概括和归纳总结。请看新大纲上的样题：

Section A

Directions: *In this section you will hear five conversations. At the end of each conversation, you will hear three questions about the conversation. The question will be spoken only once. After you hear the question, read the four possible answers marked A, B, C and D. Choose the best answer and mark the letter of your choice on the* ***ANSWER SHEET.***

Conversation One

1. A. Food packaging.

    B. Safety of processed foods.

    C. Concern about sugar intake.

    D. Maintenance of a healthy diet.

2. A. Red.   B. Orange.   C. Green.   D. Brown.

3. A. Indifference.   B. Resentment.

    C. Overreaction.   D. Undervaluation.

Conversation Two

4. A. The human emotions.

    B. The recent research on stress.

    C. The use of mind to treat the body.

D．The relation between hunger and anger.

5. A．Neural activity increases.　　　B．Blood sugar level drops.
   C．Blood pressure drops.　　　D．Heart rate increases.

6. A．They are wrongly defined.　　　B．They interact with each other.
   C．They can be confusing sometimes.　　　D．They are replaceable with each other.

Conversation Three

7. A．Choosing a hospital.　　　B．Carrying out a survey.
   C．Issuing a health policy.　　　D．Buying health insurance.

8. A．It is covered by the government.　　　B．It has limited doctor choices.
   C．It is popular in the public.　　　D．It has a wide coverage.

9. A．Saving money.　　　B．Getting better service.
   C．Being easy to manage.　　　D．Waiting for a short time.

Conversation Four

10. A．The use of MRI imaging.　　　B．The prevention of arthritis.
    C．The benefits of hand exercise.　　　D．The possible damages to knuckles.

11. A．The bubbles in joint fluid burst.　　　B．The source of infection forms.
    C．The friction of joints occurs.　　　D．The joint fluid increases.

12. A．Pop sound.　　　B．Broken finger.
    C．Pulling-apart of bones.　　　D．Cracked bone.

Conversation Five

13. A．Social media.　　　B．Animal world.
    C．Attention span.　　　D．Modern devices.

14. A．It is shorter.　　　B．It is much longer.
    C．It is misunderstood.　　　D．It is thoroughly studied.

15. A．They lack self-control.
    B．They are easily distracted.
    C．They can sustain their attention.
    D．They have an extended attention span.

答案及解析

Conversation One

1. 【答案】C
   【解析】男士说他最近一直看到过度摄入糖分的新闻，女士询问他是否有查看食品包装上的说明，最后女士说对糖分摄入不能妖魔化（demonize），因此本对话的主题是关于 sugar intake。

2. 【答案】C

   【解析】女士说，红色代表高糖分，橙色为中等糖分，绿色为低糖分。

3. 【答案】C

   【解析】女士说："Sugar is demonized. People link it to drugs. And I think this is the wrong way forward." 她认为人们将糖和毒品关联起来，是将其 demonize（妖魔化）了，她觉得这个方向是错误的。

Conversation Two

4. 【答案】D

   【解析】女士说："I was doing some research about feeling angry when you are hungry." 因此本文讨论的是 angry 和 hungry 之间的关系。

5. 【答案】B

   【解析】女士说："When we are hungry, the level of sugar in our blood is lower." 可知当我们饥饿的时候，血糖水平是下降的。

6. 【答案】B

   【解析】女士说，当我们饥饿时，大脑会分泌一种荷尔蒙，这种荷尔蒙同样会激发 anger。因此饥饿时人们也会像处于 anger 时那样做出糟糕的决策，这证明 hunger 和 anger 是相互影响的。

Conversation Three

7. 【答案】D

   【解析】对话一开始，女士就说："I need information on purchasing health insurance." 因此这段对话是关于购买健康保险的。

8. 【答案】B

   【解析】男士在解释的时候说："An HMO is a little cheaper, but you have limited choices of which doctor you choose." 即 HMO 更便宜，但是可选择的医生有限。

9. 【答案】A

   【解析】从上一题答案可知，HMO 的优势就是便宜。男士接着又解释：you save money in out-of-pocket expenses，即自付额（out-of-pocket expenses）较少。

Conversation Four

10. 【答案】D

    【解析】对话开始女士说："Don't crack your knuckles!" 即不要掰指关节，因为最后会得关节炎。因此本对话讨论的是掰指关节可能带来的伤害。

11. 【答案】A

    【解析】女士说："Now when you stretch the joint far enough, these bubbles burst, producing the 'pop' sound." 当指关节被拉得足够长时候，气泡破裂，发出"砰"的声音。

12. 【答案】C

    【解析】女士在对话最后一个轮次说，当关节被分离的时候，关节处会形成液体，从而造成对关节表面的损害。因此本题答案为 C。

Conversation Five

13. **【答案】C**

    【解析】男士在对话开始说，今天要讨论 attention span，因此 C 为正确答案。

14. **【答案】A**

    【解析】女士说，研究表明，人类的注意力集中时间已经 fallen to just eight seconds，男士接着说："Goldfish reportedly have an attention span of nine seconds."即人类的注意力时间比金鱼还短。

15. **【答案】C**

    【解析】男士在对话的最后说，智能手机使用者虽然被分散了注意力（distract），但 it doesn't mean that they don't have the ability to control and sustain their attention when they carry out another task，即他们仍可能有自控并维持注意力的能力。

▶ 录音原文

Conversation One

M: I'm always seeing in the news these days that we're eating too much sugar. And one important factor is that sugars are sometimes hidden in processed foods.

W: Do you check the information on the back of food packets, Rob?

M: Yes, I do. But it can be very confusing. There's so much information.

W: Some food products have color coding on the packaging to help you understand the information. Red for high levels of sugar, salt or fat, orange for medium, and green for low.

M: That sounds helpful.

W: But one problem we see in nutrition is sort of this focusing on any individual foods. Sugar is demonized. People link it to drugs. And I think this is the wrong way forward.

Questions number 1–3 are based on the conversation you've just heard.

1. What is mainly discussed in the conversation?

2. Which color is mentioned to represent low levels of sugar?

3. According to the woman, what is the problem with people's attitude towards sugar?

Conversation Two

W: How's your mood today? Feeling happy?

M: Very happy. I've just had lunch.

W: That's good! I was doing some research about feeling angry when you are hungry.

M: Oh, how is that?

W: When we are hungry, the level of sugar in our blood is lower. As the blood sugars drop, this causes an increase in particular hormones — hormones that the body uses to prepare us to either fight or run away from a dangerous situation. And those have an impact on brain. The neuropeptides that trigger for hunger are the same ones that trigger for anger.

M: So when we are hungry, the same emotions can run through us. We can be angry and make poor decisions. And that is hunger.

Questions number 4–6 are based on the conversation you've just heard.

4. What are the two speakers talking about?
5. According to the conversation, what will happen when we are hungry?
6. What can we say about anger and hunger according to the conversation?

Conversation Three

W: I need information on purchasing health insurance.

M: Is this the first time you have had health insurance?

W: Yes.

M: You have a choice of HMO or PPO. Do you understand the difference?

W: I am not sure what those are.

M: An HMO is a little cheaper, but you have limited choices of which doctor you choose.

W: Are the payments the same for a PPO and an HMO?

M: By going to the providers on the HMO list, you save money in out-of-pocket expenses.

W: Can you give me a comparison between a PPO and an HMO?

M: We can mail you a questionnaire and when we have all of your information, we will mail you a quote.

Questions number 7–9 are based on the conversation you've just heard.

7. What is mainly talked about in the conversation?
8. What can we learn about an HMO?
9. What is the advantage of an HMO over a PPO?

Conversation Four

W: Don't crack your knuckles! You'll end up with arthritis when you're older.

M: I don't know why I do it. It just feels nice.

W: Now we can use MRI imaging to see what is actually happening inside the joint when someone cracks their knuckles.

M: Then what is happening?

W: Well, when you crack your knuckles, it stretches the space around the joint and surrounding fluid and causes the formation of bubbles. Now when you stretch the joint far enough, these bubbles burst, producing the "pop" sound.

M: Is there any damage to the joint?

W: When the bones of the joint are pulled apart, there'll be a little bit of fluid in between, which can damage the surfaces of the joints.

Questions number 10–12 are based on the conversation you've just heard.

10. What is the conversation mainly about?

11. What happens when you stretch the joint far enough?

12. What could cause the damage to the surfaces of the joints?

Conversation Five

M: Can you stay focused for the full six minutes? Sounds easy? Maybe not, because today we're talking about our attention spans: are they shrinking?

W: Yes, a report said the average human attention span has fallen to just eight seconds.

M: Can that be true? Goldfish reportedly have an attention span of nine seconds. Human attention span is now shorter than that of a goldfish?

W: Yes. Smartphones, the Internet, and social media — these all certainly do take up a lot of our attention.

M: OK, but some psychologists said for someone distracted by their smartphone or wanting to quickly Google something, it doesn't mean that they don't have the ability to control and sustain their attention when they carry out another task.

Questions number 13–15 are based on the conversation you've just heard.

13. What is the main topic of the conversation?

14. What can we learn about the average human attention span when compared with a goldfish?

15. What did the psychologists say about some smartphone users?

（二）Section B 的主要考点及应试技巧

根据大纲要求，Section B 主要针对同一篇文章进行考查。由于听力材料比较长，且没有人物转换之间的提示，考生得到的信息会比较丰富且没有层次。那么从一堆细节中考细节的可能性就比较大，这可以测试考生获取正确信息的能力。其实，主旨大意、判断推理都是在获取正确信息的基础上进行简单的推理和概括。针对这种情况，我们将 Section B 部分的题型进行了重新划分：细节题、逻辑关系题、推理题和主旨题。下面就按照具体题型进行讲述。

细节题 这类题型对一些信息不做任何改变，或者只进行同义改写，再将其作为考核内容，以考查考生在听力过程中获得信息的能力。常常考查时间、地点、人物（关系）、事件等事实。

笔记小提示　针对数字、时间、地点、人物、价格、日期等细节，以及不断重复的名词、动词等实词做笔记。当然，在记笔记的过程中，要按照自己的习惯，使用一些类似缩写、简写、符号之类的方法，以提高笔记效果。

　　逻辑关系题　在因果关系、转折关系、比较关系、从属关系、对比关系等逻辑关系处命题，需要考生们熟悉每个类别的表达方式，以便在听材料时能迅速反应出来，并对应命题点。

　　笔记小提示　逻辑关系往往为"内容在两头，逻辑在中间"，用等式的方式来记笔记比较高效。

　　推理题　这类考题是在考听力细节的基础上要求考生进行符合逻辑的简单推理，主要测试点为推理。考生首先要理解听力细节，并且做一些简单的笔记，然后进行推理。

　　笔记小提示　细节仍然是重点。

　　主旨题　主旨常常在听力的开头处有明示、结尾处有呼应，因此文章的开头要精听，并记下关键词和词组。

　　笔记小提示　"开头就要记，末尾补缝隙"，即第一句话的主旨核心要义要记录下来，中间如果有遗漏，则在末尾尝试查缺补漏。

　　下面我们来看看最新的真题。

真题回顾

No.1

2020 年真题

Passage Two

19. A. Medical insurance in the US.
    B. Healthcare system in the US.
    C. Telemedicine services in the US.
    D. Health services for the elderly in the US.

20. A. Because they think that the doctor online is unfriendly.
    B. Because they do not have trust in online medical services.
    C. Because they are not accessible to online medical services.
    D. Because they do not know much about computer operation.

21. A. Because it can provide quality services.
    B. Because it can provide rich information.
    C. Because it can offer personalized services.
    D. Because it can cut down on healthcare cost.

▶ **听力原文**

Passage Two

The Associated Press reports that 80% of middle-sized and large US companies offered telemedicine services to their workers in 2018, but only 8% of employees used telemedicine. This seems to support what many healthcare experts say. People are often not willing to change their way of thinking about healthcare. Compared with seeing a real doctor in person, as some people may think, the quality of telemedicine is not so good. Parents, for example, may feel they are not giving their child the best care if they use a virtual doctor appointment. Older adults may also not want to see a doctor online. Experts say that one reason may be that older people don't have trust in telemedicine and services. They do not buy anything online and let alone do something as personal as seeing a doctor. It is important for them to look their doctor in the eye and shake hands. However, for some people such as young people and busy students, telemedicine might be a good choice. It can cut down on the time away from work and cut down on the cost of doctor visits.

Questions number 19–21 are based on the passage you've just heard.

19. What is the passage mainly about?
20. Why are some older adults unwilling to see a doctor online?
21. According to the passage, what is one reason that telemedicine is a good choice for young people?

第一题解析：

分析选项：四个选项均为名词＋名扩的结构，如前文所讲，当选项为名词词组时，命题可能对应主旨题。A 选项"美国的医疗保障"，B 选项"美国的保健体系"，C 选项"美国的远程医疗服务"，D 选项"美国老年人的保健服务"。

分析问题：文章的主旨大意是什么？主旨题。精听第一句：The Associated Press reports that 80% of middle-sized and large US companies offered telemedicine services to their workers in 2018, but only 8% of employees used telemedicine.（记笔记时至少应该记录：80%, telemedicine services—but 8% used），因此核心信息应该是 telemedicine 的情况。

选择答案：将核心词和各个选项一比对，Telemedicine services in the US 在文中有对应。

答案：C

第二题解析：

分析选项：四个选项均以 Because 开头，证明这是在回答 why。A 选项"因为他们认为线上的医生不友好"，B 选项"因为他们不信任线上医疗服务"，C 选项"因为他们无法获得线上医疗服务"，D 选项"因为他们不知道如何操作电脑"。

分析问题：为什么老年人不愿意使用远程医生？因果关系题。对应原文中的"Older adults may also not want to see a doctor online. Experts say that one reason may be that older people don't have trust in telemedicine and services."

选择答案：有核心词 trust 回现的为 B 选项。

答案：B

第三题解析：

分析选项：四个选项仍是以 Because 开头，证明此题仍然在回答 why。A 选项"因为它能提供高质量的服务"，B 选项"因为它能提供丰富的信息"，C 选项"因为它能提供个性化服务"，D 选项"因为它能削减保健成本"。

分析问题：对年轻人来讲，远程医疗是一个不错的选择，原因是什么？虽然题目中没有 why，但 reason 是另一个最明显的询问原因的词，这是因果关系题。文章面前讲了 old adults，可推理接下来就是拿 young people 进行对比。文中出现 however（转折后往往有重点）：However, for some people such as young people and busy students, telemedicine might be a good choice. It can cut down on the time away from work and cut down on the cost of doctor visits.

选择答案：cut down on healthcare cost 与原文有呼应。

答案：D

> 解题
> 小结
>
> ● 本文主题为 telemedicine services 在美国的发展现状、老年人和年轻人的接受状态及原因。命题题型为两道逻辑关系题、一道主旨题。原文逻辑关系简单清晰，提示词很突出，处理起来难度较低。

No.2

2021 年真题

16. A. The relationship between gardening and health benefits.
    B. The activities caused by gardening.
    C. The relationship between gardening and social association.
    D. Some kinds of outdoor activities.

17. A. The gardening people enjoy showing themselves.
    B. Gardening gives more chances of doing outdoor activities.
    C. Gardening makes young people active in socializing.
    D. Gardening is popular among all the people.

18. A. They can keep the brain calm.
    B. They can keep the brain active.
    C. They can keep the body young.
    D. They can keep the brain efficient.

1 主旨题：What is the best topic?

2 并列关系处命题：What can't gardening give us?

▶ 听力原文

Gardening is popular in many parts of the world. This outdoor activity gives us beautiful plants, pleasant smelling flowers and fresh foods and vegetables, but it also gives

> **3 因果关系处命题：** Why is it perfect to socialize with your neighbors?

us many health benefits. When you're gardening, you're outdoors, so it is the perfect time to socialize with your neighbors. People usually enjoy sharing with others their growing and sharing advice and stories about their gardens. When you garden, you must move around. Different movements for gardening, just bending, twisting, stretching and lifting work all muscles in the body. Gardening may help your brains stay young. Activities such as gardening use many repeated actions such as watering, or removing dying flowers from plants. These actions have a common effect on the brain. The brain is still active but not in the same way as it is, say, when we use computers.

> **4 细节题：** Why is gardening good for your brain to stay young?

Questions number 16–18 are based on the passage you've just heard.

16. What does it mainly talk about in the passage?
17. According to the speaker, in what way is gardening associated with socialization?
18. What effect would repeated actions in gardening have on brain?

第一题解析：

分析选项：四个选项均为名词 + 后置定语，A 选项"园艺与健康的关系"，B 选项"园艺带来的活动"，C 选项"园艺与社会联系的关系"，D 选项"一些户外活动"。预测这题是 what 类问题或者主旨题。

分析问题：题目问文章主要谈论了什么，主旨题。

选择答案：录音中说园艺不仅给我们提供美丽的植物、芬芳的鲜花、新鲜的蔬菜和水果，也对我们的健康有益。接着开始分析如何对健康有利，因此本题谈论的是园艺与健康的关系。

答案：A

第二题解析：

分析选项：选项均为完整的句子。A 选项"做园艺的人乐于展示"，B 选项"园艺提供了更多户外活动的机会"，C 选项"园艺让年轻人更乐于社交"，D 选项"园艺受到所有人的欢迎"。预测对应的问题为细节题。

分析问题：题目问到：园艺与社交以何种方式联系起来？关键词是 gardening 和 socializing。

选择答案：录音中说到园艺一般都在户外，所以做园艺是和邻居交往的绝佳时间，人们通常喜欢向邻居们展示自己种植的花花草草，分享园艺的经验和体会。看上去 C 选项既有 gardening，又有 socializing，但其核心结果 makes young people active 和原文意义不对称，录音中没有提及 young people。因此更多的户外活动是关键。

答案：B

第三题解析：

分析选项：四个选项的区别为园艺能对 brain/body 有何种效果。A 选项"让大脑冷静"，

B 选项 "让大脑活跃"，C 选项 "让身体年轻"，D 选项 "让大脑效率高"。

分析问题：题目问到：园艺中的重复活动对大脑有什么作用？问的就是 on brain，因此 C 选项先排除，答非所问，即使正确也不能作为答案。

选择答案：录音中提到 Gardening may help your brains stay young（不是 body），brain is still active, 因此本题正确答案为 keep the brain active。

答案：B

No.3 **2023 年真题**

> A detailed analysis of monkey pox case records published by the US Centers for Disease Control and Prevention on Friday offers new insight into the outbreak, which is disproportionately affecting men of certain ethnic groups. Additional analysis shows that all of the patients had a rash. However, a genital rash was more commonly reported in the current outbreak than in typical monkey pox. It was the most common location for rash, followed by arms, face and legs. More than a third of cases reported rash in four or more regions. Early warning signs of illness, however, were less common in the current outbreak. In about two in five cases, the illness started with the rash, but no reported early symptoms, such as chills, headache or malaise. About the two in five cases also did not report fever.

Questions number 19–21 are based on the passage you've just heard.

19. In which of the following groups is monkey pox more likely to occur?
20. Where was the rash most commonly found in the reported patients?
21. What was true of the early warning signs of the current outbreak?

问题分析：

19. In which of the following groups is monkey pox more likely to occur?

细节题。对应第 1 标注处，文中讲到本次猴痘暴发，certain ethnic groups（某些人种）中的男性感染率特别高（disproportionately）。

20. Where was the rash most commonly found in the reported patients?

细节题。题干关键词为 rash，most commonly found，不难对应。

21. What was true of the early warning signs of the current outbreak?

排除题。问题关键词为 early warning signs，需要对应 "Early warning signs of illness, however, were less common in the current outbreak. In about two in five cases, the illness started with the rash, but no reported early symptoms, such as chills, headache or malaise. About the two in five cases also did not report fever." 来对比每一个选项。

在 Section B 中，听力内容多，题目之间的联系较大，便于考生猜测和解题。该部分大都与医学话题和身心健康有关，因此储备一些必备知识和词汇是有必要的。下面我们来看看新大纲的 section B 全套样题，综合体会一下这三种题型。

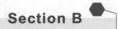

Directions: *In this section you will hear five passages. At the end of each passage, you will hear three questions about the passage. The question will be spoken only once. After you hear the question, read the four possible answers marked A, B, C and D. Choose the best answer and mark the letter of your choice on the **ANSWER SHEET.***

Passage One

16. A. The lack of vitamins.
    B. The issue of food safety.
    C. The intake of fruit and vegetable.
    D. The deficiency of basic micronutrients.
17. A. In the developing countries.　　B. In the developed countries.
    C. In the American countries.　　D. In European countries.
18. A. Unbalanced diet.　　B. Slow development.
    C. Nervous irritability.　　D. Short-term memory.

Passage Two

19. A. The harmful effects of obesity.　　B. The incidence of birth defects.
    C. Obesity in the world.　　D. Unhealthy lifestyle.
20. A. On the decline.　　B. Likely to go unnoticed.
    C. Serious enough to be fatal.　　D. Caused by an obese mother.
21. A. 20 million.　　B. 40 million.　　C. 200 million.　　D. 400 million.

Passage Three

22. A. A possible preventive for hearing loss.
    B. An attempt to develop a nutritious diet.
    C. A research on possible risks of vitamins.
    D. An effective way to reduce noise pollution.
23. A. A diet with mineral supplements.
    B. A combination of some herbal elements.
    C. A physical protection with a medication.
    D. A cocktail of vitamins plus magnesium.
24. A. Those who have hearing loss.

B．Those who work for General Motors.

C．Those who are exposed to loud noise.

D．Those who participate in the research.

Passage Four

25. A．Challenges of being a resident.

   B．Academic and clinical medicine.

   C．Importance of medical knowledge.

   D．Increased responsibility in the hospital.

26. A．You cannot afford to make a mistake.

   B．You have to be independent working.

   C．Study is placed above everything.

   D．Work comes before study.

27. A．No pain, no gain.   B．To stay or to leave.

   C．More work, less sleep.   D．More haste, less speed.

Passage Five

28. A．To persuade patients to be self-centered.

   B．To advise physicians to learn how to learn.

   C．To encourage teamwork among physicians.

   D．To urge partnerships between patients and physicians.

29. A．You are a real mentor.

   B．You practice evidence-based medicine.

   C．You have no trouble making a diagnosis.

   D．You can get all the information you need.

30. A．Hard decisions.   B．End-of-life issues.

   C．Discussion in secret.   D．Difficult medical terms.

答案与解析

Passage One

16. 【答案】D

   【解析】短文开头提到"隐性饥饿"，即 a deficiency in essential micronutrients，意为"基本微量营养素缺乏症"。全文都围绕这个话题而展开。

17. 【答案】A

   【解析】短文接着展开探讨隐性饥饿：About one-third of the world's population suffers from hidden hunger, mostly in developing countries. 可知发展中国家的隐性饥饿现象最严重。

18. 【答案】B

【解析】短文最后提到隐性饥饿对儿童的影响，它会 impede the child's ability to properly grow, learn, and ultimately reach his or her full potential，即阻碍孩子正常成长、学习，不能发挥其全部潜能，概括起来，孩子的 development 会受到影响。

Passage Two

19.【答案】A

【解析】全文讲到 obese 妈妈对新生儿的影响，还提到 obesity 会带来 2 型糖尿病、心脏病等健康问题。因此本文的主旨为肥胖的有害影响。

20.【答案】D

【解析】短文开始就讲到，专家 look at the risk of abnormalities of babies whose mothers were obese or overweight，即母亲超重或肥胖造成的婴儿畸形的风险。后面接着讲到，其风险概率是正常体重群体的两倍，同时会造成 neural defects（神经系统的缺陷）。因此 A 选项"数量下降"、B 选项"可能被忽视"都不正确。但是否都严重到致命，文中并未讲到。能确定的是这些问题都是一个体重超常的母亲所带来的，因此本题正确答案为 D。

21.【答案】D

【解析】短文中明确提到，被划为 obese 的有 4 亿人。

Passage Three

22.【答案】A

【解析】短文最开始就提出 About 10 million people in the US alone are suffering from impairing noise-induced hearing loss，即因为噪音造成听力损失的人群数量很庞大，后面接着讲一个利用 vitamin 来预防 noise 的研究。因此 A 选项"一种预防听力损失的潜在办法"是正确答案。

23.【答案】D

【解析】短文中讲到专家在研究一种方法，使用 a cocktail of vitamins and the mineral magnesium 来改变现状。

24.【答案】C

【解析】短文中讲到实验中研制的 cocktail，已经 shown promise as a possible way to prevent hearing loss caused by loud noise，同时被做成 pills，给暴露在噪音中的受试者使用。

Passage Four

25.【答案】A

【解析】短文首句为：The main challenges in residency come down to the increased responsibility. 大意是"住院医师的主要挑战来自于越来越大的责任"。因此本题正确答案为 A。

26.【答案】D

【解析】短文中先讲 medical student 的工作状态，but 之后则讲到 "as a resident, you're there to work, with learning being a secondary objective"，住院医师则不同，工作第一，

学习第二。短文中并未提到是否能犯错误、是否要独立工作，因此本题答案为D。

27. **【答案】C**

　　【解析】 短文中讲到 "Your increased responsibility also translates to many more nights on call, which means even more sleep deprivation"，即越来越大的责任通常就是夜里随叫随到，睡眠不足是常见之事。

Passage Five

28. **【答案】D**

　　【解析】 短文第一句为：I really want all of you patients to form partnerships with your physician. 即作者鼓励形成医患之间的合作关系。

29. **【答案】D**

　　【解析】 短文中说到 all the information that you need will be there if you let the patient talk and you listen，即医生听患者诉说，就会得到他／她所需要的所有信息。

30. **【答案】D**

　　【解析】 短文中讲到 "make sure the discussion is not in the big-word, top-secret language that we learned in medical school"，即交流中要确保讨论不要用big word（大词，生僻词），不要用医学院才能听得懂的语言。因此本题正确答案为D。

⊙ 录音原文

Passage One

　　To remain fit and healthy, you need a balanced diet including essential vitamins and minerals. But what if your diet consists mainly of staples like rice, bread, or corn because other foods are not available or affordable? If so, you will likely develop "hidden hunger", a deficiency in essential micronutrients.

　　Although often invisible, hidden hunger negatively impacts health and development, and ultimately, economic well-being. About one-third of the world's population suffers from hidden hunger, mostly in developing countries. This is more than the population of Europe, the America, and Australia combined.

　　Hidden hunger's impact starts early. Nutritional deficiencies during the first 1,000 days, between the start of a mother's pregnancy and the child's second birthday, impede the child's ability to properly grow, learn, and ultimately reach his or her full potential. It can be devastating for long-term health, and ultimately, society's growth and prosperity.

Questions number 16–18 are based on the passage you've just heard.

16. What is the passage mainly about?

17. Where is hidden hunger most serious in the world?

18. What is the effect of hidden hunger on a child?

Passage Two

Katherine Stothard and colleagues from Britain's Newcastle University combine data from 18 studies to look at the risk of abnormalities of babies whose mothers were obese or overweight. The study found obese women were nearly twice as likely to have a baby with neural tube defects, which are caused by the incomplete development of the brain or spinal cord. For one such defect, spina bifida, the risk more than doubled. The researchers also detected increased chances of heart defect, cleft lip and palate, water on the brain and problems in the growth of arms and legs.

The World Health Organization classifies around 400 million people around the world as obese, including 20 million under the age of five, and the number is growing. Obesity raises the risks of diseases such as type 2 diabetes, heart problems and is a health concern piling pressure on already overburdened national health system.

Questions number 19–21 are based on the passage you've just heard.

19. What is the main topic of the passage?
20. What can we learn about the birth defects in the talk?
21. According to WHO, how many people are classified as obese around the world?

Passage Three

About 10 million people in the US alone are suffering from impairing noise-induced hearing loss. The rising trend is something that researchers and physicians at the University of Michigan Kresge Hearing Research Institute are hoping to reverse, with a cocktail of vitamins and the mineral magnesium that has shown promise as a possible way to prevent hearing loss caused by loud noise. The nutrients were successful in laboratory tests, and now researchers are testing whether humans will benefit as well. The combination of vitamins A, C, and E, plus magnesium, is given on pill form to patients who are participating in the research. The medication, called Aura Quell, is designed to be taken before a person is exposed to loud noise. The preclinical translational research that led to the formulation of Aura Quell as an effective preventive was funded by General Motors and the United Auto Workers.

Questions number 22–24 are based on the passage you've just heard.

22. What is the passage mainly concerned about?
23. What did Kresge Hearing Research Institute develop to prevent hearing loss?
24. Who, according to the speaker, would benefit from the formulation of Aura Quell?

Passage Four

The main challenges in residency come down to the increased responsibility. Real patients and the attendings are fully counting on you. As a medical student, you're primarily there in the hospital to learn and you had the resident above you, who was actually responsible for the patient. If you make a mistake or don't know the answer, it isn't that big of a deal. But as a resident, you're there to work, with learning being a secondary objective. You are the primary doctor caring for the patient and sometimes that's scary, and if you don't keep on top of your study and medical knowledge, you will be doing a significant disservice to your patients. Your increased responsibility also translates to many more nights on call, which means even more sleep deprivation than when you were a medical student. Increased responsibility also often translates to being the last one to leave.

Questions number 25–27 are based on the passage you've just heard.

25. What is the main idea of the passage?
26. Which of the following can be true of a resident?
27. According to the speaker, what does the increased responsibility mean to a resident?

Passage Five

I really want all of you patients to form partnerships with your physician. This partnership requires that we think because the physician and the patient are both after the same thing and that's the truth. As physicians, we get information by listening, asking questions, observing through examinations, and touch and then we think. I heeded the words of my mentor long ago who told me all the information that you need will be there if you let the patient talk and you listen.

If you can speak with your physician easily about the simple thing, then it'll be so much better. When you come to the hard things, serious illness, addiction and end-of-life discussion, ask questions and get answers and make sure the discussion is not in the big-word, top-secret language that we learned in medical school. Make sure that you understand before making decisions.

Questions number 28–30 are based on the passage you've just heard.

28. What does the speaker intend to do in the passage?
29. What happens if you let the patient talk and you listen according to the speaker?
30. What does the speaker suggest that patient-physician communication avoid?

四、拓展场景知识

医学博士英语考试的听力对话，经常围绕普通医疗情况下的医学英语会话来命题。以下几个场景中的画线部分便是常考的考点（问诊、主诉、检查、治疗等）。熟能生巧，复习时不仅要"识字"，更要对照音频，熟悉其发音。

场景一

W: Good morning, Dr. Smith's office. <u>How can I help you?</u>

女士：早晨好，史密斯医生办公室，<u>我能为您做什么吗？</u>

M: I would like to see the doctor as soon as I can. <u>I am having trouble with my stomach again.</u> It's terrible at this moment.

男士：我要尽快看医生，<u>我的胃病又犯了，</u>现在疼得好厉害。

W: Let me see if I can get you in this afternoon. No, I am sorry. <u>It will have to be tomorrow morning, 10 o'clock, Friday.</u> <u>Will that be all right?</u>

女士：我给您看看是不是能够预约在今天下午。不行，很抱歉，<u>得到明天早晨，也就是星期五早晨十点。</u> 这样可以吗？

M: Hmm, Friday? I have other plans tomorrow morning. But I will have to go to the doctor instead. I will be there at 10 tomorrow morning. Thank you.

男士：嗯，星期五？我明天早晨还有其他安排，但是我也只好去看病了。明天早晨十点我去医院，谢谢您。

场景二

D: Good morning, Madame. <u>What seems to be bothering you?</u>

医生：早上好，女士。<u>你哪儿不舒服？</u>

P: <u>It's extremely painful in the belly. It is really killing me.</u>

病人：<u>肚子疼得厉害，难受死了。</u>

D: <u>How long have you been like this?</u>

医生：<u>这样有多久了？</u>

P: Since last night.

病人：从昨晚就开始了。

D: <u>Have you had a fever?</u>

医生：<u>发烧吗？</u>

P: Yes, I feel feverish.

病人：是的，我感觉有点发烧。

D: <u>How about your bowel movement?</u>

医生：<u>大便怎么样？</u>

P: Well, I have to tell you that I haven't had a bowel movement for two days.

病人：呃，我得告诉您我有两天没大便了。

D: <u>Have you vomited?</u>

医生：<u>呕吐吗？</u>

P: Yes, last night I threw up all the things I had eaten. I felt awful.

病人：是的，昨晚我把吃的东西都吐出来了。难受极了。

D: Let me examine you. Would you please take off your shoes and lie down on that bed over there?

医生：我给你做个检查。请脱下鞋，躺到那边的床上吧。

P: Yes. Shall I unbutton my shirt?

病人：好的。我要解开上衣扣子吗？

D: Yes, please. Does it hurt when I press the lower quadrant of your abdomen?

医生：要。我按压你右下腹部时，你觉得疼吗？

P: Yes, it hurts badly.

病人：是的，非常疼。

D: I'm afraid you've got appendicitis. You will have to have a minor operation.

医生：恐怕你得了阑尾炎，需要做一个小手术。

场景三

D: Good afternoon. What seems to be wrong?

医生：下午好，你哪里不舒服？

P: Good morning, doctor. I have a terrible headache.

病人：下午好，医生。我头痛得厉害。

D: All right, young man. Tell me how it got started.

医生：别着急，小伙子，告诉我怎么回事。

P: Yesterday I had a running nose. Now my nose is stuffed up. I have a sore throat. And I am afraid I have got a temperature. I feel terrible.

病人：昨天我老流鼻涕，现在鼻子不通，喉咙很痛，恐怕还发烧。感觉糟透了。

D: Don't worry, young man. Let me give you an examination.

医生：别担心，小伙子，我给你检查一下。

...

......

D: Look. Your throat is inflamed. And your tongue is thickly coated. You have all the symptoms of influenza.

医生：听着，你的喉咙发炎了。舌苔很厚，这些都是流感的症状。

P: What am I supposed to do then?

病人：那我怎么办呢？

D: A good rest is all you need, and drink more water. I will write you a prescription.

医生：<u>你需要好好休息，多喝水，我给你开个处方。</u>

场景四

D: <u>What's bothering you?</u>

医生：<u>你哪里不舒服？</u>

P: <u>I've got a splitting headache. More often than not every morning when I got up, I felt as if the house were moving, so I had to lie back in bed for several minutes before trying to rise again.</u>

病人：我头疼得厉害。每天早晨起床时，经常觉得房子在动，所以我又回到床上躺几分钟再起来。

D: <u>How long have you had these symptoms?</u>

医生：<u>出现这些情况多长时间了？</u>

P: <u>About four months.</u>

病人：大约四个月了。

D: <u>Can you give me a description about the character of the pain? Or in other words, which part of your head aches most?</u>

医生：<u>你能描述一下头疼的情况吗？ 或者说头部哪个部分最疼？</u>

P: The front of my head aches most.

病人：前额最疼。

D: <u>Do you think your vision is getting worse?</u>

医生：<u>你觉得视力有所减退吗？</u>

P: Only a bit.

病人：有点。

D: <u>Do you feel dizzy?</u>

医生：<u>头晕吗？</u>

P: Yes, but not very often.

病人：是的，不太频繁。

D: <u>Have you ever had swollen ankles?</u>

医生：<u>脚踝肿过没有？</u>

P: I haven't noticed that.

病人：没注意到。

D: <u>Have you got a heart disease or a kidney problem?</u>

医生：<u>有过心脏病或肾病吗？</u>

P: Not yet.

病人：没有。

D: Well, <u>let me take your blood pressure. 170 over 100.</u> It's moderately high. Well, <u>I'd like you to take a blood urea nitrogen test, urinalysis, chest X-ray and electrodiagram examination.</u>

医生：呃，<u>我来给你量量血压。170/100，</u>是有点高。<u>我希望你做一下血尿素氮测定、尿常规检查，做个胸透，再做个心电图。</u>

P: OK. I'll have these examinations immediately.

病人：好的，我马上去。

…

……

P: Hello, doctor. Here are the reports. What's wrong with me?

病人：医生，这些是检查报告。我得了什么病？

D: You don't seem to have a heart disease or any kidney problem yet, but your <u>hypertension</u> is a problem we should do something about.

医生：你似乎没有心脏病和肾病，<u>但高血压</u>得治疗一下。

P: Is it serious, doctor?

病人：严重吗，医生？

D: According to your general situation, it's not so serious. <u>As for your food, you should keep to the low-salt diet, and eat more vegetables and fruits and less meat. Besides, you have a good rest and avoid tension or stress.</u> You'll be better.

医生：根据你的总体情况来看，并不太严重。<u>至于饮食，你应吃清淡些，多吃蔬菜和水果，少吃肉。</u> 好好休息，避免紧张和焦虑。你会好起来的。

P: Thanks a lot, doctor.

病人：非常感谢您，医生。

场景五

D: Good morning. <u>What seems to be the problem?</u>

医生：早上好，<u>哪里不舒服？</u>

P: <u>I often have a pain in the abdomen.</u> It troubled me for a long time.

病人：<u>我经常肚子疼，</u>困扰我很长时间了。

D: <u>When did you begin to notice these symptoms?</u>

医生：你什么时候有这些症状的？

P: About one year ago.

病人：大概一年以前。

D: Well, can you describe the pain? Or in other words, tell me what it is like exactly.

医生：那么，你能描述一下怎么个疼法吗？也就是告诉我具体是怎么样的疼痛。

P: Yes. Here it is. It's a dull pain.

病人：这里痛，钝痛。

D: Is the pain between the two meals or after? How long does it last?

医生：两餐之间痛还是饭后痛？疼痛每次持续多长时间？

P: It usually comes one hour after the meal, and eases 1–2 hours later. But the next meal it comes again.

病人：经常是饭后一小时开始痛，一般一两个小时后缓解。下次进食又开始痛。

D: Could you tell me what else you notice when the pain comes?

医生：痛的时候你还注意到别的症状吗？

P: Sometimes I feel gastrectasia.

病人：有时候感到胃胀。

D: Well. Do you notice the color of your stool? What color is it?

医生：嗯。你注意过大便的颜色吗？是什么颜色？

P: Yes, sometimes it is black.

病人：是的，有时候是黑色的。

D: Have you ever been to other hospitals? And have you ever done any examination? What was the diagnosis?

医生：你有没有到其他医院看过？做过什么检查吗？医生说是什么病？

P: I went to a private clinic last November. The doctor told me I got a gastric ulcer, but I didn't do any examination.

病人：去年十一月份我去过一家私人诊所看过，医生说我得了胃溃疡，但是没有做任何检查。

D: Did you take any medicines? Did you feel better then?

医生：吃过什么药吗？有没有好转？

P: Yes, since then I took the medicine off and on, such as cimetidine, and I was feeling a little better but the pain recurred later.

病人：是的，自从那时候起我断断续续地服药，比如西咪替丁等，有时我感觉好一点，但后来疼痛反复发作。

D: Are there any changes in your weight since you got the disease?

医生：得病后，体重有变化吗？

P: No, there is no change in my weight.

病人：没有变化。

D: Would you please bend you knee joint? Do you feel any tenderness here? Or rebound tenderness?

医生：弯一下你的膝关节。<u>这里有压痛吗？有反跳痛吗？</u>

P: No. What am I suffering from, doctor? Do you mean I've got a gastric ulcer?

病人：没有。医生，我得了什么病，胃溃疡吗？

D: <u>Most probably, according to your case history, I think you are suffering from gastric ulcer. I suggest you have a gastroscopy.</u>

医生：<u>根据你的病史，很可能是胃溃疡，我建议你做个胃镜。</u>

场景六

D: What's wrong with you?

医生：你哪里不舒服？

P: <u>I have severe pain in my upper abdomen</u>, which may be aggravated by eating.

病人：<u>我上腹部很痛</u>，有时候因为吃饭而痛得更厉害。

D: <u>What kind of pain is it?</u>

医生：<u>是什么样的痛法？</u>

P: <u>I had the heartburn pain</u> which is off and on three years ago. It seems to be related to my bad eating habits. This time the pain got worse both in frequency and severity.

病人：三年前断断续续地痛过，<u>烧心一样地痛</u>。疼痛似乎与我的不良饮食习惯有关。最近痛得更加频繁，也更严重。

D: Could you be more specific?

医生：能更具体地说说吗？

P: It's worst after I eat spicy food or onion. And it often awakens me two or three hours after I go to sleep. After meal I feel a little better, but the pain comes on one or two hours after meals.

病人：我吃辛辣的食物和洋葱后疼痛最厉害。还有，我经常在睡后两三个小时疼醒。另外，吃完饭后我感觉舒服点，但是疼痛会在一两个小时后出现。

D: <u>Have you ever had nausea or vomiting?</u>

医生：<u>恶心或者呕吐过吗？</u>

P: Well, I vomited yesterday, some food with a little blood like coffee.

病人：嗯，昨天吐过一次，有食物和咖啡色的<u>血</u>。

D: <u>Have your stools been loose?</u>

医生：<u>大便稀吗？</u>

P: No. But I had dark stools that look like tar.

病人：不，但是有几次是黑的，像炭一样。

D: <u>I think you have gotten duodenal ulcer. I suggest you have a barium meal</u>

examination and gastroscopy.

医生：我认为你可能得的是十二指肠溃疡，建议你做个钡餐和胃镜。

场景七

D: Where is the pain exactly?

医生：具体是哪儿疼？

P: The pain is in my neck. It hurts so much that I can't move my head freely.

病人：脖子，疼得我都没法随意转头了。

D: Does the pain move about?

医生：疼痛部位是否转移？

P: No. It doesn't seem to move.

病人：不，就那一个地方疼。

D: Show me the spot that's the most painful.

医生：哪个地方最疼？

P: It's here.

病人：这里。

D: What sort of pain is it?

医生：是一种什么样的疼痛？

P: It's a pricking kind of pain.

病人：像针刺一样疼。

D: If you rub or massage it, does it help?

医生：用手揉几下或按摩几下，疼痛会减轻吗？

P: No. It actually makes it worse.

病人：不会，会更严重。

D: How long have you had this pain?

医生：疼多久了？

P: Oh, about a week . I suppose.

病人：我想大约一周。

D: Is the pain constant, or does it come and go?

医生：疼痛是持续性的还是阵发性的？

P: It's not there all the time. It comes and goes.

病人：不是一直疼，有时疼，有时不疼。

D: How long does each attack last for?

医生：每次疼痛会持续多长时间？

P: About two hours.

病人：两个小时左右。

D: Have you ever had it before?

医生：以前疼过吗？

P: Yes. I had it about three years ago.

病人：是的，三年前疼过。

场景八

D: How can I help you?

医生：你感到哪儿不舒服？

P: I feel really dizzy. It's awful.

病人：我觉得头很晕，很难受。

D: Could you describe it to me?

医生：能给我描述一下头晕时的感觉吗？

P: <u>Well, it feels like I'm on a rocking boat and I can't stand up properly.</u> I keep staggering.

病人：<u>就像坐在一条小船上，摇晃得很厉害，站立不稳。</u>我一直摇摇晃晃的。

D: Does the room appear to be moving around you?

医生：你感觉房间好像在旋转吗？

P: Yes, that's it! Everything seems to be spinning around. It helps if I close my eyes.

病人：是的，觉得一切都天旋地转似的，闭上眼睛会好一点。

D: <u>Do you have any other problems besides this dizziness?</u>

医生：<u>除了头晕，还有其他不舒服吗？</u>

P: <u>My head feels tight and distended, and there's buzzing noise in my ears. My chest feels like it's got a weight on it. And I feel nauseous, too.</u>

病人：<u>头有点胀，还有耳鸣，胸闷，恶心。</u>

D: And how do you feel emotionally?

医生：心情怎样？

P: Not very good. I get angry pretty easily.

病人：心情不太好，很容易发脾气。

D: <u>Have you ever had any head injuries?</u>

医生：<u>以前头部受过外伤吗？</u>

P: No, never, not that I can think of.

病人：没有，不记得有过。

场景九

P: I've got this buzzing and ringing sound in my ears.

病人：我感到耳内总有响声。

D: How long has it been going on?

医生：多长时间了？

P: It's just started, suddenly, yesterday afternoon.

病人：刚开始的，昨天下午突然开始的。

D: Is it loud enough to affect your hearing?

医生：耳鸣声大吗？影响听力吗？

P: Yes. It sounds like the waves breaking on the beach and when people talk to me, I don't hear them very clearly.

病人：是的，声音很大，就像海浪拍打沙滩似的，别人和我讲话我都听不太清楚。

D: Anything else going on?

医生：还有别的不舒适的地方吗？

P: Well, my eyes feel a bit swollen. And I feel tired and listless, especially in the legs.

病人：眼睛感觉有点肿，最近总是感觉乏力，疲倦，尤其是两腿没劲。

D: If you press your fingers on your ears like this, does that help?

医生：像这样用手指按压耳朵，耳鸣会有减轻吗？

P: No, no difference. It's till as loud as ever.

病人：没有区别，仍然很响。

场景十

P: I'm having awful trouble trying to sleep.

病人：我晚上总是睡不着。

D: Does this happen often?

医生：经常如此吗？

P: Yes, quite often. I have trouble falling asleep and sometimes I'm awake the entire night. So I take sleeping pills.

病人：是的，我入睡总是很困难，有时整晚都睡不着，得靠吃安眠药。

D: Do you feel like sleeping in the daytime?

医生：白天想睡觉吗？

P: No.

病人：不想。

D: How do you feel during the daytime?

医生：那白天感觉如何？

P: I'm always drowsy and really tired.

病人：白天人昏昏沉沉的，很疲劳。

D: Do you ever have a fluttering sensation in the chest, or palpitations?

医生：平时有没有心慌、心悸等感觉？

P: Yes, always, and it only takes a slight sound to set my heart off.

病人：常会感到心慌，稍微有点声响心跳就很厉害。

D: How have you been emotionally recently?

医生：最近情绪怎么样？

P: Not too good, really. I'm cranky and pretty forgetful.

病人：不是很好，总想发火，还很健忘。

D: How's your appetite been?

医生：最近胃口如何？

P: I don't feel like eating. The boating in my stomach puts me off food.

病人：不太想吃，腹胀，吃不下东西。

D: Is there anything else bothering you?

医生：还有其他不舒服吗？

P: I'm a bit dizzy and get a ringing noise in my ears sometimes.

病人：有点儿头晕，有时耳鸣。

场景十一

D: He's got a temperature and a cough. Has he had a cold?

医生：孩子发烧了，还咳嗽。他着凉了吗？

P: Yes, I didn't dress him warmly enough yesterday.

家长：是的，我昨天给他穿得不够暖和。

D: Has he had anything to eat which might be hard to digest?

医生：他吃了什么不好消化的东西吗？

P: I gave him some cold milk yesterday. Then last night he had diarrhea.

家长：我昨天给他喂了点凉牛奶，昨天晚上他就有点腹泻。

D: Has he ever had any traumatic experiences, anything to badly frighten him?

医生：孩子有没有受到什么严重的惊吓？

P: Well, yesterday we set off some fireworks, and today he's got a temperature.

家长：昨天我们放了烟花，今天他就开始发烧了。

D: Do you remember how many times did he go to the toilet?

医生：你记得孩子一天拉了几次吗？

P: I can't remember exactly. It must have been over six times.

家长：我记不太清了，肯定超过 6 次。

D: What kind of stool did you notice, watery or mucous?

医生：你注意大便是什么样的了吗？水样便还是黏液样便？

P: They are quite loose with milk curd and undigested food in them.

家长：很稀，还有奶瓣和没消化的食物。

D: Did he suffer from other diseases before?

医生：他以前有其他病史吗？

P: He is healthy always, and scarcely feel sick.

家长：他一直很健康，很少生病。

五、听力专项练习

Section A 专项练习

Directions: *In this section you will hear ten conversations. At the end of each conversation, you will hear three questions about the conversation. The question will be spoken only once. After you hear the question, read the four possible answers marked A, B, C and D. Choose the best answer and mark the letter of your choice on the **ANSWER SHEET.***

Conversation One

1. A. Eating pork.   B. Raising pigs.
   C. Eating chicken.   D. Breeding birds.
2. A. Running nose.   B. Inappetence.
   C. Pains all over.   D. Diarrhea.
3. A. To stay from crowds.   B. To see the doctor immediately.
   C. To avoid medications.   D. To go to the nearby clinic.

Conversation Two

1. A. A blood test.   B. A gastroscopy.
   C. A chest X-ray exam.   D. A barium X-ray test.
2. A. To lose some weight.   B. To take a few more tests.
   C. To take some tablets.   D. To eat smaller, lighter meals.
3. A. Ulcer.   B. Cancer.   C. Depression.   D. Hernia.

Conversation Three

1. A. White blood cell count.   B. Red blood cell count.
   C. X-ray.   D. ECG.

2.   A. Heart disease.   B. Gastric ulcer.   C. Stomach flu.   D. Pneumonia.

3.   A. Stay off work.   B. Drink plenty of liquids.

     C. Eat a lot of vegetables and fruits.   D. Postpone your exercise when sick.

Conversation Four

1.   A. He is having a physical checkup.

     B. He has just undergone an operation.

     C. He has just recovered from an illness.

     D. He will be discharged from the hospital this afternoon.

2.   A. He got an infection in the lungs.

     B. He had his gallbladder inflamed.

     C. He was suffering from influenza.

     D. He had developed a big kidney stone.

3.   A. To be confined to a wheelchair.

     B. To stay indoors for a complete recovery.

     C. To stay in bed and drink a lot of water.

     D. To move about and enjoy the sunshine.

Conversation Five

1.   A. He has got cancer in his pancreas.   B. He falls with a stomach problem.

     C. He suffers from fatigue.   D. He has a loss of weight.

2.   A. A couple of years.   B. More than 5 years.

     C. A couple of months.   D. Approximately 5 years.

3.   A. Suspicious.   B. Anxious.   C. Hesitant.   D. Factual.

Conversation Six

1.   A. He has something wrong with his blood.

     B. He has something wrong with his kidney.

     C. He has something wrong with his pancreas.

     D. He has something wrong with his case history.

2.   A. Pancreases cannot secrete insulin at all in type II.

     B. Pancreases cannot secrete enough insulin in type I.

     C. Type I is not as serious as type II.

     D. Type II is not as serious as type I.

3.   A. He should eat as much as possible to avoid blood sugar decreasing.

     B. He should remain inside the house.

     C. He should eat more vegetables.

     D. He should eat more fat to get stronger.

Conversation Seven

1. A. He has got bowel cancer. B. He has got heart disease.
   C. He has got bone cancer. D. He has got heartburn.
2. A. Thankful. B. Admitting.
   C. Resentful. D. Respectful.
3. A. It was based on the symptoms the man had described.
   B. It was prescribed considering possible complications.
   C. It was given according to the man's actual condition.
   D. It was effective because of a proper intervention.

Conversation Eight

1. A. Internet. B. Newspaper. C. Magazine. D. Books.
2. A. Fashion newspaper. B. Fashion magazine.
   C. Medical newspaper. D. Medical magazine.
3. A. A teacher. C. A journalist.
   D. A writer. D. A doctor.

Conversation Nine

1. A. Running has her ankles twisted at times.
   B. Running is making her feel hungry.
   C. Running helps little in losing weight.
   D. Running makes her feel exhausted.
2. A. They are not presently available.
   B. They mostly belong to organic foods.
   C. Many of them are low in calories.
   D. They are relatively easy to digest.
3. A. Mutton, beef and fish.
   B. Skimmed milk, eggs and bread.
   C. Hamburger, nuts and cake.
   D. Whole grains, vegetables and fruits.

Conversation Ten

1. A. Math. B. Geography.
   C. History. D. Art subjects.
2. A. Videos. B. Movies.
   C. Computers. D. Kitchenware.
3. A. Writing skills. B. Logical mind.
   C. Mathematics skills. D. Interest.

Section A 专项练习答案与解析

Conversation One

1. 【问题】什么造成人类感染猪流感？
   　　　　A．吃猪肉。　　　　B．养猪。　　　　C．吃鸡肉。　　　　D．喂鸟。
   【答案】B
   【解析】细节回现题。从对话中可知 Only people who work with pigs can catch the virus，只有接触感染病毒的猪的人，才可能感染。故 B 为正确答案。

2. 【问题】根据对话内容，下列哪一个是猪流感最常见的症状？
   　　　　A．流鼻涕。　　　　B．食欲不振。　　　C．浑身疼痛。　　　D．腹泻。
   【答案】B
   【解析】细节概括题。从文中 "The most common symptoms are fever, fatigue, lack of appetite and coughing" 可知，B 选项在最常见的症状中。

3. 【问题】讲话人对疑似猪流感患者的建议是什么？
   　　　　A．远离人群。　　　B．立刻就医。　　　C．不要用药。　　　D．就近就医。
   【答案】A
   【解析】细节概括题。对话中说："Stay home from work or school. Don't get on a place. Call your doctors to ask about the best treatment. Don't simply show up at the clinic or hospital that is unprepared for your arrival." 即不要上班或者上学，电话咨询医生诊疗方案，不要突兀直接就医。因此 A 为正确改写。

Conversation Two

1. 【问题】男士在进行什么医疗程序？
   　　　　A．验血。　　　　　　　　　　　　　B．胃镜。
   　　　　C．胸部 X 光片检查。　　　　　　　D．钡餐 X 光片检查。
   【答案】D
   【解析】细节复现题。女士说 your barium meal did not show an ulcer，即证明男士刚刚做完钡餐 X 光片检查。

2. 【问题】下列哪一个不是医生给男士的建议？
   　　　　A．减重。　　　　　　　　　　　　　B．多做几个检查。
   　　　　C．服用药片。　　　　　　　　　　　D．少食多餐，清淡饮食。
   【答案】B
   【解析】细节复现题。医生说："... if you were able to lose a bit of weight. You'll be less likely to get the pain if you can eat smaller, lighter meals regularly. Lastly, I'm going to give you some tablets ..." 可知医生建议病人减肥，"eat smaller, lighter meals" 会减少疼痛，同时还会给他开一些 tablets，因此本题正确答案为 B。

3. 【问题】医生对病人的诊断是什么？
   　　　　A．溃疡。　　　　　B．癌症。　　　　C．抑郁。　　　　D．疝。
   【答案】D

【解析】细节复现题。医生在对话开始就给出了诊断 —— 食管裂孔疝（hiatus hernia）。

Conversation Three

1. 【问题】女士的检查结果显示什么不正常？
  A．白细胞。　　　B．红细胞。　　　C．X 光片。　　　D．心电图。

  【答案】**A**

  【解析】细节复现题。医生说 But your white blood cell count is rather high，证明女士的白细胞指标不正常。

2. 【问题】医生对女士的诊断是什么？
  A．心脏病。　　　　　　　　B．胃溃疡。
  C．肠胃炎。　　　　　　　　D．肺炎。

  【答案】**C**

  【解析】细节推理题。医生说病人的白细胞指标超高，证明免疫系统在与病毒做斗争。而病人的心电图和透视检查都显示正常，由此可知 C 为最佳答案。

3. 【问题】下列哪一个不是医生的建议？
  A．不工作，休息。　　　　　B．大量饮水。
  C．多吃蔬菜水果。　　　　　D．生病时不要锻炼。

  【答案】**D**

  【解析】细节复现题。医生说 "you really shouldn't go to work. Rest as much as possible, drink plenty of liquid, and eat plenty of vegetables and fruits"，即不要工作、尽量多休息、多饮水、多摄入蔬菜和水果。只有 D 选项没有提到。

Conversation Four

1. 【问题】哪一个关于男士的描述是正确的？
  A．他在体检。　　　　　　　B．他刚做完手术。
  C．他生病初愈。　　　　　　D．他下午从医院出院。

  【答案】**B**

  【解析】细节推理题。从女士要求男士不能喝水、坐轮椅去享受阳光、日益恢复，以及说到胆结石（gall stone）的情况可以推理，男士刚刚做完手术。

2. 【问题】男士出什么问题了？
  A．肺部发炎。　　B．胆囊发炎。　　C．感冒。　　D．肾结石。

  【答案】**B**

  【解析】细节复现题。女士说 You have a pretty big gall stone and the gallbladder was quite inflamed，非常明确地告知男士的问题是胆囊发炎。

3. 【问题】根据医生指示，男士应该做什么？
  A．只能在轮椅上。　　　　　B．待在室内直到康复。
  C．卧床，多饮水。　　　　　D．多走动，享受阳光。

  【答案】**D**

  【解析】细节推理题。女士说 "the sooner we have you on the move, the quicker you start to heal",大意是"男士越快四处走动走动,就会愈合得越快"。因此 D 选项是正确答案。

Conversation Five

1. 【问题】根据医生的诊断,Scot 先生有什么问题?

    A. 胰腺癌。　　　B. 胃出了问题。　　C. 精疲力竭。　　　D. 体重减轻。

    【答案】A

    【解析】细节复现题。从最开始 got a recurrence of cancer in your pancreas 可知,男士胰腺癌复发。疲惫和体重减轻都是胰腺癌带来的症状。

2. 【问题】在医生看来,Scot 先生还能活多久?

    A. 几年。　　　　B. 5 年以上。　　　C. 几个月。　　　D. 大约 5 年。

    【答案】C

    【解析】细节复现题。根据医生说的 But I'd say it's a matter of months rather than years 可知,病人的寿命还有几个月的时间,而非几年。

3. 【问题】下列哪一个是对医生语气的最佳描述?

    A. 怀疑的。　　　B. 焦急的。　　　C. 犹豫的。　　　D. 实事求是的。

    【答案】D

    【解析】细节推理题。从医生描述病情、描述病人寿命的语气可以看出,医生的语气是平缓而实事求是的。

Conversation Six

1. 【问题】男士发生了什么问题?

    A. 血液出现了问题。　　　　　　　　B. 肾脏出现了问题。

    C. 胰腺出现了问题。　　　　　　　　D. 病历出现了问题。

    【答案】C

    【解析】细节复现题。不难得知,医生一直在解释两种糖尿病的区别,文中也明确出现了 pancreas 不能分泌胰岛素的细节,所以男士是胰腺的问题。

2. 【问题】根据对话,下列哪一项是正确的?

    A. II 型糖尿病不能分泌胰岛素。

    B. I 型糖尿病不能分泌足够的胰岛素。

    C. I 型糖尿病不如 II 型严重。

    D. II 型糖尿病不如 I 型严重。

    【答案】D

    【解析】细节复现题。医生说:"Pancreases in type I cannot secrete insulin and patients depend on the treatment of insulin all their lives, while the type II just cannot secrete enough insulin and can be treated with drugs or insulin. So, type II is not so much serious as type I." 即 I 型不能分泌胰岛素,II 型不能分泌足够的胰岛素,故 I 型更严重。

3. 【问题】男士日常生活应该注意什么？

    A．他应该多吃，避免血糖降低。

    B．他应该在室内活动。

    C．他应该多吃蔬菜。

    D．他应该多吃脂肪类食物，变得强壮些。

【答案】C

【解析】细节复现题。医生建议："Dinners should be on time, and don't eat too much. You'd better eat less sugar-rich and fatty food, eat more coarse food grain, vegetables, and take more outdoor exercise." 即按时吃饭，不要过量。少吃含糖量高的食物，少吃脂肪含量高的食物，多吃粗粮、蔬菜，多进行户外活动。故只有 C 选项是正确的。

Conversation Seven

1. 【问题】男士出什么问题了？

    A．肠癌。   B．心脏病。   C．骨癌。   D．胃灼热。

【答案】A

【解析】细节推理题。医生说他要 have an operation to remove the bowel，要切除结肠。可推理得知男士的问题在肠部。

2. 【问题】男士对医生是什么态度？

    A．感激的。   B．认可的。   C．憎恨的。   D．尊敬的。

【答案】C

【解析】细节推理题。男士对自己终身携带 colostomy bag 接受不了，埋怨医生诊断成 heartburn 是误诊：All this time you have been prescribing tablets for heart-burn, and it turns out that I got cancer of the bowel? Oh, thanks a million. What next? Will I be able to live any kind of normal life? Tell me! 语气中充满了愤怒和不满。

3. 【问题】医生如何解释之前的治疗方案？

    A．这是基于病人自述症状之上做出的。

    B．这是考虑到并发症给出的诊断。

    C．这是根据男士实际情况给出的诊断。

    D．因为有了适当干预，这是有效的。

【答案】A

【解析】细节复现题。医生解释说 I prescribed for you on the basis of the symptoms you yourself described to me，即基于病人主诉给出的治疗方案。

Conversation Eight

1. 【问题】根据对话，哪一个更有价值？

    A．互联网。   B．报纸。   C．杂志。   D．图书。

【答案】B

【解析】细节概括题。女士说"随着互联网越来越流行，看报纸杂志的人越来越少了"。男士回答，他认为报纸更有信息价值（more informative）。

2. "Rayli"和"Fashion"是什么？

    A．时尚报纸。   B．时尚杂志。   C．医学报纸。   D．医学杂志。

【答案】B

【解析】细节推理题。女士问对方是否买杂志，男士回答经常买"Rayli"和"Fashion"，可知这两份都是杂志，接着说它们能让他跟上时代潮流，可推知是时尚杂志。

3. 【问题】女士的工作是什么？

    A．教师。   B．记者。   C．作家。   D．医生。

【答案】D

【解析】细节推理题。女士说："I am reading a book about medicine history. A little boring, but it's my career." 可推知她的工作与medicine相关，做doctor的可能性更大。

Conversation Nine

1. 【问题】女士在减肥时遇到什么样的困境？

    A．跑步时经常把脚踝扭伤。   B．跑步让她感到饥饿。

    C．跑步对减重几乎无效。   D．跑步让她精疲力竭。

【答案】B

【解析】细节复现题。女士说："I'm trying to lose weight by running, but all the exercise is making me feel hungry all the time." 即运动让她感到饥饿。

2. 【问题】关于高纤维食品，男士说了什么？

    A．现在没有供应。   B．多数是有机食品。

    C．很多热量低。   D．相对比较容易消化。

【答案】C

【解析】细节复现题。男士说："... high-fiber foods are usually tight so they fill up your stomach faster and can also delay the time it takes your stomach to empty. Also, many high fiber foods are low in calories, so you can satisfy your hunger with fewer calories." 即高纤维食品密度大，饱腹感强，可延缓胃部放空的时间，同时此类食品热量低，在低热量的情况下能缓解饥饿。因此本题答案为C。

3. 【问题】下列哪种食品是纤维不错的来源？

    A．羊肉、牛肉、鱼。   B．脱脂牛奶、鸡蛋、面包。

    C．汉堡、坚果、蛋糕。   D．全麦、蔬菜、水果。

【答案】D

【解析】细节复现题。男士推荐"Whole grains, vegetables, and fruits are great sources of fiber"，可知本题正确答案为D。

Conversation Ten

1. 【问题】男士最喜欢的科目是什么？

    A．数学。   B．地理。   C．历史。   D．艺术。

【答案】A

【解析】细节概括题。男士说了不少关于学科的话："... my best subject was history and my second best was geography. However, my favorite subject was math..." 需要仔细概括一下，最喜欢的是数学，学得最好的是历史，其次是地理。

2. 【问题】女士的公司是制造什么的？

　　A．视频。　　　　B．电影。　　　　C．电脑。　　　　D．厨房用品。

【答案】C

【解析】细节复现题。男士说："I understand that you manufacture computers, prepare software and advise clients on how to use them." 即他认为女士公司是制造电脑、软件的，并给出使用建议，女士认可男士的说法。因此本题答案为C。

3. 【问题】对男士来讲，什么是对这个工作最有用的？

　　A．写作技巧。　　B．逻辑推理。　　C．数学技巧。　　D．兴趣。

【答案】B

【解析】细节概括题。男士说他被告知 working with computers needs the logical mind rather than great skills in mathematics，rather than 有否定的含义，即 logic mind 是更重要的。因此本题答案为B。

Section A 专项练习录音原文

Conversation One

W: Hello, Doctor Smith, welcome to our program "Health Journey". Could you tell us something about swine flu?

M: Well, it's a common respiratory ailment in pigs that doesn't usually spread to people.

W: Can we catch swine flu from eating pork?

M: Actually, ill pigs are not allowed to enter the market. Cooking also kills the virus. Only people who work with pigs can catch the virus.

W: How do they feel if infected?

M: The most common symptoms are fever, fatigue, lack of appetite and coughing, although some people also develop runny nose, sore throat, vomiting or diarrhea.

W: What should we do if we have these symptoms?

M: Stay home from work or school. Don't get on a place. Call your doctors to ask about the best treatment. Don't simply show up at the clinic or hospital that is unprepared for your arrival.

W: Say, the antiviral study. How is it going?

Questions 1–3 are based on the conversation you've just heard.

1. What may cause people to have swine flu?

2. According to the dialogue, which is among the most common symptoms of swine flu?

3. What does the speaker advise the suspects of swine flu to do?

Conversation Two

W: Well, your barium meal did not show an ulcer. But it did show that you have something we call a hiatus hernia. Do you know what that is?

M: I haven't much of a clue, really.

W: I think it would help if you were able to lose a bit of weight. You'll be less likely to get the pain if you can eat smaller, lighter meals regularly. Lastly, I'm going to give you some tablets that will stop your stomach from producing acid. Perhaps you could tell me what you feel about it?

M: Well, I worry that it might be difficult, because I'm a lorry driver and have to be on the road most of the day.

W: Yes, I understand you might have some problems with the diet I'm suggesting, especially as roadside cafes usually sell meals with greasy food. However, perhaps you could keep to fish and chicken, and avoid chips and fried eggs.

Questions 1–3 are based on the conversation you've just heard.

1. What medical procedure has the man undergone?
2. Which of the following is NOT among the doctor's suggestions to the man?
3. What is the doctor's diagnosis of the man?

Conversation Three

P: Here is my result, doctor.

D: Well, your ECG is perfectly normal, and there is no problem with your X-ray, either. But your white blood cell count is rather high, which is what I expected, and it shows your body is fighting the virus.

P: Is there anything here I can do so that I can feel better, doctor? I am really busy at work this week. And I have a lot of stuff to do.

D: Don't worry. I will give you some medicine for it to make you feel better. Three times a day take the white tablets as directed on the label after meals.

P: Is there anything else I can do, Doctor Hunt?

D: I know you are busy, but you really shouldn't go to work. Rest as much as possible, drink plenty of liquid, and eat plenty of vegetables and fruits. If there is no improvement after three days, come back and see me again.

P: Thank you, doctor.

Questions 1–3 are based on the conversation you've just heard.

1. According to the woman's test results, which of the following items is abnormal?
2. What is the doctor's diagnosis of the woman?
3. Which of the following is not one of the suggestions by the doctor?

Conversation Four

W: You can't drink anything at the moment.

M: The nurses have been giving me mouth washes.

W: Yes. I think you begin to pick up as the day goes on. And we'll carry on giving you something to ease the discomfort. Does it hurt much?

M: Well, it does when I move about.

W: Right. But the sooner we have you on the move, the quicker you start to heal. So we'll help you sit in the chair this afternoon. Enjoy the sunshine.

M: OK, I can't say I'm really looking forward to that.

W: You have a pretty big gall stone and the gallbladder was quite inflamed. There was a lot of infection around it and inside it. Well, it's out now. It won't cause you any more trouble. Any more questions or anything we can do for you?

M: No, I think I'm OK.

Questions 1–3 are based on the conversation you've just heard.

1. What's true about the man in the conversation?

2. What was wrong with the man?

3. What's the man supposed to do according to the doctor's orders?

Conversation Five

W: Mr. Scot, I'm afraid that you got a recurrence of cancer in your pancreas. That would explain why you've been feeling so tired, and your loss of appetite and weight.

M: Doctor Smith, do I need surgery?

W: Surgery isn't an option at this stage. There's still a lot we can do to help you. We can start you on a course of chemotherapy to help you with your symptoms. This won't cure you, but will make you feel more comfortable. I like you to see a dietician for some advice on what you eat.

M: What's my life expectancy? How long have I got?

W: One can never be certain about these issues. People with this condition vary a great deal. But I'd say it's a matter of months rather than years. I'm sorry to have to tell you all this, but my feeling is, it is always good to be honest with people.

Questions 1–3 are based on the conversation you've just heard.

1. According to the doctor's diagnosis, what's happened to Mr. Scot?

2. According to the doctor, what might be Mr. Scot's life expectancy?

3. Which of the following can best describe the tone of doctor's words?

Conversation Six

W: I suggest that you go to measure your blood sugar and urine sugar first, and then bring me the reports.

M: This is my outcomes. Are they normal?

W: Both your blood sugar and urine sugar are higher than normal. According to your case history and age, I think you are suffering from type II diabetes.

M: Is the disease serious, doctor?

W: No. There are two types of diabetes, type I and type II. Pancreases in type I cannot secrete insulin and patients depend on the treatment of insulin all their lives, while the type II just cannot secrete enough insulin and can be treated with drugs or insulin. So, type II is not so much serious as type I.

M: That's a relief. Should I pay attention to my daily life?

W: Dinners should be on time, and don't eat too much. You'd better eat less sugar-rich and fatty food, eat more coarse food grain, vegetables, and take more outdoor exercise.

Questions 1–3 are based on the conversation you've just heard.

1. What's wrong with the man?

2. According to the conversation, which of the following is TRUE?

3. What should the man do in his daily life?

Conversation Seven

W: Well, you'll probably have an operation to remove the bowel, or some of it.

M: How can I live without a bowel?

W: During the operation, they will fit you externally with a colostomy bag.

M: You mean the bag of shit hanging inside of my clothes?

W: Well, that's perhaps an unnecessarily cruel way of putting it. But it is sealed and odor-free. They'll show you how to empty it and change it for yourself. And nobody need ever know that unless you tell them.

M: All this time you have been prescribing tablets for heartburn, and it turns out that I got cancer of the bowel? Oh, thanks a million. What next? Will I be able to live any kind of normal life? Tell me!

W: I prescribed for you on the basis of the symptoms you yourself described to me. Only a colonoscopy can reveal your condition. And yes, you will be able to live a pretty normal life and go work, and everything.

Questions 1–3 are based on the conversation you've just heard.

1. What is wrong with the man?

2. What is the man's attitude towards the doctor?

3. What does the doctor say about the previous treatment for the patient?

Conversation Eight

W: As the Internet becomes more popular, fewer and fewer people like to read newspapers and magazines.

M: Really, but I think the newspaper is very informative.

W: Yes. And there is much local news and international news in it. It usually has the news section, the entertainment section, sports, and business and so on.

M: You're right. We can get current affairs from the newspaper.

W: Do you often buy magazines?

M: I buy "Rayli" and "Fashion" every month. They keep me up-to-date with all the latest trends of the fashion. I like to read a magazine in a café. By the way, what are you reading recently?

W: I am reading a book about medicine history. A little boring, but it's my career.

Questions 1–3 are based on the conversation you've just heard.

1. Which one is more worthwhile, according to the conversation?
2. What "Rayli" and "Fashion" are?
3. What is the woman's job?

Conversation Nine

W: I'm trying to lose weight by running, but all the exercise is making me feel hungry all the time. How can I feel satisfied without gaining weight?

M: You're burning more calories, so your body needs to take more in. First of all, get lots of healthy, higher-fiber foods in your diet.

W: I think that most high-fiber foods require more chewing.

M: Yes, high-fiber foods are usually tight so they fill up your stomach faster and can also delay the time it takes your stomach to empty. Also, many high fiber foods are low in calories, so you can satisfy your hunger with fewer calories.

W: I like high-fiber foods. Could you please recommend me some?

M: There are many options for you. Whole grains, vegetables, and fruits are great sources of fiber.

W: OK, I know. I'll buy these foods in a supermarket this afternoon. Have you got any other suggestions?

M: You'd better choose smaller meals in the day. If you wait for a meal for a long time, you'll be starving to eat more by the time you eat.

Questions 1–3 are based on the conversation you've just heard.

1. What kind of trouble is the woman confronted with while she is losing weight?
2. What does the man say about high-fiber foods?
3. What kind of foods have been listed as great sources of fiber?

Conversation Ten

W: Good morning. Sit down please, Mr. Johnson.

M: Thank you, ma'am.

W: I have read your letter here. You seem to have done very well at school. Can you tell me something about your school work?

M: As you can see, my best subject was history and my second best was geography. However, my favorite subject was math and the results I got in the math paper were quite reasonable.

W: That's true. Now can you tell me why you think these subjects will help you in this job?

M: Well, ma'am, I understand that you manufacture computers, prepare software and advise clients on how to use them. Is that right?

W: That's right.

M: And I've been told that working with computers needs the logical mind rather than great skills in mathematics. That's especially true, I believe, when it comes to writing programs. So I think my results show that I have some ability in logic and in mathematics as well.

Questions 1–3 are based on the conversation you've just heard.

1. What was the man's favorite subject?
2. What does the woman's company make?
3. What is viewed as the most helpful for the man in this job?

Section B 专项练习

Directions: *In this section you will hear ten passages. At the end of each passage, you will hear three questions about the passage. The question will be spoken only once. After you hear the question, read the four possible answers marked A, B, C and D. Choose the best answer and mark the letter of your choice on the **ANSWER SHEET.***

Passage One

1. A. Headaches.   B. Insomnia.
   C. Respiratory problems.   D. Digestive problems.

2. A. On Monday in Edinburgh.
   B. On Wednesday in Edinburgh.
   C. On Monday at Staffordshire University.
   D. On Wednesday at Staffordshire University.

3. A. The diarists who write of their free will.

B. The diarists who were students at Staffordshire University.

C. The diarists who had written about trauma.

D. The non-diarists who were susceptible to headaches.

Passage Two

1. A. A brief history of British pubs.

    B. Beer — the British national drink.

    C. Various attempts made to curb drinking in Britain.

    D. The frustrating opening and closing hours of British pubs.

2. A. As early as 659 AD.   B. After 659 AD.

    C. Before the Roman invasion.   D. After the Roman invasion.

3. A. The licensing hours have been extended.

    B. Old people are not allowed to drink in pubs.

    C. Children are not allowed yet to drink in pubs.

    D. Big changes have taken place in pubs.

Passage Three

1. A. The link between weight loss and sleep deprivation.

    B. The link between weight gain and sleep deprivation.

    C. The link between weight loss and physical exercise.

    D. The link between weight gain and physical exercise.

2. A. More than 68,000.   B. More than 60,800.

    C. More than 60,080.   D. More than 60,008.

3. A. Overeating among the sleep-deprived.

    B. Little exercise among the sleep-deprived.

    C. Lower metabolic rate resulting from less sleep.

    D. Higher metabolic rate resulting from less sleep.

Passage Four

1. A. She is too hard on me.

    B. She asks too many questions.

    C. She is always considerate of my feelings.

    D. She is the meanest mother in the neighborhood.

2. A. They are overconfident.

    B. Their brains grow too fast.

    C. They are psychologically dependent.

    D. Their brains are still immature in some areas.

3. A. Be easy on your teen.   B. Try to be mean to your teen.

    C. Say no to your teen when necessary.   D. Don't care about your teen's feelings.

Passage Five

1. A. Liver failure.　　　　　　　　　B. Breast cancer.
   C. Kidney failure.　　　　　　　　　D. Diabetes out of control.
2. A. Shape.　　　B. Color.　　　C. Price.　　　D. Size.
3. A. It is under a clinical trial.　　　B. It is available in the market.
   C. It is widely used in the clinic.　　D. It is in the experimental stage.

Passage Six

1. A. A hobby.　　　　　　　　　　　　B. The whole world.
   C. A learning experience.　　　　　　D. A chance to earn a living.
2. A. Her legs were broken.
   B. Her arms were broken.
   C. Her shoulders were seriously injured.
   D. Her cervical vertebrae were seriously injured.
3. A. Optimistic and hard-bitten.　　　B. Pessimistic and cynical.
   C. Humorous and funny.　　　　　　D. Kind and reliable.

Passage Seven

1. A. Life evolution.　　　　　　　　　B. Space exploration.
   C. Extraterrestrial life.　　　　　　D. Unknown flying objects.
2. A. His 50th birthday.
   B. NASA's 50th anniversary.
   C. The University's 50th anniversary.
   D. The US Cosmology Association's 50th Anniversary.
3. A. Nuclear weapons.　　　　　　　　B. Alien kidnapping.
   C. Human extinction.　　　　　　　　D. Dangerous infection.

Passage Eight

1. A. Limited living space.
   B. Crowded shopping malls.
   C. Food shortage and higher energy prices.
   D. Incidence of diabetes and cardiovascular diseases.
2. A. Over 700 million.　　　　　　　　B. Over 400 million.
   C. Over 2.3 billion.　　　　　　　　D. Over 3 billion.
3. A. Climate change.　　　　　　　　　B. The fall of food prices.
   C. A rise in energy prices.　　　　　D. An increasing demand for food.

Passage Nine

1. A. Suicide.　　　B. Obesity.　　　C. Turmoil.　　　D. Drug abuse.

2. A. Combining antidepressants and talk therapy.

   B. Promoting the transmission between neurons.

   C. Winning parental assistance and support.

   D. Administering effective antidepressants.

3. A. 65 per cent.   B. 75 per cent.   C. 85 per cent.   D. 95 per cent.

Passage Ten

1. A. 2,030 sociology students.   B. 2,300 sociology students.

   C. 2,030 psychologist students.   D. 2,300 psychologist students.

2. A. Spiritual life.   B. Image and wealth.

   C. Academic success.   D. Morality and aesthetics.

3. A. Too much texting can make you shallow.

   B. Texting is nothing but a wonder of technology.

   C. Texting has more disadvantages than advantages.

   D. Too much texting results in poorly performing students.

Section B 专项练习答案与解析

Passage One

1. 【问题】根据英国心理学家的研究，经常写日记的人更可能遭受除了＿＿＿之外的痛苦？

   A. 头疼。   B. 失眠。

   C. 呼吸系统问题。   D. 消化系统问题。

   【答案】C

   【解析】细节题。根据文章开始的"They found that people who regularly keep diaries suffer from headaches, sleeplessness, digestive problems and social awkwardness more than people who don't."可知，经常写日记的人比没有写日记习惯的人更容易遭受头痛、失眠、消化系统问题的折磨。并没有提到 C。

2. 【问题】Duncan 的研究是在何时何地发表的？

   A. 周一、爱丁堡。   B. 周三、爱丁堡。

   C. 周一、Staffordshire 大学。   D. 周三、Staffordshire 大学。

   【答案】B

   【解析】细节再现题。从文章中"... was presented on Wednesday at a meeting of the British Psychological Society in Edinburgh"可知，正确答案为 B。

3. 【问题】根据 Duncan 的研究，谁获得的健康量表分数最差？

   A. 自由记录日记的人。   B. Staffordshire 大学的学生。

   C. 记录自己创伤的人。   D. 容易犯头痛病的不记日记的人。

   【答案】C

   【解析】细节再现题。文章末尾谈到 The worst affected of all were those who had written about trauma，可知正确答案为 C。

Passage Two

1. 【问题】这篇文章的主要内容是什么？

    A．英国酒吧简要史。   B．啤酒——英国国饮。

    C．英国控制饮酒的多种尝试。   D．英国酒吧令人沮丧的营业时间。

【答案】C

【解析】细节再现题。从开始的 So is the law history to curb it 可知，本文讲的是 curb drinking 的话题。

2. 【问题】在英国，人们什么时候开始饮啤酒的？

    A．早在公元前 659 年。   B．公元前 659 年后。

    C．罗马入侵前。   D．罗马入侵后。

【答案】C

【解析】细节再现题。录音中有集中出现时间的地方，要注意区分。通过 Beer has been drunk in Britain since before the Roman invasion 可知，本题答案为 C。

3. 【问题】下列哪一个关于英国酒吧的描述是正确的？

    A．许可经营时间得以延长。   B．老年人不允许在酒吧饮酒。

    C．儿童仍然不能进酒吧喝酒。   D．酒吧发生了很大变化。

【答案】C

【解析】细节概括题。从末尾处的"Their opening and closing hours are still restricted by law although they have their recommendations recently for big changes, including extending licensing hours and admitting children. But nothing has happened yet."可知，营业时间仍然受限，尽管他们做了很多关于重大改变的建议，比如延长营业时间，允许孩子在酒吧饮酒，但是什么都没发生。由此可知 A，B，D 都不正确，只有孩子禁止入内是现状。

Passage Three

1. 【题目】Patel 的研究暗示着什么？

    A．减重和缺乏睡眠的联系。   B．增重和缺乏睡眠的联系。

    C．减重和运动的联系。   D．增重和运动的联系。

【答案】B

【解析】细节概括题。从文章首句"Here's a dreamy weight-loss plan: take a nap."可知，要想减肥，睡觉就好。后面的细节则提供证据表明，睡觉少的人容易长胖。因此本题答案为 B。

2. 【题目】Patel 的研究中有几个被试者？

    A．超过 68000。   B．超过 60800。   C．超过 60080。   D．超过 60008。

【答案】A

【解析】细节再现题。听懂了数字就能解决问题，从 His study of more than 68,000 women 可知，A 为正确答案。

3. 【题目】在 Patel 看来，体重差别背后的原因是什么？

【答案】C

【解析】细节再现题。从文中 Lower metabolic rate resulting from less sleep may be the reason behind the weight gain 可知，睡眠减少带来的新陈代谢减慢是背后的原因。

Passage Four

1. 【问题】讲话者的女儿最不可能说她妈妈什么？

    A. 她对我太严厉。   B. 她的问题太多。

    C. 她总是很考虑我的情绪。   D. 她是社区里最刻薄的妈妈。

【答案】C

【解析】细节再现题。从最开始的内容不难听到 A，B，D 的再现，这都是女儿对讲话者这个妈妈的评价，而这三个都与 C 选项是截然相反的。

2. 【问题】在科学家看来，青少年为何不能持续做出明智的决策呢？

    A. 他们过于自信。   B. 他们大脑发育太快。

    C. 他们心理上有所依赖。   D. 他们大脑的某些区域仍然不成熟。

【答案】D

【解析】细节推理题。Scientists have discovered that this has to do with the way the human brain grows. During the teen years, the brain develops rapidly, but some areas mature much earlier than others. 对青少年决策能力的质疑起源于科学家的发现：孩子大脑的某些区域发育明显早于其他区域，也就是说，某些区域不成熟。

3. 【问题】讲话者建议家长们做什么？

    A. 与孩子们轻松相处。   B. 对孩子们刻薄一点。

    C. 必要的时候对孩子们说不。   D. 不要在意孩子们的情绪。

【答案】C

【解析】细节推理题。文中说 But you have to hold the line，这里的 but 是对上文 discipline 的转折。上文讲到孩子们大脑发育不完全，无法持续做出明智的决策，因此应该有 discipline。但是纪律要有尺度（hold the line）。由此可推知 C 为正确选项。

Passage Five

1. 【问题】什么疾病不可以被闻出来？

    A. 肝脏衰竭。   B. 乳腺癌。

    C. 肾衰竭。   D. 没控制好的糖尿病。

【答案】B

【解析】细节再现题。文中说 a patient who had diabetes that is not well controlled，即没控制好的糖尿病患者是可以被闻出来的，有甜味。同时文中又说到 That means I can walk into a room and tell if a patient has kidney failure or liver failure，即肾脏和肝脏有问题的也能被闻出来。只有乳腺癌未被提及。

2. 【问题】过去的机器有什么问题？

    A. 形状。   B. 颜色。   C. 价格。   D. 尺寸。

【答案】D

【解析】细节概括题。文中说 but they were just enormous，即太庞大了，故是尺寸问题。

3. 【问题】新机器现在处于什么阶段？

      A．临床试验阶段。   B．已经投放市场。

      C．临床上被广泛使用。   D．在试验阶段。

【答案】D

【解析】细节回现题。文中最后一句 they are very much in the experimental stage 告诉我们，新机器还在试验阶段。

Passage Six

1. 【问题】在事故发生之前，滑雪对 Jill 意味着什么？

      A．一个爱好。   B．全世界。

      C．一次学习经历。   D．谋生的机会。

【答案】B

【解析】细节复现题。Jill 说 Skiing was it — everything — my world，可知本题正确答案为 B。

2. 【问题】当 Jill 从 Alta run 冲向高空时，发生了什么？

      A．她的腿摔坏了。   B．她的胳膊摔坏了。

      C．她的肩膀受伤了。   D．她的颈椎受伤了。

【答案】D

【解析】细节复现题。文章中讲到 "Her fourth, fifth, and sixth cervical vertebrae were broken"，即她的颈椎摔断了。

3. 【问题】Jill 个性中最让人印象深刻的是什么？

      A．乐观积极，顽强不屈。   B．悲观厌世，愤世嫉俗。

      C．幽默开朗，有趣好玩。   D．善良好心，值得依赖。

【答案】A

【解析】细节归纳题。Jill 遭遇事故，颈椎受伤，从肩部以下瘫痪。但她没有放弃，学会了语言和艺术，追求自己作为教师的新职业。因此她更多地体现出百折不挠、永不放弃的精神。

Passage Seven

1. 【问题】本文的主要内容是什么？

      A．生命的进化。   B．太空探索。   C．外星球生命。   D．不明飞行物。

【答案】C

【解析】细节归纳题。从文章开始的 "Life on other planets is likely, but intelligent life is less likely" 可推理得知，本文主要内容为外星球生命。

2. 【问题】霍金在华盛顿大学的演讲是针对什么事件的？

      A．他 50 岁生日。   B．NASA 的 50 周年庆。

      C．该大学 50 周年庆。   D．美国星球联合会的 50 周年庆。

【答案】B

【解析】细节复现题。文中明确提到 in honor of NASA's 50th anniversary，可知霍金的演讲是庆祝 NASA 50 周年庆的讲话。

3. 【问题】霍金对遭遇外星人时的警告是什么？

    A．核武器。   B．外星人绑架。 C．人类灭绝。   D．危险的感染。

【答案】D

【解析】细节复现题。文章最后，霍金警告说："Watch out if you would meet an alien. You could be infected with a disease to which you have no resistance."即我们要防范被感染未知疾病的可能性。

Passage Eight

1. 【问题】根据文章，下列哪一个会因为日益庞大的肥胖人群变得越来越糟？

    A．有限的生活空间。   B．拥挤的购物场所。

    C．食品短缺和更高的能源成本。   D．糖尿病和心血管疾病的概率。

【答案】C

【解析】细节推理题。从文中的第一句 Obese and overweight people require more fuel to transport them and the food they eat 可知，肥胖和超重的人需要更多的能源来行动，也需要消耗更多的食物，可推知本题答案为 C。

2. 【问题】在 WHO 看来，到 2015 年，全球肥胖人数的预测数字是多少？

    A．超过 7 亿。   B．超过 4 亿。   C．超过 23 亿。   D．超过 30 亿。

【答案】A

【解析】细节复现题。文中说："The World Health Organization (WHO) projects by 2015, 2.3 billion adults will be overweight and more than 700 million will be obese."其中 2.3 billion 是超重人数，700 million 是肥胖人数。因此本题答案为 A。

3. 【问题】在 Edwards 和 Roberts 看来，如果我们提倡 BMI 的正态分布，会带来什么样的结果？

    A．气候变化。   B．食品价格下降。

    C．能源价格的上升。   D．对食品需求的增加。

【答案】B

【解析】细节复现题。文末 Edward 和 Roberts 指出："Promotion of a normal distribution of BMI would reduce the global demand for fuel, and thus the price of ..."即促进 BMI 的正态分布将减少全球对燃料的需求，从而降低食品价格。因此本题答案为 B。

Passage Nine

1. 【问题】本文的主要内容是什么？

    A．自杀。   B．肥胖。   C．焦虑。   D．滥用药物。

【答案】A

【解析】细节归纳题。本文开始就说 Suicide is a very real risk for young people who suffer from clinical depression，后文讲到如何治疗这类人。只有 A 是最佳选项，

C 只是其中被提及的一个极小的方面。

2. 【问题】治疗该问题更好的方案是什么？
      A. 抗抑郁和谈话疗法相结合。   B. 促进神经元之间的传递。
      C. 赢得父母的支持和帮助。   D. 管理有效的抗抑郁药物。

【答案】A

【解析】细节复现题。文中说 Researches show that the most effective treatment is the combination of anti-depression and talk therapy，A 项为原文复现，可知本题答案为 A。

3. 【问题】综合治疗后有多少孩子感觉好一些？
      A. 65%。   B. 75%。   C. 85%。   D. 95%。

【答案】B

【解析】细节复现题。文中说到 75% of kids are reported feeling better and less suicidal after 3 months，因此本题答案为 B。

Passage Ten

1. 【问题】这个研究的参与者是谁？
      A. 2030 个社会学专业的学生。   B. 2300 个社会学专业的学生。
      C. 2030 个心理学专业的学生。   D. 2300 个心理学专业的学生。

【答案】D

【解析】细节复现题。从录音中 2,300 psychology students 明确可知，本题正确答案为 D。

2. 【问题】如该研究所示，频繁发信息的学生最重视的是什么？
      A. 精神生活。   B. 形象和财富。   C. 学术成就。   D. 道德和美感。

【答案】B

【解析】细节概括题。从文中 students who text frequently place less importance on moral aesthetic and spiritual goals and greater importance on wealth and image 可知，频繁发信息的人不太注意道德和精神目标（less importance），而是更关注 wealth and image（greater importance），因此本题正确答案为 B。

3. 【问题】本文主要讲什么？
      A. 发太多信息会让你变得浅薄。   B. 发信息正是科技的奇迹。
      C. 发信息的优势比劣势多。   D. 发太多信息会让学生的表现变差。

【答案】A

【解析】细节归纳题。从文章最开始的 "Teenagers who text more than 100 times a day tend to be more shallow, image-obsessed and driven by wealth." 可知，本文的主题为频繁发短信会让一个人变得更加浅薄，更注重形象和财富。比较四个选项可知，A 选项为最佳答案，B 选项与本文无关，C 选项与原文含义相反，D 选项并未直接与学生的表现进行关联，更多强调对学生价值观的影响。

Section B 专项练习录音原文

Passage One

Keeping a diary is bad for your health, say UK psychologists. They found that people who regularly keep diaries suffer from headaches, sleeplessness, digestive problems and social awkwardness more than people who don't. These findings challenge the assumption that people find it easier to get over a traumatic event if they write about it.

The study, carried out with David Sheffield of Staffordshire University, was presented on Wednesday at a meeting of the British Psychological Society in Edinburgh.

The pair studied 94 regular diarists and compared their health with that of 41 non-diarists. The researchers asked the diarists recruited to say how often they made entries and for how long they had kept diaries. They were also asked if they had written about anything traumatic.

Statistically, the diarists scored much worse on health measures than the non-diarists. The worst affected of all were those who had written about trauma.

Questions 1–3 are based on the passage you've just heard.

1. According to UK psychologists, regular diarists are more likely to suffer from the following except_____.
2. When and where was Duncan's study presented?
3. According to Duncan's study, who scored worst on the health measures?

Passage Two

Most foreigners find British pubs both fascinating and frustrating. So is the law history to curb it.

In fact, much of the law history of pub in Britain is to do with people who want to drink and others who want to stop them. The development of pubs and the law surrounding them is an interesting way of learning a little more about our social history. Beer has been drunk in Britain since before the Roman invasion. And as early as 1659 AD the king of Kent was making laws in an attempt to stop priests from getting drunk.

By the late 16th century, drunkenness was a real problem and laws were passed to restrict drinking hours. In the 19th century, cheap gin was very popular among poor people. Drunkenness again increased and more laws were passed. In spite of their various attempts to curb drinking, pubs continue to provide a major pan of British social life. Their opening and closing hours are still restricted by law although they have their recommendations recently for big changes, including extending licensing hours and admitting children. But nothing has happened yet.

Questions 1–3 are based on the passage you've just heard.

1. What is this talk mainly about?

2.　When did people start to drink beer in Britain?

3.　Which of the following is true of English pubs today?

Passage Three

Here's a dreamy weight-loss plan: take a nap. That's the message from work by Sanjay Patel at Case Western Reserve University in Cleveland, Ohio. His study of more than 68,000 women has found that those who sleep less than 5 hours a night gain more weight over time than those who sleep 7 hours a night.

Significantly, the short-sleepers consumed fewer calories than those who slept 7 hours, says Patel, who presented his results this week at the American Thoracic Society International Conference in San Diego, California. This finding overturns the common view that overeating among the sleep-deprived explains such weight differences.

Lower metabolic rate resulting from less sleep may be the reason behind the weight gain, Patel suggests. "It obviously also suggests that getting people to sleep more might be a relatively easy way to help people lose weight," he says.

Questions 1–3 are based on the passage you've just heard.

1.　What did Patel's study indicate?

2.　How many subjects did Patel have in his study?

3.　According to Patel, what might be the reason behind the weight differences?

Passage Four

I am the meanest mother in the neighborhood. I'm too strict. I ask too many questions. No one else's parents are as difficult as I am. This is the point of view of my 16-year-old daughter.

Discipline takes on a whole new meaning when your child hits adolescence. "When kids are young and do something unsafe, parents have no trouble saying no, but saying yes to your teen can almost become a reflex, because you so desperately want to avoid conflict", says Daniel Kindlon, Ph.D., assistant professor of child psychology. New research confirms that: Adolescents simply lack the ability to make smart decisions consistently. Scientists have discovered that this has to do with the way the human brain grows. During the teen years, the brain develops rapidly, but some areas mature much earlier than others.

But you have to hold the line. Your teen is secretly counting on you to do so. And too much is at stake if you don't.

Questions 1–3 are based on the passage you've just heard.

1.　What would the speaker's daughter least likely say about her mother?

2.　Why are adolescents not able to make smart decisions consistently, according to scientists?

3. What would the speaker advise parents to do?

Passage Five

A lot of doctors can tell what's wrong with you by sleeping, and I can do this by smelling. This actually goes back to the day of ancient Greece. For example, you can walk into a room or get close to a patient who had diabetes that is not well controlled. There is a kind of sweetish smell. That means I can walk into a room and tell if a patient has kidney failure or liver failure. And now there is a machine that can do that too. It is fascinating that there have been these machines in the past, but they were just enormous. So, in the past, they were not used in therapy. But the newly-invented ones are very small and concise. They use new laser technology and now are available given the size of the machine. However, they are very much in the experimental stage.

Questions 1–3 are based on the passage you've just heard.

1. What disease can't be smelt?
2. What was the problem of the machine in the past?
3. What stage of the new machine is now?

Passage Six

Jill Kinmont was an avid skier, competing and winning numerous titles in junior and senior national skiing events. As Jill says, "Skiing was it — everything — my world." Jill's world collapsed on Jan 30th 1955 when she skied off the Alta run and landed helplessly on the slope. Her fourth, fifth, and sixth cervical vertebrae were broken. For days, Jill hovered between life and death. By April, it became clear that she would be paralyzed from the shoulders down. Jill underwent rehabilitation therapy with cheerful determination. She learned to write, to type, and to feed herself. She studied art, German, and English. By this time, Jill had chosen a new career goal: teaching elementary school children. When her family moved to Seattle, Jill was able to fulfill her new dream. She attended the School of Education at the University of Washington and began her new life's work as a teacher.

Questions 1–3 are based on the passage you've just heard.

1. What did skiing mean to Jill before the accident?
2. What happened to Jill when she skied from the Alta run?
3. What is the most impressive about Jill's personality?

Passage Seven

Life on other planets is likely, but intelligent life is less likely. Famed astrophysicist, Stephen Hawking has been thinking a lot about the cosmic question: Are we alone? "The answer is probably not," he says. "If there is life elsewhere in the universe," Hawking asks, "why haven't we stumbled onto some alien broadcasts in space? Maybe something like 'alien quiz show'?" Hawking's comments were part of the lecture at George Washington University on Monday in honor of NASA's 50th anniversary. He theorized that there are possible answers to whether there is extraterrestrial life. Should you worry about aliens? Alien abduction claims come from the "weirdos" and are unlikely. However, because alien life might not have DNA like us, Hawking warned, "Watch out if you would meet an alien. You could be infected with a disease to which you have no resistance."

Questions 1–3 are based on the passage you've just heard.

1. What is the passage mainly about?
2. What is the event when Hawking delivered his lecture at the George Washington University?
3. What is Hawking's warning to the encounter of an alien?

Passage Eight

Obese and overweight people require more fuel to transport them and the food they eat, and the problem will worsen as the population literally swells in size. This adds to the food shortage and higher energy prices, a team at the London School of Hygiene & Tropical Medicine says.

The World Health Organization (WHO) projects by 2015, 2.3 billion adults will be overweight and more than 700 million will be obese.

In their model, the researchers pegged 40 percent of the global population as obese with a body mass index of near 30.

BMI is a calculation of height to weight, and the normal range is usually considered to be 18 or 25, with more than 25 considered overweight and above 30 obese.

The next step is quantifying how much a heavier population is contributing to climate change, higher fuel prices and food shortage.

"Promotion of a normal distribution of BMI would reduce the global demand for fuel, and thus the price of, food," Edwards and Roberts wrote.

Questions 1–3 are based on the passage you've just heard.

1. According to the talk, which of the following can be made worse by the growing obese population?
2. According to WHO, by 2015, what would be the estimated figure of the global obese population?
3. According to Edwards and Roberts, what would happen if we promote a normal distribution of BMI?

Passage Nine

Suicide is a very real risk for young people who suffer from clinical depression.

In fact, during the past two years suicide has increased among youths between the ages of 10 and 19, but there aren't treatments that can help. Researches show that the most effective treatment is the combination of anti-depression and talk therapy. Anti-depressants work by increasing chemicals which facilitate communications between neurons in the brain. "Anti-depressants are the most effective treatment for most adults. But when it comes to teenagers, it's not enough," says Doctor Richard, a psychiatrist in a university medical center. 13 years are full of turmoil, emotions and changes. And anti-depressant medications may not be able to deal with all of those problems. "Psycho therapy, specifically problem-behavioral therapy needs to be combined," he says. In his recent major study, with the therapy in use along with anti-depressants, 75% of kids are reported feeling better and less suicidal after 3 months.

Questions 1–3 are based on the following passage you've just heard.
1. What is the passage mainly about?
2. What way is the better alternative now to treat the problem?
3. What is the percentage of the kids who feel better after the combined-therapy?

Passage Ten

Teenagers who text more than 100 times a day tend to be more shallow, image-obsessed and driven by wealth. The study from the University of Winnipeg suggests that a lot can be learned about a person's personality simply from the number of texts they send.

The data was gathered over a period of three years from 2,300 psychology students at the University of Winnipeg. The theory the university study tried to test was that constant use of twitter and texting for communication results in a world where people have quick and shallow thoughts. The results indicate that students who text frequently place less importance on moral aesthetic and spiritual goals and greater importance on wealth and image. Strikingly the study states those who text more than 100 times a day were 30 per cent less likely to feel strongly that leading an ethical, principled life was important, in comparison to those who texted 50 times or less a day.

Questions 1–3 are based on the following passage you've just heard.
1. Who are the participants of the study?
2. As indicated by the study what do the students who text frequently value most?
3. What is the main idea of this talk?

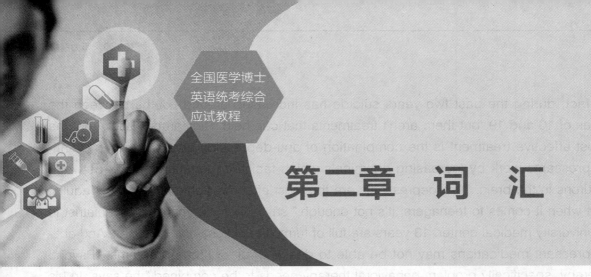

全国医学博士
英语统考综合
应试教程

第二章　词　汇

一、考试大纲的要求及试卷结构

　　根据考试大纲的要求，词汇用法部分旨在测试考生对英语词汇和短语的理解及使用能力。从试卷结构来看，这部分考试分为两个部分：Section A 和 Section B。考试时间约为10 分钟。

Section A

　　这部分考题的题干中有一处空白，要求考生从四个备选项中选出一个最佳答案，使得题干语法正确、逻辑合理、意义完整。此部分一共 10 题，每题 0.5 分，共计 5 分。例如：

This environment can also affect a person's mental and _____ health.

A. conventional　　　　　　　　B. personal

C. physical　　　　　　　　　　D. impersonal

（答案：C）

Section B

　　这部分考题的题干有一个词或短语下面画有横线。要求考生从四个备选项中选出一个与画线部分的意义相同或近似的最佳答案。本部分测试的词或词组不超出考试大纲所要求掌握的单词、词组表。这部分一共有 10 题，每题 0.5 分，共计 5 分。例如：

The queer woman kept over one hundred cats in her house.

A. odd　　　　　　　　　　　　B. energetic

C. generous　　　　　　　　　　D. subtle

（答案：A）

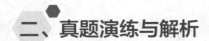

二、真题演练与解析

Part II   Vocabulary (10%)

Section A

Directions: *In this section all the sentences are incomplete. Four words or phrases, marked A, B, C and D, are given beneath each of them. You are to choose the word or phrase that best completes the sentence. Then, mark your answer on the* **ANSWER SHEET.**

1. There was no ____ but to close the road until February.
    A. dilemma   B. denying
    C. alternative   D. doubt

2. I ____ when I heard that my grandfather had died.
    A. fell apart   B. fell away
    C. fell out   D. fell back

3. I'm ____ passing a new law that helps poor children get better medicine.
    A. taking advantage of   B. standing up for
    C. looking up to   D. taking hold of

4. In front of the platform, the students were talking with the professor over the quizzes of their ____ subject.
    A. compulsory   B. compulsive
    C. alternative   D. predominant

5. The tutor tells the undergraduates that one can acquire ____ in a foreign language through more practice.
    A. proficiency   B. efficiency
    C. efficacy   D. frequency

6. The teacher explained the new lesson ____ to the students.
    A. at random   B. at a loss
    C. at length   D. at hand

7. I shall ____ the loss of my reading-glasses in newspaper with a reward for the finder.
    A. advertise   B. inform   C. announce   D. publish

8. The poor nutrition in the early stages of infancy can ____ adult growth.
    A. degenerate   B. deteriorate   C. boost   D. retard

9. She had a terrible accident, but ___ she wasn't killed.
   A. at all events
   B. in the long run
   C. at large
   D. in vain

10. His weak chest ___ him to winter illness.
    A. predicts
    B. preoccupies
    C. prevails
    D. predisposes

Section B

Directions: *Each of the following sentences has a word or phrase underlined. There are four other words or phrases beneath each sentence. Choose the word or phrase which would best keep the meaning of the original sentence if it were substituted for the underlined part. Mark your answer on the* **ANSWER SHEET.**

11. The company was losing money, so they had to <u>lay off</u> some of its employees for three months.
    A. owe
    B. dismiss
    C. recruit
    D. summon

12. The North American states agreed to sign the <u>agreement</u> of economical and military union in Ottawa.
    A. convention
    B. conviction
    C. contradiction
    D. confrontation

13. The statue would be perfect but for a few small <u>defects</u> in its base.
    A. faults
    B. weaknesses
    C. flaws
    D. errors

14. When he finally emerged from the cave after thirty days, John was <u>startlingly</u> pale.
    A. amazingly
    B. astonishingly
    C. uniquely
    D. dramatically

15. If you want to set up a company, you must <u>comply with</u> the regulations laid down by the authorities.
    A. abide by
    B. work out
    C. check out
    D. succumb to

16. The school master <u>applauded</u> the girl's bravery in his opening speech.
    A. praised
    B. appraised
    C. cheered
    D. clapped

17. The local government leaders are making every effort to <u>tackle</u> the problem of poverty.
    A. abolish
    B. address
    C. extinguish
    D. encounter

18. This report would be <u>intelligible</u> only to an expert in computing.
    A. intelligent
    B. comprehensive
    C. competent
    D. comprehensible

19. Reading a book and listening to music <u>simultaneously</u> seems to be a problem for them.

A. intermittently　　　B. constantly　　　C. concurrently　　　D. continuously

20. He was given a laptop computer in <u>acknowledgement</u> of his work for the company.
　　A. accomplishment　　B. recognition　　C. apprehension　　D. commitment

答案及解析

1. 【答案】C
　　【解析】dilemma 困境，进退两难；denying 否认，拒绝；alternative 选择；doubt 怀疑。
　　　　　　but 表示"除了……"。there was no denying or doubt 的含义为"毋庸置疑"，
　　　　　　不符合句意。
　　题干译文：除了等到二月份封路，此外别无选择。

2. 【答案】A
　　【解析】fall apart 破碎，破裂，崩溃，例如：My bike is falling apart. 我的自行车要散架
　　　　　　了。fall away 减少，消散，例如：All our doubts fell away gradually. 我们的一
　　　　　　切疑虑逐渐消失了。fall out 掉落，脱落，例如：Due to extreme fatigue, his hair
　　　　　　is falling out. 由于极度疲劳，他的头发在脱落。fall back 后退，撤退，例如：
　　　　　　The army received the order that they would fall back tomorrow. 部队接到明天撤
　　　　　　退的命令。
　　题干译文：当我听说我祖父去世的时候，我崩溃了。

3. 【答案】B
　　【解析】take advantage of 利用，例如：He took advantage of every opportunity to show
　　　　　　himself in public. 他利用每一次机会在公众场合展示自己。stand up for 支持，
　　　　　　维护，例如：You should learn to stand up for your rights. 你应该学会维护自己
　　　　　　的权益。look up to sb. 钦佩，仰慕，例如：He is the only president looked up to
　　　　　　by all people. 他是唯一受所有人钦佩的总统。take hold of 抓住，握住，例如：
　　　　　　Let's move the table. You take hold of that end. 我们来把桌子移开，你抓住那
　　　　　　一端。
　　题干译文：我支持通过一项新的法律，帮助穷苦的孩子获得更好的药品。

4. 【答案】A
　　【解析】compulsory 必修的；compulsive 强制的，强迫的；alternative 选择性的；
　　　　　　predominant 卓越的，支配的，突出的。
　　题干译文：在讲台前，学生们正在和教授讨论他们必修科目的测验。

5. 【答案】A
　　【解析】proficiency 熟练，精通；efficiency 效率；efficacy（药物，治疗）功效；
　　　　　　frequency 频率。此题关键的突破点在于题干中的介词 in，以上这些词只有
　　　　　　proficiency 与介词 in 连用，表示"在……方面熟练"，例如：proficiency in
　　　　　　English 精通英语。
　　题干译文：辅导教师告诉本科生，通过不断的练习，一个人就能精通一门外语。

6. 【答案】C

【解析】at random 随意地，任意地，胡乱地，例如：Names were chosen at random from the list. 名字是从名单上随意选择的。at a loss 不知所措，例如：His comments left me at a loss for words. 他的评论让我不知道该说什么好。at length 详尽地，例如：Please tell me what happened to you at length. 请详尽地告诉我你发生了什么事情。at hand 接近，例如：Help is always at hand. 援助总是近在咫尺。

题干译文：老师给学生详细地讲授新课。

7. 【答案】A

【解析】advertise 作为动词的含义是"登广告"。inform 通知某人某事，常用表达式为：inform sb. of sth.；announce 宣布；publish 出版。

题干译文：我要在报纸上刊登眼镜的寻物启事，寻得者将有奖金。

8. 【答案】D

【解析】degenerate 退化；deteriorate 使恶化；boost 促进；retard 阻碍，妨碍。infancy 幼年；nutrition 营养。

题干译文：幼年早期营养不良会阻碍成年成长。

9. 【答案】A

【解析】at all events 不管怎么样，无论如何，例如：At all events you should listen to your parents' opinions. 无论如何你应该听听你父母的意见。in the long run 最终，从长远观点来看，例如：In the long run, it is worthwhile to make an investment in education. 从长远来看，在教育上投资是值得的。at large 整个，全部，未被捕获的，例如：A few years ago there was unrest in the country at large. 几年前这个国家处于动荡中。The killer is still at large. 这个杀手仍然逍遥法外。in vain 徒劳，白费力气，例如：He tried to persuade her not to go out, but in vain. 他试图劝说她不要出去，但没用。

题干译文：她发生了可怕的意外，但不管怎么样，她没死。

10. 【答案】D

【解析】predict 预测；preoccupy 使全神贯注，迷住；prevail 流行，盛行；predispose 使预先有……倾向，易于感染，常与介词 to 连用，例如：Frustration predisposes him to look at things pessimistically. 挫折使他很悲观地看待事物。Fatigue predisposes one to cold. 疲劳使人容易感冒。此题的关键在于题干中的介词 to。

题干译文：他肺部很脆弱，冬天容易患病。

11. 【答案】B

【解析】题干中画线词组 lay off 的含义为"解雇"。owe 欠（债）；dismiss 解散，开除；recruit 招募；summon 召集。

题干译文：公司资金流失，他们不得不让一些员工停职 3 个月。

12. 【答案】A

　　　　【解析】题干中画线词 agreement 的含义是"协议，协定"。convention 惯例，习俗，协定；
　　　　　　　conviction 深信，定罪；contradiction 反驳，矛盾；confrontation 面对。

　　　　题干译文：北美国家同意在渥太华签署经济和军事联盟协议。

13.　【答案】C

　　　　【解析】题干中画线词 defect 的含义是"瑕疵"。fault 故障，毛病；weakness 弱点；
　　　　　　　flaw 瑕疵；error 过失，错误。题干中 statue 的含义是"雕像"，but for 意思是"要
　　　　　　　不是"，例如：But for your help, I couldn't have finished the work on time. 要不
　　　　　　　是你帮忙，我不可能按时完成工作。

　　　　题干译文：要不是底座上的一些小瑕疵，这个雕像会很完美。

14.　【答案】B

　　　　【解析】题干中画线词 startlingly 意思是"令人吃惊地，大吃一惊地"。amazingly 令人
　　　　　　　惊讶地，令人惊奇地；astonishingly 惊讶的程度比 amazingly 强，与 startlingly 意
　　　　　　　思相近；uniquely 独特地，独一无二地；dramatically 极大地，相当地。故 B 为
　　　　　　　正确选项。

　　　　题干译文：约翰 30 天后终于从洞穴中出来，他脸色苍白，让人大吃一惊。

15.　【答案】A

　　　　【解析】题干画线词组 comply with 的意思是"顺从，遵从"。abide by 坚持，遵守，
　　　　　　　例如：It is very necessary to abide by your promises. 遵守你的承诺十分必
　　　　　　　要。work out 锻炼身体，计算出，例如：I used to work out regularly to keep
　　　　　　　fit. 过去我常常定期运动，保持身体健康。She was very disappointed because
　　　　　　　she couldn't work out the math problem. 因为没能解出这道数学题，她很失
　　　　　　　望。check out 调查，核实，例如：The police are checking out evidence they
　　　　　　　found. 警察正在核实他们发现的证据。succumb to 屈服，屈从，例如：At
　　　　　　　last he succumbed to cancer and died. 他最终放弃抗癌，去世了。

　　　　题干译文：如果要成立公司，就必须遵守权力机构制定的条规。

16.　【答案】A

　　　　【解析】题干画线词 applaud 的意思是"鼓掌，赞许"。praise 表扬；appraise 估量，估价；
　　　　　　　cheer 兴高采烈；clap 鼓掌（表示赞许或欣赏），通常与 for 连用。

　　　　题干译文：学校校长在公开讲话中称赞这个女孩很英勇。

17.　【答案】B

　　　　【解析】题干画线词 tackle 的意思是"解决（问题）"。abolish 废除，废止（制度，法律等）。
　　　　　　　address 作为名词，意思是"地址；演说"；作为动词，意思为"写地址；发
　　　　　　　表演说；处理，对付"；extinguish 熄灭；encounter 遭遇。

　　　　题干译文：当地政府领导正千方百计解决贫穷问题。

18.　【答案】D

　　　　【解析】题 干 画 线 词 intelligible 的 意 思 是 " 易 懂 的 "。intelligent 聪 明 的；
　　　　　　　comprehensive 综合的；competent 有能力的，能胜任的；comprehensible 可理
　　　　　　　解的。

题干译文：这篇报道只有计算方面的专家容易懂。

19. 【答案】C

【解析】题干画线词 simultaneously 的意思是"同时发生地"。intermittently 断断续续地，间歇地；constantly 经常地；concurrently 并存地，同时发生地；continuously 连续地。

题干译文：同时看书和听音乐对他们来说似乎是个问题。

20. 【答案】B

【解析】题干画线词 acknowledgement 的意思是"承认"，题干词组 in acknowledgement of 的意思是"感谢，谢礼"，例如：I was rewarded a medal in acknowledgement of my contribution to our company. 我被授予一枚奖章，以表彰我对公司的贡献。题干中的 laptop 指的是笔记本电脑。accomplishment 成就，完成；recognition 承认；apprehension 忧虑，担心；commitment 承诺，允诺，奉献。

题干译文：为感谢他为公司所做的贡献，公司奖励他一台笔记本电脑。

三、考查内容及相应的应试技巧

（一）考查内容与解题步骤

医学考博英语词汇部分主要测试考生对单词和词组的识别和应用能力。Section A 与 Section B 两部分的考查内容分别具有以下特点：

Section A（填空题）

1）考查考生对句意的理解和词汇含义的记忆能力。这类考题选项方面的特点是：备选词汇多为较高级词汇或较高级的高频词，要求考生选择与句意吻合的单词，例如上面试题中的第 1、4、8、10 题。

2）考查考生对形近词的辨别能力，这类考题的选项特点鲜明：备选词汇在拼写上很相似或者都具有相同的前缀或后缀，例如上面试题中的第 5、10 题。

3）考查考生对同义词、近义词的识别能力，这类考题的选项往往是意思相近的单词，例如上面试题中的第 7 题。

4）考查考生对短语或词组的熟悉程度，例如上面试题中的第 3、9 题。

5）考查考生对短语或词组搭配的掌握，这类考题的选项具有的特点是：四个备选项的动词都是同一个单词，如 go, come, fall, break 等，但它们各自的介词、副词不同；或者四个选项的介词、副词相同，但与之搭配的名词或动词不同，例如：上面试题中的第 2、6、9 题。

Section A 部分的解题步骤：

1）仔细阅读题干，理解句子的大概含义，推测所填单词的含义；

2）通过题干所提供的信息，看是否涉及搭配关系；

3）根据对选项单词的掌握，先选择一个可能的答案，并放入题干中，通读全句，以验证所选词汇是否符合句意和题干中的搭配；

4）如果题干存在某种逻辑关系，如因果、转折、对比等，还要注意自己的选择是否符合这些逻辑关系的表述；

5）如果遇到选项中有自己不认识的单词，不要轻言放弃，要利用排除法解题。寻找题干中的解题信息，然后看看自己所熟悉的单词是否符合，如果不符合就可以排除，然后再在不熟悉的单词中判断最佳答案，例如：

Mary was so ___ with her money that she never spent a single extra penny.

A. rich   B. frugal   C. pretentious   D. stupid

【解析】根据对选项的分析，考生有可能不熟悉 B 选项，而可以通过构词法猜测 C 选项的大概含义，然后根据题干中的句型 so...that...（如此……以至……）来判断所熟悉的 A，C 和 D 是否符合句意。然后就可以排除这三个选项，因而答案为 B。

Section B（画线替换题）

1）题干中画线词汇考生较为熟悉，但四个备选词汇中有的单词较生僻。或者题干画线词汇为常用单词，但在题中的含义是考生不熟悉的。

2）题干中画线词汇考生不熟悉，但四个备选词汇多为考生认识的单词，例如上面试题中的第 15、18、19、20 题。

3）选项中经常出现形近词，例如上面试题中的第 12、18 题。

4）选项中可能出现近义词，例如上面试题中的第 13、14 题。

根据两部分词汇测试的不同特点，考生应该采用不同的解题步骤。

Section B 部分的解题步骤：

1）先看画线单词或词组是否熟悉；

2）然后再通读题干，确定画线部分的含义；

3）最后根据自己对选项词义的理解，选择与画线部分含义最接近的一个，此部分注意解题要领为画线词的近义词，而不是哪一个符合句意；

4）同样，如果出现不认识画线单词的情况，一定要沉着冷静，在题干中寻找解题信息。例如：

Applicant will be asked to provide information on how they will <u>disseminate</u> information to other students at their university or college.

A. disclose   B. deliver   C. spread   D. analyze

【解析】 考生可能不熟悉画线单词，但是在题干中，我们可以判断这个单词为动词，它所在的句子部分为 they + V. information to other students... 这样，我们就可以判断大概含义就是他们给其他学生信息，因而画线部分有可能是"传递"的意思，可以判断选项应该在 B 和 C 中，最后再区分两个近义词的含义，B 的含义为"递送"，如递送包裹、报纸等，因而正确答案应该为 C。

（二）考生复习提示

无论掌握了什么样的解题技巧，在词汇测试中，考生的词汇知识毋庸置疑是解题的根本。因而各位考生应该加强自己对词汇知识的掌握。但是，考生们在进行词汇部分复习的时候，并非要机械简单地按照大纲词汇表记忆每个单词的拼写和含义，这样的复习收效也不会很好，而是要注意以下几个方面：

1. 根据自身水平，合理安排复习进度。在复习过程中，切忌按照大纲词汇表，从字母 A 开始，一个一个单词地进行。应该根据自己的词汇水平和词汇难易程度、考查范围有的放矢地进行复习。词汇难易程度和考查范围级别可以参看本丛书的词汇巧战通关。

2. 词汇的具体复习要做到广而精。根据上述考查内容的分析，考生在记忆单词含义和拼写的时候，要额外注意一词多义、派生词等。对于考试中的重点词汇，不能仅停留在认识的层次，要对这样的单词做到全面掌握。

3. 注意单词、词组之间的关系。复习过程中，要学会联想，也就是说要关注同义词、反义词以及形近词或词组。这样，复习的单词就不是单一、零散的，这对考试解题也大有帮助。

4. 记忆单词的方法要多样且有效。记忆单词的拼写绝对不意味着是死记硬背单词的字母组合，要寻求甚至自己创造记忆单词的方法，目的是能够准确且牢固地记住单词。本章下面的内容将会介绍几种单词记忆的方法。

5. 固定搭配要记牢。单词搭配，尤其是介词、副词的搭配尤为重要，这在解题时有可能是关键点。

6. 培养自己对词汇语境含义的理解和认识。任何单词都不是孤立存在的，都会在一定的语境中充当一定成分，体现某个含义。这就需要考生在语境中理解单词的含义，这样不仅能更加准确地理解单词，而且对于阅读也有很大帮助。

7. 对于常用医学词汇要注意积累。虽然词汇测试部分不涉及医学词汇的考查内容，但是我们也要注意词汇在医学博士英语考试中的服务作用。考生有必要积累常用医学词汇，这对于其他考试部分尤其是阅读、写作都有很大帮助。

8. 勤复习、多运用。记忆单词绝对不是一遍就可以做到的，考生在记忆单词的时候要根据自身情况分阶段反复进行复习。此外，还要借助各种手段来巩固单词的拼写、发音和使用。

四、词汇记忆方法

这里介绍几种记忆单词的方法，供各位考生参考。

（一）词根词缀记忆法

在英语中，有很多词根是单词含义的根本，在词根的基础上增加前缀或者后缀，使得这个单词的含义发生变化。例如：cycl 相当于 circle，意思是"圆圈"，在这个词根的基础上增加前缀或后缀，就可以记忆很多词，如：

前缀 bi- 的含义是 two（两个），因而 bicycle 就是指两个圆圈，即为自行车。

cycle 作为名词含义为"周期"。

cyclic，后缀 -ic 为形容词的词缀，因而含义就是"周期的"。

recycle 是动词，前缀 re 的含义为 again（再次），因而这个单词的含义为"再生，回收"。

在复习中，考生要掌握一些常用词根、词缀，这样记忆单词就不再会毫无头绪，而是有规律可循，同时也可以减轻需要记忆的单词量。此外，这种记忆方法也有助于考生熟悉形近词。本节稍后会罗列一些常用词根、词缀。

（二）联想法

联想的形式和方法很多，比如派生词、形近词、同义词，这些都会帮助考生按照单词群去记忆。例如：

imagine, image, imaginable, imaginative, imaginary

（三）拆分法

拆分法就是将单词根据特定的特点拆分，利用它们之间的意义进行联想，从而达到记忆的效果。例如：

status — state + us   bonus — bone + us   campus — camp + us

这几个单词在进行拆分后，我们可以知道这几个词都和美国（US）有关，state + us 就是"美国的状态地位"，所以 status 的含义就是"地位"；bonus 就是"美国的骨头"，含义为"奖金，红利"；camp + us 就是"美国的营地"，含义为"校园（很轻松，没有围墙）"。

这样的方法没有一定之规，考生可以根据自己的理解，形成记忆。

（四）口诀法

顾名思义，就是考生可以像编故事一样，将毫无关系的单词串联起来，例如：

绵羊（sheep） 走陡峭（steep） 哭泣（weep） 打扫（sweep） 再睡觉（sleep）

五、常用词根和词缀

↘ 词根

fer	带来	confer refer	offer transfer	differ suffer	infer	prefer
form	形状，形式	inform formal formation	perform former	platform information	transform format	uniform formula

（续）

pose	摆放	compose oppose	dispose propose	deposit purpose	expose suppose	impose
fin	结束，范围	define finite	refine finish	confine	infinite	
quire	寻求，得到	require	inquire	acquire		
vis	看	vision revise	visual devise	visible advise	television supervise	visit
scribe	写	describe	prescribe	script		
port	搬运	export passport	import portable	transport portion	opportunity proportion	support
pend	悬挂	expend	depend	suspend	expenditure	
sume	拿，取	assume	consume	presume	resume	
press	压，按	depress pressure	express	impress	compress	oppress
spect	看	aspect	respect	perspective	suspect	prospect
vail	强有力	available	prevail			
lect	选择	select dialect	elect reflect	collect	neglect	intellect
verse	转变	adverse	diverse	universe	reverse	converse
volve	转	revolve	involve	evolve		
mit	送，放出	commit summit	omit submit	transmit	permit	emit
tract	拉，拖	attract tractor	distract	contract	abstract	subtract
ceed	前行	exceed	succeed	proceed		
sist	站	assist	consist	resist	persist	insist
tain	拿住	attain entertain	contain retain	obtain maintain	stain	sustain
gress	前行	progress	regress	aggressive	congress	
dic	说话	contradiction indicate		dictation	predict	dictionary
tribute	给予	contribute	attribute	distribute		
lev	提高	elevator				
claim	大喊	exclaim	proclaim	declaim		

（续）

voc	叫喊	advocate vocabulary vocation provoke evoke
vac	空的	vacation vacancy vacant
audi	听觉	audience audio audit auditor audition auditorium
cent	百	percent accent innocent decent incentive
celer	快	accelerate
cur	跑	current currency curriculum curtain occur excursion
demo	人	demonstrate democracy demon
duct	带来	product conduct
dur	持续	endure procedure during
fect	作用	perfect effect affect infect defect
fess	说	confess professor profession
gene	出产，产生	gene generate generation general genius generosity generous
ject	扔，投	object subject project inject reject
jud	判断	prejudice judge judicial
manu	手	manufacture manufacturer manual
seque	跟随	subsequence consequence sequence
rupt	断裂	interrupt bankrupt corrupt abrupt erupt
sent	感觉	sentimental sensitive sensible sensational sense sensibility
count	数字	account counter encounter discount county country
vey	看	survey convey
ply	重叠	apply reply imply multiply comply supply
prove	试验，验证	approve improve
tend	延伸，延展	attend contend pretend intend extend tendency tender
clude	关闭	conclude include exclude
rect	正	correct direct erect

↘ 前缀

anti-	反抗，反对	anti-corruption	anti-war
auto-	自己的，自动的	automation	autobiography
bi-	双的	bilingual	bilateral
dis-	相反	dishonest	disapprove
en-	使	enforce	encode
ex-	向外	export	external
im-	向内	import	implant
im-, in-	不	immortal	immature
inter-	相互，在内	interact	intertwine
mal-	坏，不良	malnutrition	maltreat
micro-	微小	microscope	microphone
mis-	错的	mislead	mischoice
out-	超过，过度	outweigh	outgrow
over-	过度	overweight	overdo
sub-	次的，亚于	submarine	subhealth
trans-	转换，横过	transform	transcontinental
tri-	三倍的	triangle	triagonal
un-	否定	unrest	unacceptable
under-	在下，不足	underabundant	underappreciated
uni-	单一的	uniform	unique
ab-	相反，变坏	abnormal	abuse
by-	副的，在旁的	byproduct	bypass
co-	共同	cooperate	coexist
cor-, col-	共同	collate	correspond
com-, con-	共同	combine	contemporary
de-	去掉	deforest	decode
em-, en-	包围；使……进入状态	embrace	empower
il-; ir-	不，否定	irregular	illegal

↘ 后缀

-ability -able	表能力	disability	capable
-er	动作执行者	examiner	employer
-ee	动作接受者	examinee	employee
-ality	性质，状态	personality	nationality
-ant	表示人	assistant	accountant
-ess	阴性的，雌性的	princess	hostess
-hood	表示身份，性质	neighborhood	childhood
-ify	使……化	simplify	purify
-ish	似……的	childish	selfish
-ism	主义，学说	capitalism	impressionism
-ize -ise -yze	……化	analyze	modernize
-less	不，没有	doubtless	valueless
-ogy	学科	biology	stomatology
-ness	性质，状态	carelessness	kindness
-ous -eous -ious	充满	hazardous	courteous
-ant	表示形容词	resistant	significant
-ance	表示名词	resistance	significance
-ary -ory	表示形容词	honorary	illusory
-tive	表示形容词	competitive	imaginative
-en	表示动词，变成；表示形容词	quicken	wooden
-ence	表名词	existence	competence
-ial	表示形容词	beneficial	commercial
-ic	表示形容词	fantastic	cosmic
-ward	表示方向	upward	eastward
-ics	学科	physics	mathematics
-itude	性质，状态	solitude	fortitude
-ive	表示形容词	expensive	comprehensive
-ment	表示名词	encouragement	judgment
-or	表示人	actor	vendor

六、常用词组

↘ break

1. break away from

   The prisoner **broke away from** his guards. 犯人从看守者手中逃脱了。（挣脱，逃脱）

   This organization wished to **break away from** the committee and form a new one. 该组织想脱离委员会后自立门户。（脱离）

   She **broke away from** the others and opened up a two-second lead. 她甩掉其他人，领先大约 2 秒的距离。[（尤指赛跑）甩掉]

2. break down

   Our car **broke down** on the highway. 我们的车子在高速公路上抛锚了。（出故障）

   Negotiations between the two sides have **broken down.** 双方谈判失败了。（失败）

   Her health **broke down** under the pressure of work. 在工作压力下，她的身体垮了。（垮掉）

   He **broke down** and wept when he heard the news. 他听到这个消息时不禁痛哭起来。（感情失去控制）

   Expenditure on the project **breaks down** as follows: raw materials $5,000, wages $4,000. 该项目开支如下：原材料 5000 美元，工资 4000 美元。（划分成部分）

   Firefighters had to **break** the door **down** to reach the people trapped inside. 消防员必须砸破这扇门才能营救困在里面的人。[打倒，砸破（某物）]

   He tried every means to **break down** her daughter's reserve, but in vain. 他竭尽所能去消除与她女儿之间的隔阂，但无济于事。（驱除，瓦解，消除）

   Break down your expenditure into bills, food and other. 将支出细分为现金、食物和其他。[将（金钱等）分类]

   Sugar and starch are **broken down** in the stomach. 糖和淀粉在胃里被分解。（使分解）

3. break for

   She had to hold him back as he tried to **break for** the door. 他突然冲向门跑去，她不得不拉住他。[（试图逃脱时）突然冲向]

4. break in

   Burglars **broke in** while we were away. 我们不在家时，盗贼闯入屋内行窃。（强行进入）

   Every April, the company will have a four-day orientation project to **break in** new recruits. 每年四月，公司会举办为期 4 天的新员工培训。（培训）

   She longed to **break in on** their conversation but didn't want to appear rude. 她想打断他们的谈话，但不想那么粗鲁。（打断）

5. break into

   As the professor stepped on the stage, all students **broke into** loud applause. 教授走上讲台时，所有学生爆发出热烈的掌声。（突然开始）

He **broke into** a run when he saw the police. 看见警察，他撒腿就跑。[撒腿就跑（突然开始快跑）]

I had to **break into** a $20 to pay the bus fare. 我不得不破开这张 20 美元的钞票付公交车费。（破开大面值钞票）

They had to **break into** the emergency food supplies because of the flood. 因为水灾，所以他们不得不动用应急储备的食物。（启用应急用品）

The company is having difficulty **breaking into** new markets. 公司打入新市场时遇到了困难。（顺利打入，成功参与）

6.　break off

The back section of the plane **broke off**. 飞机座舱的后面脱落了。（折断，脱落）

He **broke off** in the middle of a sentence. 在句子中间他停顿了一下。（停顿，中断）

The country's government threatened to **break off** diplomatic relations. 该国政府以断绝外交关系相威胁。（断绝外交关系）

break off one's engagement 解除婚约

7.　break out

She needed to **break out** of her daily routine and do something exciting. 她需要摆脱日常那些琐碎的工作，做一些有趣的事。[摆脱（状况），逃离（境地）]

Her face **broke out** in a rash. 她的脸突然长出皮疹。（突然布满某物）

He **broke out** in cold sweat. 他惊出了一身冷汗。（冒出）

8.　break through（*n.* breakthrough）

The sun **broke through** at last in the afternoon. 下午，太阳终于从云层后面钻出来了。（冲破，突破）

a major **breakthrough** 重大突破

9.　break up

The ship **broke up** on the rock. 船在礁石上撞得粉碎。（粉碎，破碎）

Their marriage has **broken up** / come to an end. 他们离婚了。（结束）

Sentences can be **broken up** into clauses. 句子可以分成从句。（分解，拆分）

↘ **bring**

1.　bring about

What **brought about** the change in your attitude towards English study? 是什么原因导致你改变了学习英语的态度？（导致）

Most people are against **bringing about** the death penalty. 大多数人都反对恢复死刑。（恢复，重新使用）

2.　bring back

Please **bring back** all library books by the end of the week. 请在本周末前归还所有从图书馆借的书。（归还）

The photo **brought back** many pleasant memories. 这张照片勾起许多美好的回忆。

（使回忆起）

3. bring down

The scandal may **bring down** the government. 这个丑闻可能导致政府垮台。（打垮，击败）

We aim to **bring down** prices on all our computers. 我们打算降低我们所有计算机的价格。（降低，减少）

4. bring forth

trees **bringing forth** fruit 结果的树

5. bring in

Experts were **brought in** to advise the government. 让专家参与进来，为政府提建议。（让……参与）

Two men were **brought in** for questioning. 两个男子被带到警察局问话。（逮捕）

They want to **bring in** a bill to limit arms exports. 他们想提出限制武器出口的议案。（提出）

His freelance work **brings** him **in** about $20,000 a year. 他是自由职业者，每年差不多有 2 万美元的收入。（挣得，获利）

6. bring off

It was a difficult task but we **brought** it **off**. 任务很困难，不过我们顺利渡过了难关。（顺利渡过难关）

7. bring up

We were **brought up** to respect authority. 我们受到的教育是要尊重权威。（抚养，养育）

↳ call

1. call for

The government **called for** the immediate release of the hostages. 政府要求立即释放人质。（公开要求）

2. call forth

His speech in public **called forth** an angry response. 他在公众场合的演讲引起了众怒。（引起，产生）

3. call in

Cars with serious faults have been **called in** by the manufacturers. 厂家召回了有严重问题的汽车。（召回）

4. call off

The game was **called off** because of the bad weathers. 因为天气不好，所以比赛取消了。（取消）

5. call on / upon

I now **call upon** the chairman to address the meeting. 现在我邀请主席为会议致辞。（邀请，恭请）

6. call up

The smell of the sea **called up** memories of her childhood. 海的味道让她回忆起童年时光。（使回忆起）

I **called** his address **up** on the computer. 我在电脑中调出他的地址。（调出地址/调用储存）

She **called up** her last reserves of strength. 她用尽最后一些力气。（使尽最后一点力气）

↘ carry

1. carry sb. back to = recall

The smell of the sea **carried her back to** the childhood. 海的味道让她回忆起童年时光。（回忆起）

2. carry off

Joan **carried off** all the prizes. 琼赢得了全部奖品。（赢得，获得）

3. carry out

Our planes **carried out** a bombing raid on enemy targets. 我们的飞机执行了一项轰炸敌方目标的任务。（执行，贯彻）

4. carry over

The confidence gained in remedial classes **carried over** into the children's regular school work. 孩子们在辅导班上获得的自信持续到他们正常的学校学习中去了。（延续）

5. carry sb./sth. through

His strong determination **carried him through** the ordeal. 他是靠自己坚强的决心渡过了难关。（帮助······渡过难关）

Despite powerful opposition, they managed to **carry their reforms through.** 尽管遇到了强大的阻力，他们还是设法进行了改革。（现实，完成）

↘ come

1. come about = happen

Can you tell me how the accident **came about**? 你能告诉我事故是如何发生的吗？（发生）

2. come across

Your speech **comes across** very well. 你的演讲相当受欢迎。（产生效果）

She **came across** some old photos in a drawer. 她在一个抽屉中偶然发现几张老照片。[（偶然）发现，遇见]

I hoped she would **come across with** some more information about the missing child.

我希望她会提供失踪孩子的一些信息。（提供，给予）

3. come along

When the right opportunity **comes along**, you should seize it. 当机遇出现时，你应该抓住。（到达，出现）

Your English has **come along** a lot recently because of your diligence. 因为你很勤奋，所以你的英语水平进步很大。（进步，进展）

4. come around / round

Your mother hasn't yet **come round** from the anesthetic. 你母亲尚未从麻醉状态中苏醒过来。（恢复知觉）

5. come by

Jobs are hard to **come by** now. 工作现在很难找。（得到，获得）

6. come out

When will her new book **come out**? 她的新书什么时候出版？（出版，发行）

The truth **came out** at the trial. 经过审讯，真相终于大白了。（真相大白）

7. come up

The daffodils are just beginning to **come up**. 水仙花就要破土而出了。（破土而出，长出地面）

I'm afraid something urgent has come up. 我想是发生了紧急事件。（发生）

We'll let you know if any vacancies **come up**. 如果有空缺职位，我们会通知你。（出现）

The question is bound to **come up** at the meeting. 会上一定会讨论这个问题。（被提及，被讨论）

She **came up with** a new idea for increasing sales. 她想出了促进销售的新点子。（想出）

His performance didn't really **come up to** his usual high standard. 他的表演没有达到平时的高水平。（达到）

We expect to **come up against** a lot of opposition to the plan. 我们预计这个计划会遭到很多人的反对。（面对／遭到反对）

➷ die

1. die away

The sound of their laughter **died away**. 他们的笑声渐渐远去。（逐渐减弱，逐渐消失）

2. die back（植物）枝头枯萎（但根部仍活着）

3. die down

The flames finally **died down**. 火焰终于熄灭了。（熄灭）

4. die off

As she got older and older, her relatives all **died off**. 随着她越来越老，她的亲属都相继去世了。（相继死去）

5. die out

This species has already **died out** because its habitat had been destroyed. 这一物种已经灭绝，因为它们的栖息地被毁掉了。（灭绝）

➷ fall

1. fall apart

The deal **fell apart** when we failed to agree on the price. 由于我们双方没有就价格达成一致，生意没有做成。（破裂，告吹）

2. fall away

His supporters **fell away** as his popularity declined. 因为他的声望下降了，所以支持他的人数在减少。（减少）

The market for their products **fell away** to almost nothing. 他们产品的市场占有率几乎减到零。（消散）

3. fall behind

We can't afford to **fall behind** our competitors in using new technology. 我们再也不能在使用新技术方面落在竞争对手的后面了。（落后）

4. fall down

That's where the theory **falls down**. 那便是该理论的不足之处。（失败，不起作用）

5. fall on / upon sb. or sth.

The children **fell on** the food and ate it greedily. 孩子们向食物扑去，贪婪地吃了起来。（扑向）

The full cost of the wedding **fell on** her parents. 婚礼的全部费用都落到她父母身上。（由……负担）

6. fall out

Jane and Paul **fell out** with each other. 简和保罗争吵不休。（争吵）

7. fall over

I rushed for the door and **fell over** the cat in the hallway. 我冲向门，在走廊上绊倒在一只猫身上。（跌倒，摔倒）

8. fall through

Our plan **fell through** because of lack of money. 我们的计划因缺钱而落空了。（失败）

➥ **give**

1. give away

He **gave away** most of his money to charity. 他把大部分钱都捐赠给了慈善机构。（捐赠）

The principal **gave away** the prizes at the school sports day. 校长在学校运动会上颁奖。（颁发）

They've **given away** two goals already. 他们已经白白送给对方两个球了。（白送）

She **gave away** state secrets to the enemy. 她向敌人泄露了国家机密。（泄露机密）

2. give in

give sth. in to sb. = hand over sth. to sb. 呈上，交上

3. give off

The flowers **gave off** a fragrant perfume. 花散发出香味。（散发，放出）

4. give out

After a month their food supplies **gave out**. 一个月后，他们的食物耗尽了。（用完，耗尽）

Her legs **gave out** and she collapsed. 她的腿残疾了，她整个人崩溃了。（坏掉）

The teacher **gave out** the exam papers. 老师分发考试卷。（分发）

The radiator **gives out** a lot of heat. 暖气片散发出大量的热量。（散发）

5. give up

After a week on the run, he **gave himself up to** the police. 逃亡一周之后，他向警方投案自首了。（投案自首）

I have **given up on** you. 我对你已不抱希望。（对……不抱希望）

➴ go

1. go about

Despite the threat of war, people **went about** their business as usual. 尽管受到战争的威胁，人们还继续忙着自己的事，一如往常。（继续做，忙于某事）

How should I **go about** finding a job? 我该如何着手去找工作？（着手做）

2. go after

She left the room in tears so I **went after** her. 她流着泪离开了房间，我追了出去。（追赶）

Unfortunately both my best friend and I are **going after** the same job. 不幸的是，我和我最好的朋友应聘的是同一份工作。（追求某人，谋求某事）

3. go against sb.

He would not **go against** his parents' wishes so he went abroad for further study. 他不愿违背父母的意愿，于是他出国深造去了。（违背，不相符）

4. go along

I'd **go along with** you there. 在那一点上我赞同你的意见。（赞成，支持）

5. go at

John **went at** Bob when the class was over. 约翰一下课就扑向了鲍勃。（攻击某人）

He **went at** his breakfast as if he hadn't eaten for days. 他吃早餐时的样子就像多日没吃东西似的。（拼命干）

6. go by

Things will get easier as time **goes by**. 随着时间的推移，事情会变得越发简单。（时间流逝）

He always **goes by** the rules. 他总是根据规则办事。（遵循，依照）

7. go for

They have a high level of unemployment—but the same **goes for** many other countries. 他们失业率很高，不过其他很多国家也是这样。（适用于）

go for sth.

I hear you're **going for** that job. 我听说你准备争取那个职位。（争取获得）

8. go in for

Several people **went in for** the race. 有几个人参加了赛跑。（参加考试或比赛等）

She doesn't **go in for** team games. 她对团队比赛项目不感兴趣。（对……感兴趣）

9. go through

   He's amazingly cheerful considering all he's had to **go through**. 想到自己经历过的一切，他欣喜若狂。（经历）

   Have you **gone through** all your money? 你把所有的钱都花光了吗？（用完，耗尽）

10. go with

    Disease often **goes with** poverty. 疾病和贫穷常相伴而生。（与某物相伴而生）

    It is very common that the color of green doesn't **go with** red. 一般说来，绿色与红色不相配。（与……相配）

11. go without

    There wasn't time for breakfast, so I had to **go without**. 没时间吃早饭了，所以只好不吃了。（将就，没有……也行）

➥ hand

1. hand down to sb.

   These skills used to be **handed down** from father **to** son. 这些手艺在过去常常是以父传子的方式传承。（传承）

2. hand in

   Please **hand in** your papers. 请交卷。（上交，提交）

3. hand over

   He resigned and **handed over** his work to his colleague. 他辞职了，并把工作移交给了同事。[（权力、责任）移交]

➥ hold

1. hold back

   The police were unable to **hold back** the crowd. 警察无法拦住人群。（阻拦）

   You could become a good musician, but your lack of practice is **holding** you **back**. 你有可能成为一名优秀的音乐家，但是缺少练习正在妨碍你的发展。（妨碍发展）

   hold back information 隐瞒信息

   hold back one's anger 压住怒火

   hold back tears 忍住泪水

   hold sb. **back** from doing sth. 阻止某人做某事

2. hold down

   It took three men to **hold** him **down**. 三个人才将他制服。（制服）

   The people are **held down** by a repressive regime. 人们受到残酷政权的压迫。（压迫）

   The rate of inflation must be **held down**. 通货膨胀率必须控制在较低的水平。（控制在低水平）

   He was unable to **hold down** a job after the accident. 事故发生后他无法保住自己的

工作了。（保住）

3. hold forth 喋喋不休，大发议论

4. hold on

They managed to **hold on** until help arrived. 他们一直坚持到救援时来。（坚持住，顶住）

These nuts and bolts **hold** the wheels **on**. 这些螺栓和螺母将车轮固定住。（固定住）

5. hold off

We could get a new computer now or **hold off** until prices are lower. 我们可以现在就买台新电脑或者推迟到价格低一些再买。（推迟）

He **held off** all the last-minute challengers and won the race in a new record time. 他与其他选手保持一定距离并赢得了比赛，创造了一项新纪录。（战胜，克服）

6. hold out

We can stay here as long as our supplies **hold out**. 只要给养充足，我们就留在这里。（维持，坚持）

The doctor **held out** little hope of her recovery. 医生对她康复不抱多大希望。（提供机会，给予希望，使有可能）

7. hold up

She is **holding up** well under the pressure. 她能很好地承受压力。（承受住）

An accident is **holding up** traffic. 事故阻碍了交通。（阻碍）

My application was **held up** by the postal strike. 邮政系统罢工把我的申请耽误了。（耽搁）

His idea was **held up** to ridicule. 他的想法被当成笑料。（举出例子；提出）

↘ keep

1. keep away from

His illness **kept** him **away from** work for several weeks. 他生病了，几周都无法工作。（阻止）

2. keep back

She was unable to **keep back** her tears. 她无法抑制住自己的泪水。（抑制或阻止感情等流露）

He **kept back** half the money for himself. 他将一半的钱留给自己。（保留或扣留某物一部分）

I'm sure they are **keeping** something **back** from me. 我确信他们有事瞒着我。（隐瞒）

3. keep down

The people have been **kept down** for years by a brutal regime. 人们已在暴政下被奴役多年。（压制，奴役）

The government is trying to **keep down** inflation. 政府正试图控制通货膨胀。（控制，防止）

4. keep off

I'm trying to **keep off** fatty foods. 我正在试着不吃脂肪多的食物。（回避，避免）

They lit a fire to **keep off** wild animals. 他们点燃火把以使野生动物无法靠近。（使某

人 / 某物不接近）

5. keep on 继续

6. keep to sth.

He **kept to** his room for the first few days of term. 这个学期的头几天，他一直待在自己的房间里。（留在某个位置，不离开）

I'm resigning — but **keep** it **to** yourself! 我会辞职——但你自己知道就行了，不要说出来。（遵守，信守，对……保守秘密）

7. keep up

The rain **kept up** all afternoon. 整个下午都在下雨。（持续不变）

The high cost of raw materials is **keeping** prices **up**. 较高的原材料价格使商品价格居高不下。（居高不下）

keep sb. up 使某人熬夜

➜ pay

1. pay back

I'll **pay** him **back** for making me look like a fool in front of everyone. 他让我在大家面前像个傻子，我要报复他。（报复）

2. pay in

Have you **paid** the cheque **in** yet? 你把支票存入银行了吗？（存入）

3. pay off

We **paid** him **off** at the end of the week. 我们周末给他算清工资后就把他解雇了。（付清工资解雇）

4. pay out

I **paid out** a lot of money for that car. 我为那辆车付出了一大笔钱。（付出大笔款项）

5. pay up 偿还（欠款），全部付清

➜ pick

1. pick at 磨蹭着吃；揪，扯

2. pick off

Snipers were **picking off** innocent civilians. 狙击手逐个瞄准无辜百姓射杀。（逐个瞄准射击）

3. pick out

She **picked out** a scarf to wear with the dress. 她挑选了一条围巾以配她穿的连衣裙。（精心挑选）

4. pick up

Sales have **picked up** 14% this year. 今年的销售增加了 14%。（好转，改善）

All I seem to do is cook, wash and **pick up** after the kids. 我要做的全部工作是做饭、

洗衣以及在孩子屁股后收拾。（收拾，整理）

The bus **picks up** passengers outside the airport. 公共汽车在机场外接旅客。（接载）

A lifeboat **picked up** survivors. 救生艇在营救生还者。（营救，搭救）

He was **picked up** by the police and taken to the station for questionings. 他被警察逮捕，并被带到派出所审问。（逮捕，抓捕）

He **picked up** the phone and dialed the number. 他拿起电话拨号。（拿起）

We were able to **pick up** the BBC World Service. 我们能收听到 BBC World Service 的节目。（接收信号、节目）

She **picked up** French when she was living in Paris. 她在巴黎生活期间学会了法语。（学到，得到）

Scientists can now **pick up** early symptoms of the disease. 科学家现在能辨认疾病的早期症状。（辨认）

I **picked up** my coat from the cleaner on the way home. 我在回家的路上从洗衣店取回衣服。（取回）

I seemed to have **picked up** a terrible cold from somewhere. 我好像从什么地方染上了重感冒。（感染）

pick up the trails of animals 追寻动物的踪迹

pick up the theme again 又回到主题

I **picked up** the faint sound of a car in the distance. 我觉察到远处汽车微弱的声音。（察觉，发现）

➥ **pull**

1. pull back

   Their sponsors **pulled back** at the last minutes. 他们的赞助人在最后一刻打了退堂鼓。（打退堂鼓）

   They **pulled back** a goal just before half-time. 下半场结束前他们扳回一球。（挽回局势）

2. pull down 拆毁

3. pull through

   The doctors think she will **pull through**. 医生认为她会痊愈的。（恢复，痊愈）

   It's going to be tough but we'll **pull through** it together. 这件事会很困难，不过我们会协力完成的。（完成，做成）

➥ **put**

1. put sth. aside

   They decided to **put aside** their differences. 他们决定将分歧搁在一边。（搁置，不理睬）

2. put away

   She has a few thousand dollars **put away** for her retirement. 她攒了几千美元，留作退休后使用。（积攒）

He must have **put away** a bottle of whisky last night. 他昨晚一定是喝了一瓶威士忌。（猛吃，喝）

3. put back

Poor trading figures **put back** our plans for expansion. 贸易数据极差，我们扩张的计划因此推迟。（延迟，推迟）

Remember to **put** your clock **back** tonight because the time has officially changed. 记得今晚把时钟拨慢，因为官方时间已更改。（拨慢时间）

4. put down

The novel is so interesting that I couldn't **put** it **down**. 小说很精彩，我一看起来就无法释卷。（放下）

The meeting's on the 22nd. **Put** it **down** in your diary. 会议日期是 22 号，把它记在日记里。（写下）

The military government is determined to **put down** all opposition. 军人政府决定镇压所有反对者。（镇压，平定）

The cat is so miserable that we had to have it **put down**. 这只猫现在太痛苦了，我们不得不用药物将它结束生命。（用药物结束生命）

5. put forward 拨快时钟；提出（建议）

6. put off

The match had to be **put off** because of the heavy rain. 比赛因大雨而推迟。（推迟）

The sudden noise **put** me **off** my game. 突然的噪声让玩游戏的我分神了。（使分神）

7. put on

Due to lack of regular exercise, I have **put on** several kilos. 因为缺乏有规律的锻炼，我增重了几公斤。（增加体重）

A foreign drama club is **putting on** a new drama in Beijing. 一个外国戏剧俱乐部在北京上演一场新戏剧。（举办，上演）

8. put out

Firefighters soon **put** the fire **out**. 消防员很快扑灭了大火。（扑灭）

The plant **puts out** 500 new mobile phones a week. 工厂一周可以生产 500 部新手机。（生产，制造）

Police have **put out** a description of the man at large. 警察公布了这名逃犯的情况。（公布）

↘ **take**

1. take after （在外貌、性格等方面）与（父、母等）相像

2. take apart 拆（机器）

3. take away

I was given some pills to **take away** the pain on the back. 给我开了一些药，可以消

除我的背痛。（解除，消除）

4. take back

The picture **took** me **back** to my childhood. 这张图片让我回忆起童年时光。（使回想起）

5. take down 拆除；写下，记录

6. take in

The old woman **took in** those homeless children. 这位老妇人收留了那些无家可归的孩子。（收留）

He listened very attentively, **taking in** every word the professor said. 他听得十分认真，把教授说的每一句话都领会了。（吸收）

7. take off 起飞；脱下；模仿

8. take on

The city has taken great changes recently and **takes on** a new look. 这座城市近来变化巨大，呈现出崭新的面貌。（呈现）

She was **taken on** as a trainee. 她被雇为实习生。（雇用）

9. take out

The fine will be **taken out** of your salary. 罚款将从你的工资中扣除。（扣除）

It is very awful for me to **take out** teeth. 对我来说，拔牙真是太可怕了。（切除，摘除）

10. take over 接管

11. take to

I've **taken to** go to bed very early. 我养成了早睡的习惯。（养成……习惯）

He hasn't **taken to** his new school. 他还没有对他的新学校产生好感。（对……产生好感）

12. take up

Lap tops will not **take up** much room. 笔记本电脑占用空间较小。（占地方）

七、词汇专项练习及最新真题解析

Section A

Directions: *In this section all the sentences are incomplete. Four words or phrases, marked A, B, C and D, are given beneath each of them. You are to choose the word or phrase that best completes the sentence. Then, mark your answer on the **ANSWER SHEET**.*

1. He had always had a good opinion of himself, but after the publication of his best-selling novel he became unbearably _____.

   A. cordial   B. proud

   C. conceited   D. exaggerated

2. An enormous number of people in the world's poorest countries do not have clean

water or adequate sanitation _____.

    A. capacities   B. facilities   C. authorities   D. warranties

3. Pleasure, or joy, is vital to _____ health.

    A. optimistic   B. optional   C. optimal   D. operational

4. I haven't met anyone _____ the new tax plan.

    A. in honor of   B. in search of   C. in place of   D. in favor of

5. At the party we found the shy girl _____ her mother all the time.

    A. harmonizing with   B. clinging to   C. depending on   D. adjusting to

6. This software can be _____ to the needs of each customer.

    A. tailored   B. administrated   C. entailed   D. accustomed

7. If the cells cannot use sugar, the body begins to _____ its own tissues for food.

    A. break through   B. break down   C. break out   D. break over

8. If you are a member of the company, you must _____ to its rules.

    A. approach   B. conform   C. respond   D. abide

9. It is the only problem requiring special techniques and _____.

    A. qualification   B. therapies   C. specification   D. expertise

10. Some officials insist that something be done to _____ inflation.

    A. curb   B. sue   C. detoxify   D. condemn

11. Human beings are _____ creatures, designed to be on the move.

    A. distinctive   B. dynamic   C. intrinsic   D. mysterious

12. The fall in production over the past year has caused 200 workers to be made redundant and a further 500 have been _____ temporarily.

    A. laid off   B. laid down   C. laid out   D. laid away

13. The black clouds and the lightning suggest that a big storm is _____.

    A. eminent   B. imminent   C. immense   D. immanent

14. Stories in this novel seem to have happened in the real world. However, all characters and plots are _____.

    A. imaginable   B. imaginative   C. imaginary   D. imaging

15. He has a very _____ plan: he wants to master three foreign languages and travel abroad in three years.

    A. arbitrary   B. aggressive   C. ambitious   D. abundant

16. The local government decided to gave the top _____ to education.

    A. authority   B. protection   C. profession   D. priority

17. When a psychologist does a general experiment about the human's attitudes towards pressure, he selects interviewees _____ and asks them questions.

    A. at random   B. in essence   C. at heart   D. in bulk

18. He was _____ of a crime he didn't commit. He fought for many years to prove his

innocence.

    A. convicted   B. convinced   C. conceived   D. condemned

19. Finding out information about these universities has become easy for anyone with Internet _____.

    A. entrance   B. admission   C. access   D. entry

20. The disrespectful sons began to concern about the ultimate _____ of the family's property.

    A. proposal   B. disposal   C. removal   D. refusal

21. Two decades ago a woman who shook hands with others on her own _____ was usually viewed too forward.

    A. endeavor   B. initiative   C. motivation   D. preference

22. He wanted to stay at home, but at last he agreed, very _____ though, to go to the cinema.

    A. decisively   B. reluctantly   C. willingly   D. deliberately

23. His parents blamed his son for his _____ the younger children in school.

    A. imitating   B. intimating   C. intimidating   D. emigrating

24. Eating too much fat can _____ heart diseases and cause hypertension.

    A. distribute to   B. attribute to   C. devote to   D. contribute to

25. The soccer team has had five _____ victories in the last three years.

    A. successive   B. excessive   C. subsequent   D. eventual

26. The Car Club couldn't _____ to meet the demands of all its members.

    A. ensure   B. guarantee   C. insure   D. assure

27. In the Chinese household, grandparents and other relatives play _____ roles in raising children.

    A. incapable   B. insensible   C. indispensable   D. infinite

28. None of us expected the chairman to _____ at the party. We thought he was still in hospital.

    A. turn in   B. turn over   C. turn up   D. turn down

29. The European Union countries were once worried that they would not have _____ supplies of petroleum.

    A. proficient   B. efficient   C. potential   D. sufficient

30. His wife is constantly finding _____ with him, which makes him very angry.

    A. errors   B. weakness   C. fault   D. flaw

31. His neighbors became _____ of his behavior and contacted the police.

    A. suspicious   B. doubtful   C. susceptible   D. dubious

32. It is suggested that criticism without any tips for improvement is not _____ and should be avoided.

    A. constructive   B. destructive   C. productive   D. descriptive

33. It is _____ that the Internet is exerting a growing important influence on people's lives.
    A. indistinctive   B. indissoluble   C. indispensable   D. indisputable
34. He _____ on her new dress without even looking at it.
    A. complemented   B. complimented   C. praised   D. appraised
35. AIDS is becoming the top threat to people's health, and the _____ fatal disease claimed many lives.
    A. deceptively   B. invariably   C. imperatively   D. transiently
36. He is an extremely arbitrary leader, so everything must be done in _____ with his ideas.
    A. appliance   B. compliance   C. defiance   D. reliance
37. When he realized that he had been _____ to sign the contract, he threatened to take legal actions to cancel the agreement.
    A. adduced   B. induced   C. deduced   D. produced
38. Local people are encouraged to _____ their homes to save energy.
    A. insulate   B. insane   C. assault   D. insult
39. During the Olympics, the emergency services were _____ in the Olympic Village.
    A. by hand   B. in hand   C. at hand   D. on hand
40. In order to pursue the click rate, the Internet media reported _____ social news deliberately.
    A. sensitive   B. sensible   C. sensational   D. sensory
41. They set up a(n) _____ training schedule for the candidates for the final competition.
    A. ridiculous   B. rigorous   C. ambiguous   D. anonymous
42. The new traffic regulations of "even-and odd-numbered license plates on alternate days" will make a(n) _____ difference to most people.
    A. appreciative   B. appreciable
    C. comprehensive   D. comprehensible
43. At _____ Smith received a medal as a reward for his prominent achievements in research.
    A. compliment   B. complement   C. commitment   D. commencement
44. As the most outstanding writer in the 20th century in America, Hemingway created lots of _____ works.
    A. impartial   B. immortal   C. immemorial   D. immoral
45. We have arranged to go to the cinema on Friday, but we can be _____ and go another day.
    A. probable   B. reliable   C. flexible   D. feasible
46. Some people apparently have an amazing ability to _____ the right answer.
    A. come up with   B. look up to   C. put up with   D. clear up
47. On behalf of our school, I'm _____ to your generous help in the earthquake.

A. subject   B. inclined   C. liable   D. obliged

48. The appearance of this used car is quite _____, and it is much newer than it really is.

   A. descriptive   B. impressive   C. deceptive   D. indicative

49. All the information we have collected in relation to that case _____ very little.

   A. adds up to   B. comes up with   C. puts up with   D. keeps up with

50. We now obtain more than two-thirds of our protein from animal sources, while our grandparents _____ only one-half from animal sources.

   A. originated   B. digested   C. deprived   D. derived

51. The new secretary has written a remarkably _____ report in a few pages but with all details.

   A. concise   B. clear   C. precise   D. elaborate

52. Expected noises are usually more _____ than unexpected ones of the like magnitude.

   A. manageable   B. controllable   C. tolerable   D. perceivable

53. With prices _____ so much, it's hard for the company to plan a budget.

   A. fluctuating   B. waving   C. swinging   D. vibrating

54. Please do not be _____ by his bad manners since he is merely trying to attract attention.

   A. disregarded   B. distorted   C. irritated   D. intervened

55. Sam assured his boss that he would _____ all his energies in doing this new job.

   A. call forth   B. call at   C. call on   D. call off

56. Care should be taken to decrease the length of time that one is _____ loud continuous noise.

   A. subjected to   B. filled with   C. associated with   D. attached to

57. The news item about the earthquake is followed by a detailed report made _____.

   A. on the spot   B. on site

   C. on location   D. on the ground

58. Mother who takes care of everybody is usually the most _____ person in each family.

   A. considerate   B. considerable

   C. considering   D. constant

59. If you know what the trouble is, why don't you help them to _____ the situation?

   A. simplify   B. modify   C. verify   D. rectify

60. I tried very hard to persuade him to join our group but I met with a flat _____.

   A. disapproval   B. rejection   C. refusal   D. decline

61. He has failed me so many times that I no longer place any _____ on what he promises.

   A. faith   B. belief   C. credit   D. reliance

62. The wealth of a country should be measured _____ the health and happiness of its people as well as the material goods it can produce.
    A. in line with   B. in terms of
    C. regardless of   D. by means of

63. His _____ and unwillingness to learn from others prevent him from being an effective member of the team.
    A. arrogance   B. dignity   C. humility   D. solitude

64. An ambulance must have priority as it usually has to deal with some kind of _____.
    A. urgency   B. danger   C. emergency   D. crisis

65. The old man _____ defended the right of every citizen to freedom of choice in religion, which enabled him to win the respect of all people.
    A. peculiarly   B. indifferently   C. vigorously   D. inevitably

66. The _____ difference in Chinese dialect has become a problem in mutual communication among people.
    A. enormous   B. immense   C. imminent   D. eminent

67. In the family where the roles of men and women are not sharply separated and where many household tasks are shared to a greater or lesser extent, notions of male _____ are hard to maintain.
    A. privilege   B. predominance
    C. prevalence   D. priority

68. After years of being exposed to the sun and rain, the sign over the shop had become completely _____.
    A. illegal   B. eligible   C. illegible   D. unreasonable

69. It's time you _____ some reading or the other students will leave you behind.
    A. got down to   B. adapted to   C. held on to   D. attended to

70. Geologists maintain that a mountain is a mountain _____ its geological structure though it may not reach an altitude of 3,000 feet above sea level.
    A. by virtue of   B. in the way of   C. by way of   D. for the sake of

71. Find out how researchers will inform you about the trial's progress or _____ you of any problem.
    A. denounce   B. secure   C. notify   D. ensure

72. America simply does not have enough prisons to _____ all its criminals.
    A. cope with   B. put up to   C. hold up   D. dispose of

73. Dying patients receive some small hope that the new treatment may _____ the course of disease but risk experiencing severe side effects.
    A. prolong   B. identify   C. alter   D. expose

74. The thief was caught because of the neighbors' _____.
    A. vigilance   B. aggregate   C. varnish   D. visage

75. A body that produces its own light waves, like the sun or an electric bulb, is said to be _____.

    A. illuminative   B. flashy   C. luminous   D. flaming

76. True, he couldn't see the tears, yet she was afraid that voice would _____ her emotion.

    A. give off   B. give away   C. give over   D. give out

77. Shops _____ the do-it-yourself craze by offering consumers bits and pieces which they can assemble at home.

    A. ask for   B. send for   C. run for   D. cater for

78. A new technique, called electronic dental anaesthesia could soon _____ the need for the dreaded dentist's needle.

    A. amplify   B. decrease   C. stimulate   D. meet

79. Shortness of breath often goes hand in hand with _____, the kind that sweeps over the whole body and isn't confined to one area.

    A. infection   B. fatigue   C. syncope   D. suffocation

80. At the national level, the National Institutes of Health and especially the National Institute on Aging are _____ many types of research programs on aging.

    A. allocating   B. expanding   C. sponsoring   D. summing

81. HIV and AIDS may threaten the fundamental values of society, and any attempt to deal with them presents a _____ challenge.

    A. formidable   B. fatal   C. favorable   D. fantastic

82. Kelley's publicists abruptly _____ a planned seven-city publicity tour, announcing that their "publishing objectives have been accomplished".

    A. called off   B. called down   C. called up   D. called for

83. Crowding as an environmental variable is only beginning to be seriously examined and the data so far is _____.

    A. informative   B. inconclusive

    C. inconspicuous   D. indisputable

84. During the sterilization process which follows, the cans are _____ to steam or boiling water with the temperature and duration varying according to the type of food.

    A. proportional   B. subjected   C. susceptible   D. liable

85. But research can have no economic impact if the new scientific discoveries are not _____ into marketable goods and services.

    A. launched   B. translated   C. dissected   D. conveyed

86. Nature never ceases to surprise us. Molecules with _____ structures and properties turn up in the laboratory all the time.

    A. bioactive   B. miniature   C. bizarre   D. invisible

87. Since patients cannot always tell the difference between psychologically induced

chest pain and heart attack, the physician should _____ the possible causes of the pain.

A. rule out　　　　B. divide up　　　C. bring apart　　D. sort out

88. David L. Rinion of School of Medicine, the University of California, Los Angeles says that such a test, if it _____ expectations could usher in a new area of prenatal diagnosis.

A. meets up with　　B. comes up with　C. sheds light on　D. lives up to

89. Suffering from his leg illness, Tom is very _____ nowadays.

A. emaciated　　　B. eligible　　　C. elastic　　　　D. exceptional

90. Today investigators are still far from _____ a master map of the vasculature of the heart.

A. constituting　　B. decoding　　　C. drafting　　　D. encoding

91. I have never seen a more caring, _____ group of people in my life.

A. emotional　　　B. impersonal　　C. compulsory　　D. compassionate

92. As we need plain, _____ food for the body, we must have serious reading for the mind.

A. wholesome　　　B. diet　　　　　C. tasteful　　　D. edible

93. The best exercise should require continuous _____, rather than frequent stops and starts.

A. compassion　　B. acceleration　　C. frustration　　D. exertion

94. Salk won _____ as the scientist who developed the world's first effective vaccine against polio.

A. accomplishment　B. qualification　C. eminence　　D. patent

95. A coronary disease is the widely-used term _____ insufficiency of blood supply to the heart.

A. denoting　　　B. donating　　　C. relating　　　D. resorting

96. It is the builder's job to make sure that the house conforms to the architects' _____ in every way.

A. regulations　　B. specialities　　C. essentials　　D. specifications

097. Publicly, they are trying to _____ this latest failure, but in private they are very worried.

A. put off　　　　B. laugh off　　　C. pay off　　　D. lay off

098. The poor nutrition in the early stages of infancy can _____ adult growth.

A. degenerate　　B. deteriorate　　C. boost　　　　D. retard

099. During rush hour, downtown streets are _____ with commuters.

A. scattered　　　B. condensed　　　C. clogged　　　D. dotted

100. I'm afraid that you'll have to _____ the deterioration of the condition.（2008 年真题）

A. account for　　B. call for　　　C. look for　　　D. make for

101. Twelve hours a week seemed a generous _____ of your time to the nursing home. （2008 年真题）

    A. affliction   B. alternative   C. allocation   D. alliance

102. Every product is _____ tested before being put into the market. （2008 年真题）

    A. expensively   B. exceptionally   C. exhaustively   D. exclusively

103. Having clean hands is one of the _____ rules when preparing food. （2008 年真题）

    A. potent   B. conditional   C. inseparable   D. cardinal

104. The educators should try hard to develop the _____ abilities of children. （2008 年真题）

    A. cohesive   B. cognitive   C. collective   D. comic

105. Mortgage _____ had risen in the last year because the number of low-income families was on the increase. （2008 年真题）

    A. defects   B. deficits   C. defaults   D. deceptions

106. The symptoms may be _____ by certain drugs. （2008 年真题）

    A. exaggerated   B. exacerbated   C. exceeded   D. exhibited

107. Her story was a complete _____ from start to finish, so nobody believed in her. （2008 年真题）

    A. facility   B. fascination   C. fabrication   D. faculty

108. The police investigating the traffic accident have not ruled out _____. （2008 年真题）

    A. salvage   B. safeguard   C. sabotage   D. sacrifice

109. The government always _____ on the background of employees who are hired for sensitive military projects. （2008 年真题）

    A. takes up   B. checks up   C. works out   D. looks into

110. The _____ conditions and places are likely to cause diseases. （2009 年真题）

    A. unsanitary   B. insidious   C. insane   D. inefficacious

111. The witness was _____ by the judge for failing to answer the question. （2009 年真题）

    A. abstained   B. acquitted   C. admonished   D. adduced

112. He has _____ two cars this year because of traffic accidents. （2009 年真题）

    A. pulled of   B. worn out   C. passed out   D. written off

113. People are much better informed since the _____ of the Internet. （2009 年真题）

    A. convenient   B. advent   C. interface   D. aftermath

114. All instruments that come into contact with the patient must be _____ before being used by others. （2009 年真题）

    A. sterilized   B. labeled   C. quarantined   D. retained

115. By adopting this cunning policy, the clinic risks _____ many of its patients. （2009 年真题）

    A. acquitting   B. allocating   C. alleviating   D. alienating

116. Diabetes upsets the _____ of sugar, fat and protein. （2009 年真题）

A. metastasis   B. metabolism   C. malaise   D. maintenance

117. The muscular _____ can affect the way we feel mentally.（2009 年真题）

A. potency   B. fiber   C. lethargy   D. synthesis

118. Evidence is widespread that HIV-infected persons show to _____ their unsafe behavior.（2009 年真题）

A. respond to   B. reflect on   C. wipe out   D. put off

119. A number of black youths have complained of being _____ by the police. （2010 年真题）

A. harassed   B. distracted   C. sentenced   D. released

120. Despite his doctor's note of caution, he never _____ from drinking and smoking. （2015 年真题）

A. retained   B. dissuaded   C. alleviated   D. abstained

121. People with a history of recurrent infections are warned that the use of personal stereos with headsets is likely to _____ their hearing.（2015 年真题）

A. rehabilitate   B. jeopardize   C. tranquilize   D. supplement

122. Impartial observers had to acknowledge that lack of formal education did not seem to _____ Larry in any way in his success.（2015 年真题）

A. refute   B. ratify   C. facilitate   D. impede

123. When the supporting finds were reduced, they should have revised their plan _____. （2015 年真题）

A. accordingly   B. alternatively   C. considerably   D. relatively

124. It is increasingly believed among the expectant parents that prenatal education of classical music can _____ future adults with appreciation of music.（2015 年真题）

A. acquaint   B. familiarize   C. endow   D. amuse

125. If the gain of profit is solely due to rising energy prices, then inflation should be subsided when energy prices _____.（2015 年真题）

A. level out   B. stand out   C. come off   D. wear off

126. Heat stroke is a medical emergency that demands immediate _____ from qualified medical personnel.（2015 年真题）

A. prescription   B. palpation   C. intervention   D. interposition

127. Asbestos exposure results in Mesothelioma, asbestosis and internal organ cancers, and _____ of these diseases is often decades after the initial exposure.（2015 年真题）

A. offset   B. intake   C. outlet   D. onset

128. Ebola, which spreads through body fluid or secretions such as urine, _____ and semen, can kill up to 90% of those infected.（2015 年真题）

A. saline   B. saliva   C. scabies   D. scrapes

129. The newly designed system is _____ to genetic transfection, and enables an incubation

period for studying various genes. (2015 年真题)

  A. comparable   B. transmissible

  C. translatable   D. amenable

130. Employers have a legal obligation to pay _____ to their workers for injuries. (2016 年真题)

  A. compensation   B. compromise   C. commodity   D. consumption

131. The argument between the two patients became so fierce that the doctor had to _____. (2016 年真题)

  A. alleviate   B. aggravate   C. extinguish   D. intervene

132. But despite all the legal hustle and bustle, they don't actually expect to _____ death sentences to life terms without parole. (2016 年真题)

  A. induce   B. convert   C. revive   D. swerve

133. To maintain physical well-being, a person should eat _____ food and get sufficient exercise. (2016 年真题)

  A. integral   B. gross   C. wholesome   D. intact

134. The Central Government's pledge to maintain the _____ and stability of Hong Kong at all costs is a great encouragement to the local finance. (2016 年真题)

  A. provision   B. prosperity   C. privilege   D. preference

135. It is pointed out that patients must be reassured that "their lives will not be _____ as a result of bed shortages". (2016 年真题)

  A. facilitated   B. forfeited   C. fulfilled   D. furnished

136. The cause of his death has been a mystery and _____ unknown so far. (2016 年真题)

  A. exclusively   B. superficially   C. utterly   D. doubtfully

137. It is known that some ways of using resources _____ can destroy the environment as well as the people living in it. (2016 年真题)

  A. recklessly   B. sparingly   C. sensibly   D. incredibly

138. Cholera is a preventable waterborne bacterial infection that is spread through _____ water. (2016 年真题)

  A. filtered   B. distilled   C. contaminated   D. purified

139. We welcome him not _____ as a new broom but rather as a very old friend. (2016 年真题)

  A. by the way   B. at all events   C. by no means   D. in any sense

140. Chronic high-dose intake of vitamin A has been shown to have _____ effects on bones. (2017 年真题)

  A. adverse   B. prevalent   C. instant   D. purposeful

141. Drinking more water is good for the rest of your body, helping to lubricate joints and _____ toxins and impurities. (2017 年真题)

A. screen out　　　B. knock out　　　　C. flush out　　　　D. rule out

142. Rheumatologist advises that those with ongoing aches and pains first seek medical help to _____ the problem.（2017 年真题）

A. affiliate　　　　B. alleviate　　　　C. aggravate　　　　D. accelerate

143. Generally, vaccine makers _____ the virus in fertilized chicken eggs in a process that can take four to six months.（2017 年真题）

A. penetrate　　　B. designate　　　　C. generate　　　　D. exaggerate

144. Danish research shows that the increase in obese people in Denmark is roughly _____ to the increase of carbon dioxide in the atmosphere.（2017 年真题）

A. equivalent　　　B. temporary　　　　C. permanent　　　　D. relevant

145. Ted was felled by a massive stroke that affected his balance and left him barely able to speak _____.（2017 年真题）

A. bluntly　　　　B. intelligibly　　　C. reluctantly　　　　D. ironically

146. In a technology-intensive enterprise, computers _____ all processes of the production and management.（2017 年真题）

A. dominate　　　B. overwhelm　　　　C. substitute　　　　D. imitate

147. Although most dreams apparently happen _____, dream activity may be provided by external influences.（2017 年真题）

A. homogeneously　　　　　　　　B. instantaneously

C. spontaneously　　　　　　　　D. simultaneously

148. We are much quicker to respond, and we respond far too quickly by giving _____ to our anger.（2017 年真题）

A. vent　　　　　B. impulse　　　　C. temper　　　　D. offence

149. By maintaining a strong family _____, they are also maintaining the infrastructure of society.（2017 年真题）

A. bias　　　　　B. honor　　　　　C. estate　　　　D. bond

150. The medical team discussed their shared _____ to eliminating this curable disease.（2017 年真题）

A. obedience　　　B. susceptibility　　C. inclination　　　D. dedication

答案及解析

1. 【答案】C

【解析】此题考点为备选词是否符合句意。cordial 热诚的，衷心的；proud 自豪的；conceited 自负的；exaggerated 夸张的，夸大的。此题解题的关键在于题干中所给的信息。have a good opinion of oneself 意思是"自视过高"。unbearably 意思是"不堪忍受的"。只有 C 符合句意。

题干译文：他一向自视过高，但在他最畅销的小说出版后，他又开始变得自负，让人无法忍受。

2. 【答案】B

【解析】此题考点为备选词是否符合句意。capacity 容量，能力，才能；facility 设施，设备；authority 权威；warranty 正当理由，保证。此题解题的关键在于题干中所给的信息。enormous 庞大的；adequate 适当的，足够的；sanitation 卫生。故只有 B 符合句意。

题干译文：在世界上最穷困的国家里，许多人没有清洁的水或者足够的卫生设施。

3. 【答案】C

【解析】此题考点为形近词辨析。optimistic 乐观的；optional 可选择的；optimal 最佳的，最理想的；operational 操作的，运作的。只有 C 符合句意。

题干译文：愉悦或快乐，是保持理想健康状态的关键。

4. 【答案】D

【解析】此题考点为词组辨析。in honor of 的含义是"为纪念……"，例如：The monument is in honor of soldiers losing lives for the country. 这个纪念碑是为了纪念为国家牺牲的士兵们。in search of 的含义是"寻找"，例如：He went in search of a doctor for his sick son. 他为他生病的儿子寻找医生。in place of 的含义是"替代"，例如：Nothing can be used in place of love of mother. 没有什么可以用来替代母爱。in favor of 的含义是"赞同，支持"，例如：Those who are in favor of my suggestion nodded. 那些赞同我的建议的人们点着头。只有 D 符合句意。

题干译文：我还没遇到一个支持新税计划的人。

5. 【答案】B

【解析】此题考点就是备选词组的含义是否符合句意。harmonize with 的含义是"与……和谐，协调"，例如：The colors harmonize well with the decorations on the wall. 这些颜色和墙上的装饰很协调。cling to 的含义是"依附，依靠，坚持"，例如：I was caught in the heavy rain and wet clothes clung to my body. 我挨大雨淋了，湿衣服紧贴在身上。depend on 的含义是"依靠，依赖"，例如：He hasn't found a job so he has to depend on his parents. 他还没找到工作，所以他得依靠父母生活。adjust to 的含义是"适应，调节"，例如：You should adjust yourself to the new environment as soon as possible. 你应该尽快适应新环境。

题干译文：在聚会上我们发现这个害羞的女孩一直黏着她妈妈。

6. 【答案】A

【解析】此题考点为备选词是否符合句意。tailor 做名词时的含义是"裁缝"，做动词时的含义是"定做，专门制作"，例如：Special courses are tailored to the needs of specific groups. 制定特殊课程，以满足特殊群体的需要。administrate 管理，支配；entail 使必要，使承担；accustom 使习惯于，固定搭配是 be accustomed to。此题解题的关键在于题干中的介词 to，根据固定搭配可以排除 B 和 C，再根据题干句意要求排除 D。

题干译文：这个软件可以为顾客量身定做。

7. 【答案】B

【解析】此题考点为词组辨析。break through 突破，克服，例如：They have broken through in the fight against AIDS. 他们在抗击艾滋病方面已经有所突破。In front of the platform, he managed to break through his reserve. 在讲台前，他成功地克服了拘谨。break down 使……分解，出故障，例如：Sugar and starch are broken down in the stomach. 糖和淀粉在胃里被分解。Our car broke down on the way home. 我们的车在回家路上抛锚了。break out 的含义是"爆发"，例如：Fire broke out last night. 昨晚上发生了火灾。break over 这个搭配极为少见，意思是"破例"。

题干译文：如果细胞不能使用糖，身体就开始分解自身的组织来提供养分。

8. 【答案】B

【解析】此题解题的关键在于题干中的介词 to，根据四个备选单词各自的含义以及介词搭配就可以解题。approach 做动词的含义是"临近"，例如：The winter is approaching. 冬季即将来临。做名词，且与介词 to 连用，含义是"方式，方法"，例如：I support his approach to the problem. 我支持他解决这个问题的方法。conform "顺应，遵守（法律、规则等），相符合"，例如：You should conform to the local customs when you are in foreign countries. 在外国你应该遵从当地风俗。Every driver is required to conform to traffic laws. 每一个驾驶员都必须遵守交通法规。This building doesn't conform to the style of this city. 这座建筑物与这个城市的风格不一致。respond 的含义是"回答"，例如：He hasn't responded to my letter. 他还没给我回信。abide 的含义是"忍受，容忍"，常与 by 连用，意为"遵守"，例如：It is the students' responsibility to abide by regulations in school. 遵守学校规章制度是学生的责任。故本题选 B。

题干译文：如果你是公司成员，就必须遵守公司的规章。

9. 【答案】D

【解析】此题解题的关键在于题干所给的信息。qualification 资格；therapy 治疗；specification 规格，说明书；expertise 专门的知识或技能。

题干译文：这是唯一一个要求特殊技巧和技能的问题。

10. 【答案】A

【解析】此题解题的关键在于题干中的动宾搭配。curb 控制，遏制；sue 起诉，控告；detoxify 使解毒；condemn 谴责，判刑。

题干译文：一些官员建议要采取措施遏制通货膨胀。

11. 【答案】B

【解析】此题解题的关键在于题干所给的信息。题干中 on the move 的含义是"在活动中，在进行中"，例如：Science is always on the move. 科学总是在进步。根据这个词组的含义就可以解题。四个选项含义如下：distinctive 有特色的；dynamic 动态的，有活力的；intrinsic 本质的，本身的；mysterious 神秘的。

题干译文：人类是富有活力的生物，总是在前进。

12. 【答案】A

【解析】此题的考点是固定搭配的辨析，解题的关键在于题干所给予的信息。题干中 redundant 的含义是"多余的"。to be made redundant 的含义就是"冗员而被裁减"。lay off 的含义是"解雇"，例如：Many workers were laid off last year. 去年许多工人被解雇了。lay down 的含义是"放下"，例如：The killer surrendered and laid down his arms. 凶手投降，放下了武器。lay out 的含义是"布局，安排，展示"，例如：The living room is poorly laid out. 客厅布局很差。lay away 的含义是"储备"，例如：Many animals always lay away food for winter. 许多动物都会为冬天储存食物。

题干译文：去年生产力下降使得 200 名工人被裁员，还有 500 名工人被暂时解雇。

13. 【答案】B

【解析】此题考点为形近词辨析。四个选项含义如下：eminent 著名的，卓越的；imminent 即将发生的；immense 广大的，无边无际的；immanent 内在的，固有的。

题干译文：乌云和闪电说明暴风雨即将来临。

14. 【答案】C

【解析】此题考点为形近词辨析。四个选项含义如下：imaginable 可以想象的，可能的；imaginative 富有想象力的；imaginary 虚构的，想象的；imaging 为名词，意为"成像"。

题干译文：这本小说里面的故事似乎在现实世界发生过，但所有人物和情节都是虚构的。

15. 【答案】C

【解析】此题解题关键在于题干提供的信息。四个选项含义如下：arbitrary 专横的；aggressive 侵略的；ambitious 有野心的，雄心勃勃的；abundant 丰富的，充裕的。

题干译文：他有一个很雄心勃勃的计划：三年中要掌握三门外语，以及出国旅行。

16. 【答案】D

【解析】此题考点是固定搭配。各选项含义如下：authority 权威，威信；protection 保护；profession 职业，表白，宣布；priority 优先权。give the top priority to 给予……优先权。

题干译文：当地政府决定优先发展教育。

17. 【答案】A

【解析】此题考点是词组含义。各选项含义如下：at random 随意地；in essence 本质上；at heart 实际上，在内心；in bulk 大批地。

题干译文：当一个心理学家要就人类对压力的态度进行试验时，他会随意选择被访问者，问他们一些问题。

18. 【答案】A

【解析】此题解题关键在于题干中的介词 of 以及句意。be convicted of 的含义是"被控……罪"，例如：The young man was convicted of theft. 这个年轻人被控盗窃罪。be convinced of 的含义是"确信"，例如：I am fully convinced of his honesty. 我完全相信他的诚实。conceive of 的含义是"构思，想到"，例如：Unfortunately, he didn't conceive of the possibility of any difficulty. 不幸的是，他没能想到任何困难的可能性。condemn 的含义是"谴责，判刑"。

题干译文：他被判刑，但其实他并没有犯罪。他多年来一直为证明自己的清白而斗争。

19. 【答案】C

【解析】此题考点为近义词辨析。entrance 的含义是广义的"入口"；admission 的含义是"允许进入"；access 符合句意的"互联网入口"；entry 的含义是"入口，通道"。

题干译文：对于能上网的人来说，找到关于这些大学的信息很容易。

20. 【答案】B

【解析】此题考点为形近词辨析，解题的关键在于题干所提供的信息。四个选项含义如下：proposal 提议，建议；disposal 处置，安排；removal 移动，切除；refusal 拒绝。题干中 disrespectful 的含义是"无礼的"。

题干译文：不孝之子开始关注家产如何处置了。

21. 【答案】B

【解析】此题考点为固定搭配。on one's own initiative 的含义是"主动地"，例如：I felt very surprised that he came to help on his own initiative. 他主动来帮忙，我感到很意外。其他三项：endeavor 努力；motivation 动机；preference 偏爱。题干中的 decade 指"十年"。

题干译文：二十年前主动与别人握手的女士通常被认为太超前了。

22. 【答案】B

【解析】此题解题的关键在于题干提供的信息。四个选项的含义为：decisively 果断地；reluctantly 不情愿地；willingly 自愿地；deliberately 故意地。题干中的转折词是解题的信号词。

题干译文：他想待在家里，但最终还是不情愿地同意去看电影。

23. 【答案】C

【解析】此题考点为形近词辨析。imitate 模仿；intimate 形容词的含义是"亲密的"，动词的含义为"提示，通告"；intimidate 威胁，恐吓；emigrate 移民。

题干译文：因为儿子在学校威胁年龄较小的孩子，父母批评了他。

24. 【答案】D

【解析】此题考点为形近词组辨析。distribute to 的含义是"分发，分配"，例如：They distributed new clothes to those orphans. 他们把新衣服分发给那些孤儿。attribute to 的含义是"归因于"，例如：He attributed his success to diligence.

他把成功归功于勤奋。devote to 的含义是"致力于"，例如：The scientist devoted himself to his research. 这位科学家致力于他的研究。contribute to 的含义是"贡献，造成，导致"，例如：His living habits contributed to his poor health. 他的生活习惯导致他健康不佳。

题干译文：吃太多脂肪会导致心脏病和高血压。

25. 【答案】A

【解析】此题考点为四个备选单词的含义与题干句意。四个选项含义如下：successive 连续的，继承的；excessive 过多的，过分的；subsequent 后来的，并发的；eventual 最终的。

题干译文：这个足球队在过去三年里连续取得了五场胜利。

26. 【答案】B

【解析】此题考点为形近词辨析。ensure 的含义是"保证，担保"，例如：The pills ensure that you can have a good sleep tonight. 这药片保证你今晚能睡个好觉。guarantee 的含义是"保证"，例如：We guarantee to deliver the goods in three weeks. 我们保证三周后交货。insure 的含义是"为……投保险"，例如：He insured himself against illness. 他为自己投保了疾病险；assure 的含义是"向……保证"，例如：I assure you that I didn't mean to hurt you. 我向你保证我没打算要伤害你。

题干译文：汽车俱乐部不能保证满足所有会员的需求。

27. 【答案】C

【解析】此题考点为四个备选单词的含义与题干句意。四个选项含义如下：incapable 无能的；insensible 无知觉的；indispensable 不可缺少的；infinite 无限的，无穷的。

题干译文：在中国家庭里，祖父母以及其他亲戚在抚养孩子上起着不可或缺的作用。

28. 【答案】C

【解析】此题考点是词组辨析。turn in 的含义是"归还"，例如：You are required to turn in your pass when you leave here. 你离开这里的时候要交还通行证。turn over 的含义是"翻转"，例如：She turned over in the bed and couldn't fall asleep. 她在床上辗转反侧无法入睡。turn up 的含义是"到来，出现"，例如：She is still hoping that good luck will turn up. 她仍旧希望好运出现。turn down 的含义有：①拒绝，例如：She turned down his invitation politely. 她礼貌地谢绝了他的邀请。②把……调小，例如：He turned the lights down in the room. 他把房间里的灯光调暗了。

题干译文：我们没人料到主席会出现在聚会上，我们以为他还在住院。

29. 【答案】D

【解析】此题考点为形近词辨析。四个选项含义如下：proficient 精通的；efficient 有效率的；potential 潜在的；sufficient 充足的。

题干译文：欧盟国家曾担心他们不会有充足的石油供应了。

30. 【答案】C

【解析】此题考点为固定搭配，find fault with sb. 的含义是"挑某人的毛病"。

题干译文：他妻子总是在挑他的毛病，这让他很生气。

31. 【答案】**A**

【解析】此题考点为固定搭配。根据提干信息可以推断，所填词的含义为"可疑"。A 项 suspicious 的含义为"感觉可疑的，令人怀疑的"，通常与介词 of 或者 about 连用，例如：I am suspicious of his intention. 我怀疑他的用意。B 项 doubtful 的含义是"不确定的"，例如：I am doubtful about accepting extra work. 我对接受额外的工作不确定。C 项 susceptible 的含义是"易受影响的"，与介词 to 连用，例如：These plants are susceptible to frost damage. 这些植物易受霜冻危害。D 项 dubious 的含义是"不可信的，没把握的"，通常与介词 about 连用。例如：I am dubious about the whole idea. 我对整个想法持怀疑态度。

题干译文：他的邻居对他的行为表示怀疑，因此通知了警察。

32. 【答案】**A**

【解析】此题考点为形近词辨析。四个选项的含义如下：constructive 有建设性的；destructive 破坏性的；productive 生产的；descriptive 描述性的。此题解题的关键在于题干空白处所需的含义。备选项可以通过词根，如 construct，destroy，produce，describe 了解含义。

题干译文：没有任何改进建议的批评是没有建设性的，应该避免。

33. 【答案】**D**

【解析】此题考点为形近词辨析。四个选项的含义如下：instinctive 没有特色的；indissoluble 不能分解的；indispensable 不可或缺的；indisputable 无可争辩的。

题干译文：毋庸置疑，互联网对人们生活的影响越来越大。

34. 【答案】**B**

【解析】此题考点为形近词辨析。解题的关键在于动词和介词搭配。complement 是名词也是动词，做动词时含义为"补充（使完美）"，例如：The couple should complement each other. 夫妇应该互补（达到完美）。做名词时含义有：①补充物，与介词 to 连用，例如：a complement to your diet 饮食上的补充。②足数，足额，例如：We've taken our full complement of employees this year. 今年我们招入的职员已经满员了。compliment 可以做动词和名词，含义为"称赞"。做动词时要与介词 on 连用，例如：The teacher complimented him on his diligence. 老师称赞了他的勤奋。praise 表示"表扬"，词组为 praise sb. for sth.。appraise 是及物动词，含义为"评价"。

题干译文：他甚至都没看一眼就称赞了她的新衣服。

35. 【答案】**B**

【解析】此题考点为四个备选单词的含义与题干句意。deceptively 的含义是"迷惑地，虚伪地"；invariably 的含义是"总是，始终如一"，例如：This acute infection of the brain is almost invariably fatal. 这种急性大脑传染病几乎总是致命的。imperatively 的含义是"命令式地";transiently 的含义是"瞬时地，短暂地"。只有 B 符合句意。在题干中，claim 的含义是"导致死亡"，而不是"索取或宣称"，例如：The car crash claimed three lives. 撞车事故夺走三条生命。

题干译文：艾滋病成为人类健康的最大威胁，这个一贯致命性的疾病夺去很多人的生命。

36. 【答案】B

【解析】此题考点为形近词辨析，解题的关键在于题干中的 arbitrary。这个单词的含义为"专断的，独裁的"，因而可以推断空白处的含义。appliance 的含义是"器具，用具"；compliance 的含义为"顺从，遵从"，与介词 with 连用，例如：Compliance with the regulations is expected of all students. 所有学生都要遵守规章制度。defiance 的含义是"违抗"；reliance 的含义是"依靠，信任"，与介词 on 或者 upon 连用，例如：Too much reliance on the teacher is not beneficial to students. 过分依赖老师对学生不利。

题干译文：他是一个极其独断专行的领导，所以任何事情都必须遵从他的想法。

37. 【答案】B

【解析】此题考点为形近词辨析。adduce 的含义是"引证，举出例证"；induce 的含义是"劝诱，引诱，诱发"，例如：These pills will induce sleep. 这些药片会引起困意。deduce 的含义是"推论，演绎出"；produce 的含义是"生产，产生"。

题干译文：当他意识到被诱使签署合同的时候，他威胁要采取法律手段取消协议。

38. 【答案】A

【解析】此题考点为四个备选单词的含义与题干句意。insulate 的含义是"使隔热，使绝缘"，常用词组为 insulate sth. from / against sth.，例如：The room is insulated against noise. 这个房间隔音。insane 的含义是"精神失常的"；assault 的含义是"攻击"；insult 的含义是"侮辱"。

题干译文：当地居民被鼓励去给房屋加隔热装置以节约能源。

39. 【答案】D

【解析】此题考点为形近词组辨析。by hand "手工的，手写的"，例如：The fabric is made by hand. 这个织品是手工制作的。in hand 的含义是"在手头，在进行中"；at hand 的含义是"（时间或距离上）接近"，例如：Winter is close at hand. 冬天就要到了；on hand 的含义是"（尤指服务）现有"。

题干译文：奥运会期间，在奥运村随时都有急诊服务。

40. 【答案】C

【解析】此题考点为形近词辨析。sensitive 是形容词，意为"敏感的，过敏的"，与介词 to 连用，例如：I am sensitive to sea food. 我对海鲜过敏。sensible 意为"明智的"，例如：It is sensible for you to buy a relatively cheap house. 对你来说买一个相对便宜的房子是明智的。sensational 意为"轰动性的"；sensory 意为"感官的，感觉的"，sensory organs 意为"感觉器官"。

题干译文：为了追求点击率，网络媒体故意报道轰动性的社会新闻。

41. 【答案】B

【解析】此题考点为形近词辨析。四个选项含义如下：ridiculous 荒谬可笑的；rigorous 严格的；ambiguous 不明确的，模棱两可的；anonymous 匿名的。

题干译文：他们为参加决赛的选手制订了很严格的训练计划。

42. 【答案】B

【解析】此题考点为形近词辨析。四个选项含义如下：appreciative 有欣赏力的，感激的；appreciable 相当于 considerable，含义为"相当多的，相当大的"；comprehensive 全面广泛的；comprehensible 可以理解的。根据题干信息，空白处需要一个表示量多少的形容词。故 B 正确。

题干译文：对大多数人而言，新的"单双号限行"交通法规作用很大。

43. 【答案】D

【解析】此题考点为形近词辨析。compliment 的含义是"称赞，恭维"；complement 的含义是"补足"；commitment 的含义有：①许诺，承担义务，与介词 to 连用，例如：make a commitment to providing best service 提供最佳服务的承诺。②奉献，投入，与介词 to 连用，例如：Whatever you do, you are required 100% commitment to your career. 无论你做什么，都应该百分之百地投入工作。commencement ①开始；②毕业典礼。

题干译文：在毕业典礼上，史密斯因为他在研究方面的卓越贡献获得一枚奖章，以示奖励。

44. 【答案】B

【解析】此题考点为形近词辨析。impartial（根据构词法可以得知 im + partial）意为"公平的，不偏不倚的"；immortal 意为"不朽的"；immemorial 可以联想到 memory，因而意为"古老的，远古的"；immoral（根据构词法可以得知 im + moral）意为"不道德的"。

题干译文：作为美国 20 世纪最杰出的作家，海明威创作了许多不朽之作。

45. 【答案】C

【解析】此题考点为形近词辨析。各选项含义如下：probable 很可能的，大概的；reliable 可信赖的，可靠的；flexible 灵活的；feasible 切实可行的。

题干译文：我们已经定好了周五去看电影，但我们可以灵活一点，改天去。

46. 【答案】A

【解析】此题考点为词组辨析。come up with 的含义是"提出，想出"，例如：The young man finally came up with a good idea of increasing sales. 这个年轻人最终想出增加销量的好主意。look up to sb. 的含义是"钦佩，仰慕某人"；put up with 的含义是"忍受，容忍"，例如：I can't put up with his bad temper any more. 我再也忍受不了他的坏脾气了。clear up 是指"天气放晴；（疾病）痊愈；清理，打扫；解决，解释，解答"，例如：clear up the mystery 揭开谜团。

题干译文：显然，有些人有一种惊人的能力，很快能得到正确答案。

47. 【答案】D

【解析】此题考点为固定搭配以及词组辨析。be subject to 的含义有：①易遭受，例如：Flights are subject to delay because of fog. 航班因大雾可能延误。②取决于，例如：The article is subject to your approval. 这篇文章等你的批准。③服从于，例如：He is not subject to discipline. 他不守纪律。incline 的含义是"有……趋势，倾向于"，例如：I incline to the view that we should be more careful now. 我倾向于我们现在应该更小心谨慎的观点。be liable to 的含义有：①可能受……影响，例如：You are more liable to injury if you don't take regular exercise. 如果你没能定期锻炼，你更容易受伤。②负有责任，例如：People with high income are liable to high tax. 高收入者必须缴纳高税收。be obliged to sb. for sth. 的含义是"感激，感谢"，例如：I'm much obliged to you for helping us. 承蒙相助，本人不胜感激。

题干译文：我代表学校感谢你在地震中的慷慨相助。

48. 【答案】C

【解析】此题考点为形近词辨析。四个选项含义如下：descriptive 描述性的；impressive 印象深刻的；deceptive 欺骗性的；indicative 指示的。

题干译文：这辆旧车的外表相当具有欺骗性，比实际要新很多。

49. 【答案】A

【解析】此题考点为词组辨析。题干中的词组 in relation to 的含义是"和……有关的"。四个选项含义为：add up to 合计；come up with 提出，想出；put up with 忍受，容忍；keep up with 跟上。

题干译文：我们收集的和那个案子有关的所有信息太少了。

50. 【答案】D

【解析】此题考点为备选单词是否与句意符合。解题的关键在于：while 表示对比，因而空白处应该为 obtain 的同义词。originate from 的含义是"起源于"，例如：The hot dog did not originate in the United States, but in Germany. 热狗不是起源于美国，而是起源于德国。digest 的含义是"消化"；deprive 的含义是"剥夺"，与介词 of 连用，例如：If you don't drive carefully, I will deprive you of your license. 如果你不谨慎驾驶的话，我就要没收你的驾照了。derive from 的含义是"从……获得"，例如：You can derive great pleasure from travel. 你可以从旅行中获得很多乐趣。

题干译文：现在我们从动物身上获得超过三分之二的蛋白质，而我们的祖父母们只能从动物身上获得一半。

51. 【答案】A

【解析】此题考点为备选单词含义是否符合句意。解题的关键在题干，题干是个由 but 连接的转折并列句，根据转折关系就可以推断空白处单词的含义。各选项含义为：concise 简明的；clear 清楚的；precise 精确的；elaborate 精心制作的，详细阐述的。

题干译文：这位新秘书写了一份仅几页的相当简洁的报告，但却包含了所有信息。

52. 【答案】C

【解析】此题考点为备选单词含义是否符合句意。解题的关键在题干，题干是由两个互为反义的单词构成的对比。各选项含义为：manageable 易管理的，易处理的；controllable 可以控制的；tolerable 忍受的；perceivable 可知觉的。

题干译文：预料之中的噪声通常比预料之外的同等强度的噪声更容易忍受。

53. 【答案】A

【解析】此题考点为近义词辨析。各选项含义为：fluctuate 一般指价格上下波动；wave 挥舞，摇曳；swing 摇摆（如钟摆的摆动）；vibrate 震动（如汽车经过，房屋震动）。

题干译文：由于价格波动较大，这个公司很难做预算。

54. 【答案】C

【解析】此题考点为备选单词是否与句意搭配。四个选项含义如下：disregard 漠视，不理会；distort 歪曲，曲解；irritate 恼怒；intervene 干涉，介入。

题干译文：请不要因为他的不礼貌而恼怒，因为他只是试图引起注意。

55. 【答案】A

【解析】此题考点为词组辨析。call forth 的含义是"唤起，引起"，例如：The song called forth sad memories. 这首歌唤起了伤心的回忆。call at 的含义是"停靠，停留"，例如：This train called at the small village. 这辆火车停靠在这个小村庄。call on 的含义是"请求，要求"，例如：The government called on citizens to save energies as possible as they could. 政府要求公民们尽可能地节约能源。call off 的含义是"取消"，例如：The game was called off because of bad weather. 比赛因恶劣天气而取消了。

题干译文：山姆向老板保证他会尽全力做好这份新工作。

56. 【答案】A

【解析】此题考点为词组辨析。四个选项的含义是：be subjected to 遭受……影响；fill with 装满；associate with 联系；attach to 把……系上，例如：Please attach the dog to the tree. 请把狗拴到树上。I attach importance to the education. 我认为教育很重要。

题干译文：要注意减少受持续噪声影响的时间。

57. 【答案】A

【解析】此题考点为词组辨析。on the spot 的含义是"当场，现场，立即，马上"，例如：Certain decisions had to be taken by the man on the spot. 某些决定必须由现场人员做出。on site 的含义是"在现场，临场"，例如：Since all the materials are on site so that work can start immediately. 既然所有材料都到了，立即开工。on location 的含义是"（电影）外景拍摄地"，例如：The movie was shot entirely on location in Rome. 这部电影的外景完全是在罗马拍摄的。on the ground 在地上。

题干译文：地震新闻报道后，紧接着就出现一份详细的现场报道。

58. 【答案】A

　　【解析】此题考点为形近词辨析。considerate 表示"细心周到的"；considerable 表示"数量上相当可观的"；considering 可以用作介词，表示"考虑到，鉴于"，例如：Considering that he is only a beginner, he did pretty well. 鉴于他只是一个初学者，他做得非常好了。constant 表示"持续的，不断的"。题干需要一个形容词修饰人。

　　题干译文：母亲要照顾家里的每个人，她们通常是每个家庭里最细心周到的人。

59. 【答案】D

　　【解析】此题考点为形近词辨析。simplify 这个单词的词根是 simple，词缀 -ify 表示"使……化"，因而单词的含义就是"使……简单化"；modify 表示"对……稍加修改使更适合，缓和"；verify 表示"核实，校验"；rectify 表示"矫正，改正"。

　　题干译文：如果你知道问题是什么，你为什么不帮助他们整顿局面呢？

60. 【答案】C

　　【解析】此题考点为近义词辨析。disapproval 是名词，其动词形式为 disapprove，含义为"不赞成"，通常与介词 of 连用，例如：I disapprove of your plan. 我不赞成你的计划。rejection 的含义为"否决，回绝"，用于拒绝提议等。例如：Her proposal met with unanimous rejection. 她的建议遭到了一致否决。refusal 的含义为"拒绝，回绝"，但通常表示拒绝别人请你做的事情，例如：the refusal of a request / an invitation 拒绝请求 / 邀请。decline 作为名词，含义为"（数量、价值上）减少，下降"，例如：economic decline 经济衰退；decline 作为动词，有"婉言谢绝"的含义，但题干上需要一个名词。题干中，前半句话已经给出了解题信息，劝说加入，因而 refusal 最合适。

　　题干译文：尽管我努力地劝说他加入我们集团，却遭到了他的断然拒绝。

61. 【答案】D

　　【解析】此题考点为近义词辨析，而解题关键在于固定搭配。四个备选单词均有"信任"的含义，但各自的用法不同。faith 的含义为"信仰，信任"，固定搭配为 have faith in sb. or sth.，例如：We have faith in the government's promises. 我们相信政府的承诺。belief 的用法与 faith 相同；credit 表示"相信"的含义时，作为动词主要用于疑问句或者否定句；reliance 的含义是"依赖，依靠，信任"，固定搭配为 place reliance on / upon sth.，例如：Students should not be encouraged too much reliance on their teachers. 不应鼓励学生过多依赖老师。

题干译文：他让我失望多次，以至于我不再相信他的承诺。

62. 【答案】B

【解析】此题考点为词组辨析。in line with 的含义如下：①与……成一排，例如：An eclipse happens when the earth and moon are in line with the sun. 地球、月亮、太阳成一条直线，日食就发生了。②与……一致，例如：Annual pay increases will be in line with inflation. 每年加薪将与通货膨胀挂钩。in terms of 的含义是"依据，根据"，例如：In terms of my view, I disapprove of the plan. 就我的观点看，我不同意这个计划。regardless of 的含义是"不管，不顾"，例如：He is always expressing his own views regardless of others' feeling. 他总是表达自己的观点，不顾别人的感受。by means of 的含义是"借助……手段"，例如：The load was lifted by means of a crane. 重物是借助起重机吊起来的。

题干译文：衡量一个国家的财富，应该依据国民生活健康和幸福的状况，以及能够生产的物质财富。

63. 【答案】A

【解析】此题考点为四个备选词是否符合句意。解题的关键在于题干所提供的信息。unwillingness to learn from others 为解题线索。四个选项的含义如下：arrogance 傲慢，自大；dignity 尊严；humility 谦卑；solitude 孤独。

题干译文：他傲慢自大，不愿意向他人学习，这使得他不能成为一个团队的有效成员。

64. 【答案】C

【解析】此题考点为近义词辨析。首先，题干中的关键词为 ambulance，含义为"急救车"，因而 B 项 danger 与 D 项 crisis（危机）就不适合题干语境。urgency 的含义是"时间紧迫，某事必须得到处理"，例如：The attack added a new urgency to the peace talk. 这个袭击事件使得和平谈判越发紧迫。emergency 指的是"突发事件"。

题干译文：救护车必须享有优先权，因为它通常被用于处理一些突发事件。

65. 【答案】C

【解析】此题考点为四个备选词是否符合句意。根据题干所提供的信息，空白处应该为修饰谓语动词 defend 的副词。根据题干中的后半句我们可以推断出这位长者应该是积极维护。peculiarly 表示"奇特地"；indifferently 表示"冷漠地，漠不关心地"；inevitably 表示"不可避免地"；vigorously 表示"精力充沛地"，在题干中表示"积极地"。

题干译文：这位老者积极维护每个公民自由选择宗教的权利，他因此赢得了人们的尊重。

66. 【答案】A

【解析】此题考点为近义词、形近词辨析。根据题干的信息，空白处应该是一个表示"大"的形容词来修饰名词 difference。四个选项含义分别为：enormous 巨大的，immense 是指体积或者数量大到无法衡量的地步。imminent 即将到来的，逼近的，例如：No one has given out a warning of the imminent danger. 没人为即将到来的危险发出警告。eminent 卓越的，杰出的。

题干译文：汉语方言之间的巨大差异成为人们互相交流的一个问题。

67. 【答案】B

【解析】此题考点为备选单词是否符合句意。根据题干所提供的信息，可以推断出空白处的含义为"主导地位"。notion 的含义是"观念"；四个选项含义为：privilege 特权，特别待遇；predominance（数量上）占优势或者占主导地位；prevalence 流行；priority 优先权。

题干译文：在男女角色没有明显划分，家务事由双方共同承担的家庭中，男尊女卑的观点是很难维持的。

68. 【答案】C

【解析】此题考点为形近词辨析。各选项含义如下：illegal 非法的；eligible 符合条件的；illegible 字迹模糊的，无法辨认的；unreasonable 不合理的。

题干译文：经过多年日晒雨淋，这个商店的招牌已经完全无法辨认。

69. 【答案】A

【解析】此题考点为词组辨析。get down to 的含义是"开始认真做某事"，例如：It's high time I got down to thinking about my essay. 我该开始认真思考我的论文了。adapt to 的含义是"适应"，例如：When freshmen enter the university, they should adapt themselves to the new environment soon. 大一新生入校后应该尽快适应新环境。hold on to 的含义是"保住（优势），不送，不卖（某物）"，例如：You should hold on to your oil shares. 你应该保留你的石油股份。attend to 的含义是"处理，应付"，例如：I have some urgent business to attend to. 我有些急事需要处理。只有 A 项符合句意。另外，It's time that 句型里，从句中的动词要用动词的过去式。

题干译文：该是你静下心读书的时候了，否则你会落在其他同学的后面。

70. 【答案】A

【解析】此题考点为词组辨析。by virtue of 的含义是"由于，凭借"，例如：He was exempt from charges by virtue of being so young. 他因为年龄小而免费。in the way of 的含义是"关于，就……而言"，用于疑问句或否定句，例如：There isn't much in the way of entertainment here. 这里没有什么娱乐活动。by way of 的含义是"经由，路过"，例如：I arrived in Paris by way of London. 我途经伦敦到达巴黎。for the sake of 的含义是"为了……某人起见"，例如：The couple still stayed together for the sake of children. 这对夫妇因为孩子还是住在一起。只有 A 符合句意。

题干译文：地质学家认为山是因其地质结构特点才被称为山，即使它的海拔高度不足 3000 英尺。

71. 【答案】C

【解析】此题解题关键在于题干中的 or，or 表示前后两个句子为并列关系，所以空白处需要和 inform 近义的词。denounce 的含义是"告发，公然抨击"，例如：The minister's bribery was denounced in the newspapers. 这位部长的受贿行为在报纸上受到谴责。The passer-by denounced the offenders to the police. 这个路人向警察告发了肇事者。secure 的含义是"获得，使安全"，例如：To secure the major arms deal contract, he has put substantial sum of money into the bank account of the party in power. 为了获得大宗武器交易合同，他向执政党的银行账户存入数量可观的钱。ensure 的含义是"确保"，例如：We must ensure the purity of drinking water in the flooded area. 我们必须保证洪灾地区饮用水的纯净。notify 的含义是"通知"，是题干中 inform 的近义词，故 C 项为正确答案。

题干译文：去发现研究者们是怎么通知你试验的进程的，或者通知你出现的问题的。

72. 【答案】C

【解析】此题考点为词组。cope with 的含义是"应付，处理"。dispose of 的含义是"处理，解决"，例如：His high debts forced him to dispose of his art treasures. 高额债务迫使他处理掉他的艺术珍品。hold up 的含义是"承受住，拦劫，举起"，例如：The young man was accused of holding up a pedestrian. 这个小伙子被控拦劫一个行人。All I can do is to try to hold up two of us so well. 我所能做的就是让我们两个人的感情继续发展下去。put up to 词组不存在。

题干译文：美国没有足够多的监狱容纳所有的罪犯。

73. 【答案】A

【解析】此题解题关键在于题干中的"dying patients""course of disease"等信息，意思分别为"即将死去的病人""患病期"。prolong 的含义是"延长，拖延"；identify 的含义是"辨认"；alter 的含义是"改变"；expose 的含义是"揭穿，使暴露"。

题干译文：临终的病人有了一线希望，新的治疗可以延长患病期，但要冒着产生严重副作用的危险。

74. 【答案】A

【解析】vigilance 的含义是"警惕，警觉"；aggregate 的含义是"聚集，集合"；varnish 的含义是"粉饰，装饰"；visage 的含义是"容貌"。

题干译文：因为邻里的警觉，这个小偷被抓住了。

75. 【答案】C

【解析】此题解题关键在于 produces its own light wave。illuminative 的含义是"照明的"；flashy 的含义是"闪光的，一瞬间的，浮华的"；luminous 的含义是"发光的"；flaming 的含义是"火焰般的"。

题干译文：像太阳和灯泡那样自身产生光波的物体被认为是发光的。

76. 【答案】B

【解析】此题考点为形近词组辨析。选项词组解释参见"常用词组"中 give 的解释。

题干译文：的确，他没能看见她的眼泪，然而她担心声音会暴露她的情感。

77. 【答案】D

【解析】此题考点为形近词组辨析。这道题的解题关键在于题干中适合 craze 的动词搭配。ask for 的含义是"请求，要求"，例如：As the boss of this company, I have the right to ask for an explanation. 作为这个公司的老板，我有权利要求一个解释。send for 的含义是"派人去请，召唤"，例如：He is so ill that we have to send for a doctor. 他病得太重了，我们必须派人去请个大夫了。run for 的含义是"竞选"；cater for 的含义是"迎合"，例如：TV programmes couldn't cater for different tastes. 电视节目不能迎合不同的爱好。

题干译文：商店给消费者提供能回家自己组装的零部件，迎合了他们 DIY 的狂热追求。

78. 【答案】B

【解析】解此题要依靠语境。amplify 的含义是"放大"；decrease 的含义是"减少"；stimulate 的含义是"刺激"；meet 如果与 need 搭配含义为"满足……的需要"。题干语境是"减少需求"，故 B 正确。

题干译文：一种称为牙科电子麻醉的新技术将很快能减少对可怕的牙医针的需求。

79. 【答案】B

【解析】解此题要依靠语境。infection 的含义是"感染"；fatigue 的含义是"疲劳"；syncope 的含义是"昏厥"；suffocation 的含义是"窒息"。shortness of breath 的含义是"气短"，go hand in hand with 的含义是"共同行动，紧密联系"。sweep 的含义是"横扫，席卷"。be confined to 的含义是"局限于……"。

题干译文：气短经常与疲劳紧密联系，这种情况遍布全身并且不局限于某一个部位。

80. 【答案】C

【解析】此题解题关键在于与 types of research programs 的搭配。allocate 的含义是"分派"；expand 的含义为"扩张"；sponsor 的含义是"发起，赞助，倡议"；sum 的含义是"总计，概括"。

题干译文：从国家层面上看，国家健康研究所尤其是国家老年研究所正主办许多形式的有关老年的研究项目。

81. 【答案】A

【解析】此题解题要依靠语境，尤其是句中"threaten the fundamental values of society""challenge"等词语的提示。formidable 的含义是"强大的，可怕的，难以对付的"，例如：The task is formidable and impossible to achieve without international cooperation. 这项任务很艰巨，没有国际合作不可能实现。fatal 的含义是"致命的"。favorable 的含义是"有利的"，例如：Spring is favorable to fly a kite. 春天适合放风筝。fantastic 的含义是"极好的，难以置信的"，例如：He made fantastic progress on English in the short period. 在这么短时间内他英语进步神速。题干中 fundamental 的含义是"基本的"。

题干译文：HIV 和 AIDS 可能威胁到社会的基本价值观，任何针对两者的尝试都是可怕的挑战。

82. 【答案】A

【解析】此题考点为形近词组辨析。其他选项的含义和例句参见"常用词组"。abrupt 的含义是"突然的"。

题干译文：Kelley 的公关人员突然取消七个城市的宣传巡回计划，宣布他们的"宣传目标已经完成"。

83. 【答案】B

【解析】此题解题关键在于语境，尤其是题干中 "is only beginning to be seriously examined" 的提示。informative 的含义是"见多识广的"；inconclusive 的含义是"无确定结果的"；inconspicuous 的含义是"不明显的"；indisputable 的含义是"无可争议的"。variable 的含义是"变量"。

题干译文：将拥挤作为一个环境变量来研究才刚刚开始，至今尚无结论性的数据。

84. 【答案】B

【解析】此题考点为词组含义。be proportional to 的含义是"与……成比例"，例如：The result of the exam is always proportional to your efforts. 考试结果总是和你的努力成比例。be subjected to 的含义是"使经历，使遭受"，例如：Your wages will be subjected to changes based on your performance. 你的薪水会因你的表现而有变化。be susceptible to 的含义是"易受……的感染或影响"，例如：This kind of plant is susceptible to disease. 这种植物容易受病害的侵袭。be liable to 的含义是"有……的倾向"，例如：Your silly attempt is liable to failure. 你愚蠢的尝试多半是要失败的。

题干译文：在紧接着的杀菌过程中，罐头被放入水蒸气或者沸腾的水中，温度和持续时间因食物的类别而不同。

85. 【答案】B

【解析】此题解题关键在于语境。launch 的含义是"发射，发起"，例如：The recruitment of new members has been launched this afternoon. 招募新会员的工作今天下午已经启动了。translate 的含义除了"翻译"以外，还有"转移，调动"。dissect 的含义是"解剖，详细分析"，例如：Commentators are still dissecting the result of the election. 评论家们还在详细分析选举的结果。convey 的含义是"传达"。

题干译文：但是如果新的研究发现不能转化为市场商品和服务，研究就没有经济影响。

86. 【答案】A

【解析】此题考点为语境搭配。bioactive 的含义是"生物活性的"；miniature 的含义是"小型的"；bizarre 的含义是"奇异的，怪诞的"；invisible 的含义是"看不见的"。题干中 property 的含义是"财产，性质"。all the time 的含义是"总是，一直"。

题干译文：大自然给我们的惊奇从未停止。实验室中不断发现拥有生物活性结构和特性的分子。

87. 【答案】D

【解析】此题考点为词组含义。rule out 的含义是"消除，排除"，例如：He didn't rule out the possibility to change his mind. 他没有排除改变想法的可能性。divide up 的含义是"瓜分"；bring apart 的搭配不成立；sort out 的含义是"选出，分类"，例如：She is sorting out the good apples from bad ones. 她正在把好的苹果和坏的苹果分开。

题干译文：由于病人不能总是辨别心理诱发的胸痛和心脏病发引起的胸痛，医生应该挑选出疼痛的可能原因。

88. 【答案】D

【解析】此题考点为固定搭配。meet up with 的含义是"意外碰到"。come up with 的含义是"提出，想出"，例如：They are beating their brains to come up with a solution to the sticky problem. 他们正绞尽脑汁想出这个棘手问题的解决办法。shed light on 的含义是"阐明"。live up to 的含义是"符合，达到预期标准"，例如：They will do their utmost to live up to their parents' expectations. 他们会竭尽全力，不辜负父母的期望。usher 的含义是"引导"。

题干译文：洛杉矶的加利福尼亚大学医学院的 David L. Rinion 说，如果符合预期，这样的测试能够开辟一个产前诊断的新领域。

89. 【答案】A

【解析】此题考点为单词词义。emaciated 的含义为"瘦弱的，憔悴的"。eligible 的含义是"有资格的，合格的"，例如：Everyone with an annual income of $ 100,000 may be eligible to apply for the membership of this club. 任何年收入 10 万美元的人都有资格申请成为这个俱乐部的会员。elastic 的含义是"有弹性的"。exceptional 的含义是"例外的"，例如：Forestry has advanced with exceptional speed. 植树造林以罕见的速度得到了发展。

题干译文：深受腿病折磨，汤姆最近非常憔悴。

90. 【答案】C

【解析】此题考点为固定搭配。constitute 的含义是"构成，建立"；decode 的含义是"解码"；draft 的含义是"绘制，起草"；encode 的含义是"编码，译码"。只有 draft 与 map 搭配。master 的含义是"主要的"，vasculature 的含义是"脉管系统"。

题干译文：如今调查者仍旧没能绘制出心脏脉管系统的精确图。

91. 【答案】D

【解析】此题解题关键在于 caring "关怀的"，空白处需要一个与这个词近义的词。emotional 情感的；impersonal 非个人的；compulsory 必需的，义务的；compassionate 有同情心的（与 caring 近义）。

题干译文：他们是我见过的最关心人、具有同情心的一群人。

92. 【答案】A

【解析】wholesome 的含义是"有益健康的";diet 的含义是"饮食";tasteful 的含义是"有滋味的,有品位的";edible 的含义是"可食用的"。

题干译文:正如我们的身体需要简单健康的食物一样,我们的心智发展也需要认真的阅读。

93. 【答案】D

【解析】此题通过 rather than frequent stops and starts 可以解题。compassion 的含义是"同情心";acceleration 的含义是"加速";frustration 的含义是"挫败";exertion 的含义是"努力,运用,发挥",例如:He failed to lift the rock in spite of all his exertions. 他虽竭尽全力,但仍然未能将那块石头搬起来。

题干译文:最好的锻炼要求持久的努力,而不是频繁的做做停停。

94. 【答案】C

【解析】accomplishment 的含义是"成就,完成"。qualification 的含义是"资格"。eminence 的含义是"显赫,崇高",例如:He reached eminence as a doctor. 他已成为名医。patent 的含义是"专利权"。

题干译文:Salk 作为发明世界上第一个有效的小儿麻痹疫苗的科学家赢得了显赫的声誉。

95. 【答案】A

【解析】denote 的含义是"象征,表示",例如:A smile often denotes pleasure and friendship. 微笑常常表示高兴和友善。donate 的含义是"捐赠";relate 的含义是"有关联",通常与介词 to 连用;resort 的含义是"求助,诉诸",通常与介词 to 连用。coronary disease 的含义是"冠心病"。

题干译文:冠心病是一个广泛使用的术语,表示对心脏的供血不足。

96. 【答案】D

【解析】本题考查词义辨析。regulation 意为"规定,规矩",speciality 意为"专业",essential 意为"必需品,要点",specification 意为"规格,尺寸"。满足建筑设计师的"规格"符合上下文语义。regulation 侧重于约束行为的规范,放这里不合适。

题干译文:修建者的工作是使房子在所有方面都符合设计师的规格要求。

97. 【答案】B

【解析】此题解题关键在于 but 和 worry,转折结构提示空白处需要一个与它意思相反的词。put off 的含义是"推迟";laugh off 的含义是"一笑置之",例如:An actor has to learn to laugh off bad reviews. 演员须学会对贬斥性评论一笑置之的本事。pay off 的含义是"还清(债务)";lay off 的含义是"解雇"。只有 B 项与 worry 互为反义词。

题干译文:在公开场合,他们对最近一次的失败一笑置之,但私下里他们很是担心。

98. 【答案】D

【解析】此题解题关键在于语境,尤其是短语 poor nutrition 和 adult growth,由此可知应该选择贬义的词填入空白处。degenerate 的含义是"衰退，退化"；deteriorate 的含义是"恶化"；boost 的含义是"促进，推动"；retard 的含义是"阻止，妨碍"。infancy 的含义是"婴儿期"。

题干译文：婴儿期早期阶段营养不良会阻碍成年发育。

99. 【答案】C

【解析】此题解题要注意题干中的限定成分"during rush hour"。scatter 的含义是"分散"，例如：When the tree falls, the monkeys scatter. 树倒猢狲散。condense 的含义是"浓缩，凝结；归纳"；clog 的含义是"阻塞，阻碍"；dot 的含义是"点缀"。commuter 的含义是"每日往返上班者"。

题干译文：高峰期，市区街道挤满了上下班的人。

100. 【答案】A

【解析】此题考点为形近词组辨析。account for 的含义是"解释，（在数量方面）占"；call for 的含义是"要求，接人"；look for 的含义是"寻找"；make for 的含义是"移向，有助于，造成"。

题干译文：恐怕你得就状况的恶化做出解释。

101. 【答案】C

【解析】此题考点为意思搭配。affliction 的含义是"痛苦"；alternative 的含义是"选择，备选"；allocation 的含义是"派发，分配"；alliance 的含义是"结盟，联姻"。generous 的含义是"充足的，慷慨大方的"。此题空白处的选项应该和 time 搭配，故 C 项为正确答案。

题干译文：你每周有 12 小时都在养老院，分配的时间似乎挺充裕。

102. 【答案】C

【解析】此题解题关键在于语境。expensively 的含义是"昂贵地"；exceptionally 的含义是"例外地"；exhaustively 的含义是"彻底地，无遗漏地"；exclusively 的含义是"排外地，独占地"。

题干译文：每个产品在投入市场前都是经过彻底检验的。

103. 【答案】D

【解析】此题解题关键在于语境。potent 的含义是"有效的，强有力的"，例如：I was eventually convinced by his potent arguments. 最终我被他有力的论述说服了。conditional 的含义是"有条件的"；inseparable 的含义是"不可分开的"；cardinal 的含义是"主要的"，例如：The cardinal idea of this party for the election is that everybody should enjoy equality. 这个政党竞选的主要思想就是人人享有平等。

题干译文：烹调前洗手是主要规定之一。

104. 【答案】B

【解析】此题考点为形近词辨析。cohesive 的含义是"黏性的"；cognitive 的含义是"认知的"；collective 的含义是"集体的"；comic 的含义是"喜剧的"。

题干译文：教育者应该努力发展孩子的认知能力。

105.【答案】C

【解析】此题考点为形近词辨析。defect 的含义是"缺陷"，例如：The type of cars has been withdrawn from the market because of mechanical defects. 这款车因为机械缺陷撤市了。deficit 的含义是"赤字，亏损"，例如：The current trade deficit indicates a serious imbalance between our import and export trade. 当前的贸易赤字表明我们的进出口贸易严重失调。default 的含义是"默认值，缺席，拖欠，违约"；deception 的含义是"欺诈，骗局"；mortgage 的含义是"抵押"。

题干译文：按揭借款违约在近一年里呈上升趋势，这是因为低收入家庭的数目一直增长。

106.【答案】B

【解析】此题考点为单词含义。exaggerate 的含义是"夸大"。exacerbate 的含义是"加重，恶化"，例如：Scratching exacerbates a skin rash. 抓挠后会恶化成皮疹。exceed 的含义是"超过，领先"；exhibit 的含义是"展览"。

题干译文：症状可能会因某些药物加重。

107.【答案】C

【解析】此题解题关键在于语境的提示。facility 的含义是"设施"；fascination 的含义是"魔力，魅力"；fabrication 的含义是"捏造"；faculty 的含义是"才能，全体教职员工，（大学）系"。

题干译文：她的故事彻头彻尾是捏造的，所以没人相信她。

108.【答案】C

【解析】此题考点为单词含义。salvage 的含义是"海上救助，打捞"；safeguard 的含义是"保卫，保护"；sabotage 的含义是"蓄意破坏"，例如：Owing to the sabotage, the train jumped the rails. 由于蓄意破坏，火车出轨了。sacrifice 的含义是"牺牲，祭品"，例如：Success in the job is not worth the sacrifice of health. 以牺牲健康获得工作上的成功不值得。rule out 在这里的含义为"排除"。

题干译文：调查交通事故的警察没排除蓄意破坏的可能性。

109.【答案】B

【解析】此题考点为词组含义，语境中介词 on 是解题关键。take up 的含义为"占据"；check up 的含义是"检查，调查，核查"，例如：He was careful enough to check up every detail. 他非常仔细，把每一个细节都核对过了。The police are checking up on him. 警方正在调查他。work out 的含义是"解决，算出"；look into 的含义为"调查，观察"。

题干译文：政府总是会对受雇于敏感军事项目的员工的背景进行调查。

110.【答案】A

【解析】此题解题关键在于语境，尤其是短语 cause disease 的提示。unsanitary 的含义是"不洁净的"。insidious 的含义是"阴险的，隐伏的"，例如：That insidious man bad-mouthed me to almost everyone else. 那个阴险的家伙几乎

见人便说我的坏话。Bleeding may be chronic and insidious or brisk and life-threatening. 出血可能是慢性的、隐伏的或者是活跃的、危及生命的。insane 的含义是"精神错乱的"；inefficacious 的含义是"无效力的"。

题干译文：不卫生的条件和环境可能引起疾病。

111.【答案】C

【解析】此题考点为单词含义。abstain 的含义是"放弃，戒除"，例如：The doctor asked the patient to abstain from smoking. 医生让这个病人戒烟。acquit 的含义是"释放，开释"，例如：He was acquitted of the crime. 他被宣告无罪。admonish 的含义是"训诫，提醒"，例如：His wife admonished him not to drive too fast. 他妻子警告他开车不要太快。adduce 的含义是"引证，举出"，例如：I can adduce several reasons for his strange behavior. 我可以列举出几个他行为古怪的原因。根据词义以及语境，我们可以判断 C 项正确。

题干译文：证人因为没能回答问题而受到法官的警告。

112.【答案】D

【解析】此题考点为词组含义。pull of 的搭配不成立；wear out 的含义是"穿破，磨损，耗尽"；pass out 的含义是"昏倒，失去知觉"。write off 的含义是"注销，报废"，例如：He wrote off three cars in a year because of his dreadful driving. 因他可怕的驾车技术，他一年内报废了三辆车。根据 because of traffic accidents 我们可以推断他的车不是用坏了，而是报废了，故答案 D 正确。

题干译文：因为交通事故，今年他已经报废了两辆车。

113.【答案】B

【解析】此题考点为固定搭配。advent 的含义是"到来"，因而 advent of the Internet 的含义就是"互联网的到来"。convenient 是形容词，含义是"便利的"；interface 的含义是"界面，接口"；aftermath 的含义是"（不幸事件的）后果"。

题干译文：自从有了互联网，人们信息更灵通了。

114.【答案】A

【解析】此题根据已知语境我们可以知道空白处的含义应该是消毒。sterilize 的含义是"消毒"；label 的含义是"贴标签"；quarantine 的含义是"隔离，检疫"，例如：This is a highly infectious disease. All the patients must be put under quarantine. 这是一种传染性极大的病，所有病人都必须采取隔离措施。retain 的含义是"保留"，例如：You have to retain your ticket for inspection. 你应该留票以备验票。

题干译文：所有病人接触过的器具必须在他人使用前进行消毒。

115.【答案】D

【解析】此题解题关键在于题干中 risk 的提示，表示"诊所冒着……的风险"，所以空白处应该选取贬义的词。acquit 的含义是"释放，开释"；allocate 的含义是"分配"；alleviate 的含义是"缓解，减轻（疼痛或痛苦）"；alienate 的含义是"使疏远"。cunning 的含义是"狡猾的"。

题干译文：诊所采取了这个狡猾的政策，这样做的风险是可能会减少患者资源。

116. 【答案】B

【解析】此题考点为单词词义。metastasis 的含义是"转移"；metabolism 的含义是"新陈代谢"；malaise 的含义是"身体不适"；maintenance 的含义是"维护，保持"。upset 的含义是"打乱，搅乱"。

题干译文：糖尿病破坏了糖、脂肪和蛋白质的代谢机制。

117. 【答案】C

【解析】此题解题关键在于 affect，这个词通常表示产生不好的影响。potency 的含义是"效力，力量"，例如：The doctor says that he will not wake until the anesthetic loses potency. 医生说要等麻醉剂的药劲过了他才能醒。fiber 的含义是"纤维"；lethargy 的含义是"没精打采，昏睡"；synthesis 的含义是"合成"。只有选项 C 可以产生不好的影响，故答案是 C。

题干译文：肌肉无力会影响我们的精神感知方式。

118. 【答案】B

【解析】respond to 的含义是"对……回应"，例如：I will respond to your message when I return. 我回来后会回复你的信息。reflect on 的含义是"反思，仔细思考"；wipe out 的含义是"消除"，例如：Medical experts are trying to wipe out the malaria in some countries. 医学专家正设法消除一些国家的疟疾。put off 的含义是"推迟"。

题干译文：大量事实表明，HIV 病毒感染者在反思他们不安全的行为。

119. 【答案】A

【解析】此题解题关键在于语境提示，complain of 的含义是"抱怨，控诉"，所以空白处需要表示贬义的词。harass 的含义是"骚扰"，例如：The court ordered him to stop harassing his ex-wife. 法庭命令他停止骚扰他的前妻。distract 的含义是"使分心"，常与介词 from 连用，例如：The noise outside distracted me from my work. 门外的噪声使我分心,不能集中精力工作。sentenced 的含义是"宣判，判决"；release 的含义是"释放"。

题干译文：很多黑人年轻人抱怨曾被警察骚扰过。

120. 【答案】D

【解析】选项 A 为"滞留"；选项 B 为"劝阻"；选项 C 为"减轻"；选项 D "戒除，远离"。根据题意，本题答案为 D。

题干译文：尽管医生有警示，但他从未戒烟戒酒。

121. 【答案】B

【解析】选项 A 为"康复"；选项 B 为"伤害，使……危险"；选项 C 为"使平静"；选项 D 为"补充"。根据题意，本题答案为 B。

题干译文：医生警告，有感染复发病史的人使用头戴式耳机随身听可能会伤害他们的听力。

122. 【答案】D

【解析】选项 A 为"驳斥";选项 B 为"批准";选项 C 为"促进";选项 D 为"妨碍"。根据题意,本题答案为 D。

题干译文:公正的观察者不得不承认,正规教育的欠缺似乎并未妨碍 Larry 取得成功。

123. 【答案】A

【解析】选项 A 为"相应地";选项 B 为"有选择地";选项 C 为"巨大地";选项 D 为"相关地"。根据题意,本题答案为 A。

题干译文:支持性的成果减少了,他们应该随之修改计划。

124. 【答案】C

【解析】选项 A 为"使……认识";选项 B 为"使……熟悉";选项 C 为"赋予";选项 D 为"使娱乐,逗乐"。根据题意,本题答案为 C。

题干译文:期望值很高的父母们越来越相信,古典音乐的胎教会赋予未来成年人对音乐的欣赏能力。

125. 【答案】D

【解析】选项 A 为"平坦,达到平衡";选项 B 为"突出";选项 C 为"成功";选项 D 为"磨损,逐渐消失"。根据题意,本题答案为 D。

题干译文:如果收益仅仅来自于上升的能源价格,那么当能源价格下调时,通货膨胀应该会下降。

126. 【答案】C

【解析】选项 A 为"处方";选项 B 为"触诊";选项 C 为"干预";选项 D 为"插嘴,提出异议"。根据题意,本题答案为 C。

题干译文:热中风是一种医学紧急情况,需要合格的医疗人员立刻干预。

127. 【答案】D

【解析】选项 A 为"抵消,补偿";选项 B 为"吸入";选项 C 为"发泄";选项 D 为"启动,发病"。根据题意,本题答案为 D。

题干译文:接触石棉能导致间皮瘤、石棉沉滞症和内脏癌症,并且这些疾病的发病都是在首次感染的几十年后。

128. 【答案】B

【解析】选项 A 为"盐溶液";选项 B 为"唾液";选项 C 为"疥疮";选项 D 为"摩擦"。根据题意,本题答案为 B。

题干译文:埃博拉病毒通过体液或者像尿液、唾液和精液这样的排泄物传播,可以杀死多达 90% 的感染者。

129. 【答案】D

【解析】选项 A 为"可比拟的";选项 B 为"可传递的";选项 C 为"可转换的,可翻译的";选项 D 为"易控制的,经得起检验的"。根据题意,本题答案为 D。

题干译文:新设计的系统能经受基因传染的抗击,还能留出潜伏期,以便研究各种基因。

130. 【答案】A

【解析】compensation 赔偿;compromise 折中,妥协;commodity 商品;consumption 消耗,消费。

题干译文：雇主在法律上有义务支付给工人工伤赔偿金。

131.【答案】D

【解析】alleviate 减轻，缓和（痛苦或困难）；aggravate 使加重，使恶化；extinguish 熄灭（火或光），使消亡，使（想法或希望）破灭；intervene 干预，介入，例如：The army will have to intervene to prevent further fighting. 部队不得不介入以阻止战争继续。The police don't usually like to intervene in disputes between husbands and wives. 警察通常不想介入夫妻之间的争吵。

题干译文：两位患者的争吵很激烈，医生不得不出面干涉。

132.【答案】B

【解析】induce 劝诱，诱导；引产，催生；诱发（身体反应）。convert 与 to 连用，意思是"转变为"；revive 使复兴、复原、复苏。swerve ①突然转向，例如：The car swerved sharply to avoid the dog. 汽车突然改变方向以避开狗。②改变，背离（主意、做法、目的等），例如：swerve from the truth 违背真理。hustle and bustle 的含义为"熙熙攘攘，喧闹繁忙"，例如：He wants a cottage far away from the hustle and bustle of city life. 他想要一座远离喧嚣的城市生活的小屋。

题干译文：尽管法律上仍有争论，但他们并不期望死刑改为不可假释的无期徒刑。

133.【答案】C

【解析】integral 不可缺少的，例如：Vegetables are an integral part of our diet. 蔬菜是我们饮食中不可缺少的部分。（用于名词前，作为组成部分的，内置的）。gross ①总共的，例如：gross income 总收入；②（仅用于名词前）恶劣的，糟糕的，例如：gross violation。wholesome 对健康有益的；intact 完好无损的。

题干译文：为了保持身体健康，人应该吃对健康有益的食物并且保证足够的锻炼。

134.【答案】B

【解析】provision 条款，规定，粮食；prosperity 繁荣；privilege 特权，特殊待遇；preference 偏好；优待。

题干译文：中央政府不惜一切代价保证香港的繁荣和稳定，这极大地刺激了当地金融业。

135.【答案】B

【解析】facilitate 促进，使便利；forfeit 没收；丧失；fulfill 实现（希望、目标等）；履行，执行；furnish 配备家具；提供，供应。

题干译文：必须向患者保证他们不会因为床位紧张而丧命。

136.【答案】C

【解析】exclusively 仅仅，唯独；superficially 表面地，不重要地；utterly 完全地；doubtfully 不确定地。

题干译文：他的死因一直以来都是谜，至今全然未知。

137.【答案】A

【解析】recklessly 不计后果地；sparingly 节省地；sensibly 明智地；incredibly 不可思议地。

题干译文：众所周知，一些不计后果利用资源的方式会破坏环境，影响人们的生活。

138.【答案】C

【解析】filtered 过滤的；distilled 蒸馏的；contaminated 被污染的；purified 纯净的。

题干译文：霍乱是一种可预防的、经水传播的细菌性感染疾病，细菌通过污水得以传播。

139.【答案】D

【解析】by the way 顺便说一下；at all events 无论如何；by no means 决不；in any sense 从任何意义上说。

题干译文：从任何意义上说，我们欢迎他，不是把他当作新成员，而是一个老朋友。

140.【答案】A

【解析】adverse 不利的；prevalent 流行的；instant 立刻的，即时的；purposeful"有目的的，故意的"。根据题意，本题选择 adverse。

题干译文：维生素 A 的慢性高剂量摄入已证明对骨骼有不利影响。

141.【答案】C

【解析】screen out 筛查；knock out 击倒；flush out 冲刷掉；rule out 排除。根据题意，本题正确答案为 C。

题干译文：多喝水对身体是有益的，有助于润滑关节并冲洗掉毒素和杂质。

142.【答案】B

【解析】affiliate 加入，为……工作；alleviate 减少，减缓；aggravate 使严重，使恶化；accelerate 使加速。根据题意，正确答案为 B。

题干译文：风湿病学家建议，那些持续疼痛和痛苦的人首先应该借助医疗来缓解问题。

143.【答案】C

【解析】penetrate 穿透；designate 指定；generate 生产，产生；exaggerate 夸张。根据题意，正确答案为 C。

题干译文：一般来说，疫苗制造者可以在受精的鸡蛋中生产病毒，这个过程会持续四到六个月。

144.【答案】A

【解析】equivalent to 相当于，等同于；temporary 暂时的；permanent 永恒的；relevant 相关的。根据题意，本题正确答案为 A。

题干译文：丹麦的研究表明，丹麦肥胖人数的增加大致相当于大气中二氧化碳的增加。

145.【答案】B

【解析】bluntly 直言地；intelligibly 清晰地；reluctantly 不情愿地；ironically 讽刺地。根据题意，正确答案为 B。

题干译文：泰德得了一次严重的中风，平衡受到影响，连话都难以说清楚了。

146.【答案】A

【解析】dominate 主导，控制；overwhelm 压倒，淹没；substitute 代替；imitate 模仿。根据题意，正确答案为 A。

题干译文：在技术密集型企业中，计算机控制着生产和管理的所有过程。

147.【答案】C

【解析】homogeneously 同类地；instantaneously 立即地；spontaneously 自发地；simultaneously 同时地。根据题意，正确答案为 C。

题干译文：虽然大多数梦是明显的自发行为，但梦境可能是由外部影响造成的。

148.【答案】A

【解析】give vent to sth. 发泄（愤怒）；impulse 脉搏；temper 脾气；offence 防卫。根据题意，正确答案为 A。

题干译文：我们更快地做出了回应，通过发泄愤怒而做出的这种回应方式过于迅速了。

149.【答案】D

【解析】bias 偏见；honor 荣誉；estate 财产；bond 联系，联结。根据句意，正确答案为 D。

题干译文：通过维持强有力的家族纽带，同时也维持了社会的基层结构。

150.【答案】D

【解析】obedience 顺从；susceptibility 易受影响（或伤害）的特性；inclination 倾向；dedication 贡献。根据句意，此题选择 D。

题干译文：医疗队讨论了他们对消除这种可治愈疾病的共同贡献。

Section B

Directions: *Each of the following sentences has a word or phrase underlined. There are four other words or phrases beneath each sentence. Choose the word or phrase which would best keep the meaning of the original sentence if it were substituted for the underlined part. Mark your answer on the **ANSWER SHEET**.*

1. It would be wildly optimistic to believe that these advances offset such a large reduction in farmland.
   A. take in   B. make up   C. cut down   D. bring about

2. To study the distribution of disease within an area, it is useful to plot the cases on the map.
   A. mark   B. allocate   C. erase   D. pose

3. The temperature of the atmosphere becomes colder as elevation increases.
   A. altitude   B. aptitude   C. latitude   D. longitude

4. I have no idea of fashion, so my choice of clothes seems quite arbitrary.
   A. assertive   B. decisive   C. optional   D. tasteful

5. This child was so obstinate that he refused to admit to his mistakes.
   A. obsessive   B. furious   C. stubborn   D. rebellious

6. The indomitable spirit displayed by athletes embodies the new look of this nation.
   A. brave   B. unsubdued   C. determined   D. industrious

7. The two sides had an in-depth exchange of views on how to enhance their further cooperation.
   A. specific   B. shallow   C. profound   D. thorough

8. Children should be carefully <u>insulated</u> from harmful experiences.
   A. isolated   B. seceded   C. absent   D. distinguished

9. <u>In the light of</u> the current situation, I have to review my plans.
   A. Throwing light on   B. In line with
   C. In accordance with   D. In terms of

10. In today's competitive job market, people, especially young men are required to be <u>aggressive</u> and industrious.
    A. invasive   B. belligerent   C. progressive   D. enterprising

11. <u>Assimilating</u> the report in computing requires much time, for I'm not specialized in this field.
    A. Digesting   B. Incorporating   C. Imitating   D. Compiling

12. As a member of the society, a person should <u>be responsible for</u> and dedicate to the society.
    A. answer for   B. account for
    C. charge for   D. compensate for

13. To my surprise, the young man was <u>resourceful</u> enough to find infinite ways to express his emotions with gestures.
    A. imaginary   B. imaginative   C. plentiful   D. versatile

14. To lower the risk of <u>secondary diseases</u> of pregnancy, it may be required that you have a change in your lifestyle as soon as you confirm you are pregnant.
    A. complication   B. complexity   C. knottiness   D. hindrance

15. This treaty gave an <u>impetus</u> to the trade between the two countries and the respective development in industry.
    A. impetuous   B. impulse   C. hindrance   D. impasse

16. He suffered a <u>hideous</u> torment when the enemy caught him, but he didn't surrender himself at all.
    A. painful   B. inhumane   C. horrid   D. brutal

17. The average commercial business can shut down in such an emergency but a hospital doesn't dare, for lives are <u>at stake</u>.
    A. on hand   B. in circulation
    C. under consideration   D. at risk

18. We never wondered whether some other dish might be an equally tasty <u>substitute</u> for dumplings on the eve of Spring Festival.
    A. alternative   B. allusion   C. alteration   D. altercation

19. The sales representative was dismissed as he <u>was accused of</u> cheating customers.
    A. was accustomed to   B. adhered to
    C. was charge with   D. stuck to

20. The middle-aged man killed his wife and his children in person. Nothing can extenuate such <u>appalling</u> behavior.

    A. appealing   B. dreadful   C. imprudent   D. displeasing

21. Don't trust the speaker any more, since his deeds are never <u>compatible with</u> his ideology.

    A. suitable for   B. consistent with

    C. in harmony with   D. in favor of

22. Juveniles are more <u>vulnerable to</u> negative influences and outside pressures, including peer pressure.

    A. susceptible to   B. favorable to   C. relevant to   D. capable of

23. Is there anything at work that might subject you to <u>dangerous</u> chemicals?

    A. vicious   B. insidious   C. hazardous   D. notorious

24. Ginger tea may also help <u>alleviate</u> the misery of colds by increasing circulation.

    A. expel   B. diminish   C. endure   D. chop

25. Thousands of people became victims and many children became orphans in the <u>deadly</u> quake.

    A. brutal   B. terrible   C. horrible   D. lethal

26. When she thought no one was looking at she opened the cupboard and took a few sweets <u>on the sly</u>.

    A. secretly   B. punctiliously   C. dilatorily   D. cunningly

27. We no longer keep up the close friendship of few years ago, though we still visit each other <u>on occasion</u>.

    A. at times   B. at a time   C. at all times   D. at one time

28. The British people belong to one of the <u>wealthy</u> countries of Europe and enjoy a high standard of living compared to the rest of the world.

    A. powerful   B. affluent   C. promising   D. almighty

29. <u>Without question</u>, people's lives here have improved dramatically in the past twenty years.

    A. Out of the question   B. Apparently

    C. Undoubtedly   D. Naturally

30. Workers were <u>indignant</u> at the unfair treatment and the indifferent attitudes of their boss.

    A. imprudent   B. wrathful   C. tenacious   D. impatient

31. He was unwilling to press her with questions about her health, since she seemed to make light of the <u>indisposition</u>.

    A. aliment   B. situation   C. ailment   D. incompetence

32. It is an important responsibility for the government to provide safe and <u>wholesome</u> food to the society and the public.

    A. decent   B. wholesale   C. moral   D. salubrious

33. It is <u>absurd</u> that women must be paid less than men for doing the same work.

    A. unreasonable   B. immoral   C. ridiculous   D. abnormal

34. It is believed that this taxi driver is <u>upright</u> and he has never charged extra money for services.

    A. vertical   B. honest   C. modest   D. incorruptible

35. Safety officials have <u>earnestly</u> questioned whether the increased use of synthetic materials heightens the risk of fire.

    A. cautiously   B. severely   C. accurately   D. seriously

36. The senator agreed that his support of the measure would <u>jeopardize</u> his chances for reelection.

    A. benefit   B. endanger   C. hinder   D. disturb

37. We were very angry with his <u>ambiguous</u> views on how to tackle the problem completely.

    A. obscure   B. ambitious   C. indifferent   D. explicit

38. In the Han Dynasty, the royal government sent special envoys to the Western countries to <u>disseminate</u> the Chinese culture.

    A. disclose   B. spread   C. analyze   D. deliver

39. I shall never forget the look of intense <u>anguish</u> on the face of his parents when they knew his death.

    A. surprise   B. stress   C. dilemma   D. misery

40. Wives tend to believe that their husbands are infinitely <u>resourceful</u> and versatile.

    A. diligent   B. clever   C. capable   D. perfect

41. There is no denial that in the tropical areas there is a high <u>incidence</u> of malaria.

    A. morbidity   B. precedent   C. mobility   D. proficiency

42. We want you to report all the events of that morning <u>in sequence</u> without any delay.

    A. at length   B. in order   C. in advance   D. in earnest

43. Most lecturers find it <u>expedient</u> to use notes when addressing to the public.

    A. beneficent   B. contributive

    C. advantageous   D. profitable

44. Some people prefer to remain <u>anonymous</u> when they call the police to report a crime.

    A. undisturbed   B. unnoticed   C. unrecorded   D. unnamed

45. Young children may show a relatively precocious pattern of movement at one age and an <u>immature</u> pattern at a subsequent age.

    A. puerile   B. sophisticated   C. crude   D. worldly

46. The soldiers swore <u>allegiance</u> to their motherland before the war.

    A. truthfulness   B. loyalty   C. faith   D. endurance

47. Don't drive the car if you are drunk, because death was <u>instantaneous</u> in a fatal accident.

    A. instance   B. spontaneous   C. homogenous   D. immediate

48. Workaholics tend to have an <u>compulsive</u> and unrelenting need to work at any time.

    A. compulsory   B. obstructive   C. constructive   D. impulsive

49. We've made great efforts to <u>exterminate</u> mosquitoes and flies in the tropical areas.

    A. erase   B. eliminate   C. demolish   D. ruin

50. Poor eyesight will <u>exempt</u> you <u>from</u> military service.

    A. prevent from   B. deprive from   C. free from   D. hinder from

51. The 19th-century physiology was <u>dominated</u> by the study of the transformation of food energy into body mass and activity.

    A. boosted   B. governed   C. clarified   D. pioneered

52. Surely, it would be <u>sensible</u> to get a second opinion before taking any further action.

    A. realistic   B. sensitive   C. reasonable   D. sensational

53. The Chinese people hold their ancestors in great <u>veneration</u>.

    A. recognition   B. sincerity   C. heritage   D. honor

54. I worked to develop the <u>requisite</u> skill for a managerial staff.

    A. perfect   B. exquisite   C. unique   D. necessary

55. If exercise is a bodily maintenance activity and an <u>index</u> of physiological age, the lack of sufficient exercise may either cause or hasten aging.

    A. instance   B. indicator   C. appearance   D. option

56. The doctor advised Ken to avoid <u>strenuous</u> exercise.

    A. arduous   B. demanding   C. potent   D. continuous

57. The hospital should be held <u>accountable</u> for the quality of care it delivers.

    A. practicable   B. reliable   C. flexible   D. responsible

58. Greenpeace has been invited to <u>appraise</u> the environment costs of such an operation.

    A. esteem   B. appreciate   C. evaluate   D. approve

59. The company still hopes to find a buyer, but the future looks <u>bleak</u>.

    A. chilly   B. dismal   C. promising   D. fanatic

60. These were vital decisions that <u>bore upon</u> the happiness of everybody.

    A. ensured   B. ruined   C. achieved   D. influenced

61. Memory can be both enhanced and <u>impaired</u> by use of drugs.

    A. inhibited   B. injured   C. induced   D. intervened

62. Is it true that this is the major <u>drawback</u> of the new medical plan?

    A. defect   B. assistance   C. culprit   D. triumph

63. The physician was becoming <u>exasperated</u> with all the questions they were asking.

A. frustrated   B. perplexed   C. irritated   D. crippled

64. We were shocked at the physician's <u>callous</u> disregard for the human dimension of medicine.

    A. involuntary   B. apparent   C. deliberate   D. indifferent

65. For years, biologists have known that chimpanzees and even some monkeys produce a <u>panting</u> sound akin to human laughter.

    A. rocking   B. gasping   C. vibrating   D. resonating

66. Everybody at the party was in a very relaxed and <u>jolly</u> mood.

    A. rejoicing   B. reconciling   C. refreshing   D. resenting

67. The bacterial infection is curable with <u>judicious</u> use of antibiotics.

    A. impudent   B. imprudent   C. purulent   D. prudent

68. He tried to run, but he was <u>hampered</u> by his broken leg.

    A. endangered   B. endured   C. encountered   D. encumbered

69. The whole holiday was a <u>colossal</u> waste of money.

    A. consecutive   B. conductive   C. considerate   D. considerable

70. The idea of correcting defective genes is not particularly <u>controversial</u> in the scientific community.

    A. inevitable   B. applicable   C. disputable   D. incredible

71. She fell <u>awkwardly</u> and broke her leg.（2011 年真题）

    A. embarrassingly   B. reluctantly   C. clumsily   D. dizzily

72. Throughout most of the recorded history, medicine was <u>anything but</u> scientific.（2011 年真题）

    A. more or less   B. by and large

    C. more often than not   D. by no means

73. The students were <u>captivated</u> by the way the physician presented the case.（2011 年真题）

    A. illuminated   B. fascinated   C. alienated   D. hallucinated

74. We demand some <u>tangible</u> proof of our hard work in the form of statistical data, a product or a financial reward.（2011 年真题）

    A. intelligible   B. infinitive   C. substantial   D. deficient

75. But diets that restrict certain food groups or promise unrealistic results are difficult or unhealthy to <u>sustain</u> over time.（2011 年真题）

    A. maintain   B. reserve   C. conceive   D. empower

76. The molecular influence pervades all the traditional <u>disciplines</u> underlying clinical medicine.（2011 年真题）

    A. specialties   B. principles   C. rationales   D. doctrines

77. One usually becomes aware of the onset of puberty through <u>somatic</u> manifestations.（2011 年真题）

A. juvenile   B. potent   C. physical   D. matured

78. His surgical procedure should succeed, for it seems quite <u>feasible</u>. （2011 年真题）

A. rational   B. reciprocal   C. versatile   D. viable

79. These are <u>intensely</u> important questions about quality and the benefits of special care and experience. （2011 年真题）

A. irresistibly   B. vitally   C. potentially   D. intriguingly

80. This guide gives you information on the best self-care <u>strategies</u> and the latest medical advances. （2011 年真题）

A. tends   B. techniques

C. notions   D. breakthroughs

81. She, a crazy fan, felt a <u>tingle</u> of excitement at the sight of Michael Jackson. （2012 年真题）

A. glimpse   B. gust   C. panic   D. pack

82. She could never <u>transcend</u> her resentments against her mother's partiality for her brother. （2012 年真题）

A. discipline   B. complain   C. conquer   D. defy

83. One could neither <u>trifle with</u> a terror of this kind, nor compromise with it. （2012 年真题）

A. belittle   B. exaggerate   C. ponder   D. eliminate

84. <u>In light of</u> his good record, the police accepted defense. （2012 年真题）

A. In place of   B. In view of   C. In spite of   D. In search of

85. City officials stated that workers who lied on their employment applications may be <u>terminated</u>. （2012 年真题）

A. accused   B. punished   C. dismissed   D. suspended

86. An outbreak of swine flu outside of Mexico City was <u>blamed for</u> the deaths of more than a hundred people in April 2009. （2012 年真题）

A. attached to   B. ascribed to   C. composed of   D. related to

87. When a forest goes ablaze, it <u>discharges</u> hundreds of chemical compounds, including carbon monoxide. （2012 年真题）

A. puts out   B. passes off   C. pulls out   D. sends out

88. Unfortunately, the bridge under construction clasped in the earthquake, so they had to do the whole thing again <u>from scratch</u>. （2012 年真题）

A. from the beginning   B. from now on

C. from time to time   D. from the bottom

89. Identical twin sisters have led British scientists to a breakthrough in leukemia research that <u>promises</u> more effective therapies with fewer harmful side-effects. （2012 年真题）

A. administers   B. nurtures   C. inspires   D. ensures

90. Radical environmentalists have blamed pollutants and synthetic chemicals in pesticides for the <u>disruption</u> of human hormones.（2012 年真题）

    A. disturbance   B. distraction   C. intersection   D. interpretation

91. Christmas shoppers should be aware of the possible <u>defects</u> of the products sold at a discount.（2013 年真题）

    A. deficits   B. deviations   C. drawbacks   D. discrepancies

92. The goal of this training program is to raise children with a sense of responsibility and necessary courage to be willing to <u>take on</u> challenges in life.（2013 年真题）

    A. despise   B. evade

    C. demand   D. undertake

93. After "9.11", the Olympic Games severely <u>taxed</u> the security services of the host country.（2013 年真题）

    A. improved   B. burdened   C. inspected   D. tariffed

94. The clown's performance was so funny that the audience, adults and children alike, were all thrown into <u>convulsions</u>.（2013 年真题）

    A. a fit of enthusiasm   B. a scream of fright

    C. a burst of laughter   D. a cry of anguish

95. We raised a <u>mortgage</u> from Bank of China and were informed to pay it off by the end of this year.（2013 年真题）

    A. loan   B. payment   C. withdrawal   D. retrieval

96. The advocates highly value the "sport spirit", while the opponents devalue it, asserting that it's a <u>sheer</u> hypocrisy and self-deception.（2013 年真题）

    A. fine   B. sudden   C. finite   D. absolute

97. Whenever a rattlesnake is <u>agitated</u>, it begins to move its tail and make a rattling noise.（2013 年真题）

    A. irritated   B. tamed   C. stamped   D. probed

98. The detective had an unusual <u>insight</u> into criminal's tricks and knew clearly how to track them.（2013 年真题）

    A. induction   B. perception   C. interpretation   D. penetration

99. My little brother practices the speech repeatedly until his <u>delivery</u> and timing were perfect.（2013 年真题）

    A. presentation   B. gesture

    C. rhythm   D. pronunciation

100. In recent weeks both housing and stock prices have started to retreat from their <u>irrationally</u> amazing highs.（2013 年真题）

    A. untimely   B. unexpectedly

    C. unreasonably   D. unconventionally

101. All Nobel Prize winners' success is a process of long-term accumulation, in which lasting efforts are <u>indispensable</u>.（2014 年真题）

    A. irresistible   B. cherished   C. inseparable   D. requisite

102. The Queen's presence <u>imparted</u> an air of elegance to the drinks reception at Buckingham Palace of London.（2014 年真题）

    A. bestowed   B. exhibited   C. imposed   D. emitted

103. Physicians are clear that thyroid dysfunction is <u>manifest</u> in growing children in the form of mental and physical retardation.（2014 年真题）

    A. intensified   B. apparent

    C. representative   D. insidious

104. The mechanism that the eye can <u>accommodate</u> itself to different distances has been applied to automatic camera, which makes a revolutionary technique advance.（2014 年真题）

    A. yield   B. amplify   C. adapt   D. cast

105. Differences among believers are common; however, it was the pressure of religious persecution that <u>exacerbated</u> their conflicts and created the split of the union.（2014 年真题）

    A. eradicated   B. deteriorated   C. vanquished   D. averted

106. When Picasso was particularly poor, he might have tried to <u>obliterate</u> the original composition by painting over it on canvases.（2014 年真题）

    A. duplicate   B. eliminate   C. substitute   D. compile

107. For the sake of animal protection, environmentalists <u>deplored</u> the construction program of a nuclear power station.（2014 年真题）

    A. disapproved   B. despised   C. demolished   D. decomposed

108. Political figures in particular are held to very strict standards of moral <u>fidelity</u>.（2014 年真题）

    A. loyalty   B. morality   C. quality   D. stability

109. The patient complained that his doctor had been <u>negligent</u> in not giving him a full examination.（2014 年真题）

    A. fury   B. ardent   C. careless   D. brutal

110. She has been handling all the complaints without <u>wrath</u> for a whole morning.（2014 年真题）

    A. fury   B. chaos   C. despair   D. agony

111. Every year more than 1,000 patients in Britain die on transplant waiting lists, <u>prompting</u> scientists to consider other ways to produce organs.（2015 年真题）

    A. propelling   B. prolonging

    C. puzzling   D. promising

112. Improved treatment has changed the outlook of HIV patients, but there is still a serious <u>stigma</u> attached to AIDS.（2015 年真题）

   A. disgrace
   B. discrimination
   C. harassment
   D. segregation

113. Survivors of the shipwreck were finally rescued after their courage of persistence lowered to zero by their physical <u>lassitude</u>.（2015 年真题）

   A. depletion
   B. dehydration
   C. exhaustion
   D. handicap

114. Scientists have invented a 3D scan technology to read the otherwise <u>illegible</u> wood-carved stone, a method that may apply to other areas such as medicine.（2015 年真题）

   A. negative
   B. confusing
   C. eloquent
   D. indistinct

115. Top athletes <u>scrutinize</u> both success and failure with their coach to extract lessons from them, but they are never distracted from long-term goals.（2015 年真题）

   A. anticipate
   B. clarify
   C. examine
   D. verify

116. His <u>imperative</u> tone of voice reveals his arrogance and arbitrariness.（2015 年真题）

   A. challenging
   B. solemn
   C. hostile
   D. demanding

117. The discussion on the economic collaboration between the United States and the European Union may be <u>eclipsed</u> by the recent growing trade friction.（2015 年真题）

   A. erased
   B. triggered
   C. shadowed
   D. suspended

118. Faster increases in prices <u>foster</u> the belief that the future increases will be also stronger, so that higher prices fuel demand rather than quench it.（2015 年真题）

   A. nurture
   B. eliminate
   C. assimilate
   D. puncture

119. Some recent developments in photography allow animals to be studied in previously inaccessible places and in <u>unprecedented</u> detail.（2015 年真题）

   A. unpredictable
   B. unconventional
   C. unparalleled
   D. unexpected

120. A veteran negotiation specialist should be skillful at <u>manipulating</u> touchy situation.（2015 年真题）

   A. estimating
   B. handling
   C. rectifying
   D. anticipating

121. In any event, lethal injections are under federal <u>scrutiny</u>.（2016 年真题）

   A. sanction
   B. restriction
   C. census
   D. examination

122. The humble tomato could become a <u>potent</u> weapon in the fight against prostate cancer.（2016 年真题）

   A. inexpensive
   B. powerful
   C. conventional
   D. lethal

123. Men's perception of the amount of caregiving they do is completely <u>at odds with</u> women's.（2016 年真题）

   A. in tune with
   B. in favor of

C. for the sake of　　　　　　　　D. in disagreement with

124. Huangshan Mountain is eminent for its natural scenery and deserves a visit.（2016年真题）

　　A. renowned　　　　B. notorious　　　　C. popular　　　　D. mysterious

125. Obesity is a condition perpetuated by a diversity of factors.（2016年真题）

　　A. severity　　　　　B. reliability　　　　C. variety　　　　D. specificity

126. He is usually well-behaved; this rudeness is only a lapse.（2016年真题）

　　A. error　　　　　　B. sin　　　　　　C. guilt　　　　　D. offense

127. Did you detect a touch of jaundice in her remark?（2016年真题）

　　A. grievance　　　　　　　　　　B. sympathy

　　C. jealousy　　　　　　　　　　 D. indignation

128. In 1912, German doctors attempted to treat children who had underactive thyroids with normal thyroid cells, but to little avail.（2016年真题）

　　A. by no means　　　　　　　　B. in vain

　　C. of no account　　　　　　　　D. at stake

129. To many observers, he spent his wealth lavishly.（2016年真题）

　　A. fearlessly　　　　B. conspicuously　　C. wastefully　　　D. ferociously

130. At present, no medical therapy is known to affect progressions of rheumatic mitral stenosis.（2016年真题）

　　A. deterioration　　　B. accumulation　　C. expansion　　　D. promotion

131. Inform the manager if you are on medication that makes you drowsy.（2017年真题）

　　A. uneasy　　　B. sleepy　　　　　C. guilty　　　　D. fiery

132. Diabetes is one of the most prevalent and potentially dangerous diseases in the world.（2017年真题）

　　A. crucial　　　　B. virulent　　　　C. colossal　　　　D. widespread

133. Likewise, soot and smoke from fire contain a multitude of carcinogens.（2017年真题）

　　A. a matter of　　B. a body of　　　C. plenty of　　　D. sort of

134. Many questions about estrogen's effects remain to be elucidated, and investigations are seeking answers through ongoing laboratory and clinical studies.（2017年真题）

　　A. implicated　　B. implied　　　　C. illuminated　　　D. initiated

135. A network chatting is a limp substitute for meeting friends over coffee.（2017年真题）

　　A. accomplishment　　　　　　 B. refreshment

　　C. complement　　　　　　　　 D. replacement

136. When patients spend extended periods in hospital, they tend to become overly dependent and lose interest in taking care of themselves.（2017年真题）

　　A. extremely　　　B. exclusively　　　C. exactly　　　D. explicitly

137. Attempts to restrict parking in the city centre have further aggravated the problem of traffic congestion.（2017年真题）

　　A. ameliorated　　B. aggregated　　　C. deteriorated　　D. duplicated

138. It was reported that bacteria <u>contaminated</u> up to 80% of domestic retail raw chicken in the United States. （2017 年真题）

  A. inflamed   B. inflicted   C. infected   D. infiltrated

139. Researchers recently ran the numbers on gun violence in the United States and reported that right-to-carry-gun laws do not <u>inhibit</u> violent crime. （2017 年真题）

  A. curb   B. induce   C. lessen   D. impel

140. Regardless of our uneasiness about <u>stereotypes</u>, numerous studies have shown clear difference between Chinese and western parenting. （2017 年真题）

  A. specifications   B. sensations

  C. conventions   D. conservations

141. The truly <u>competent</u> physician is the one who sits down, senses the "mystery" of another human beings, and offers the simple gifts of personal interest and understanding. （2018 年真题）

  A. imaginable   B. capable   C. sensible   D. humble

142. The physician often <u>perceived</u> that treatment was initiated by the patient. （2018 年真题）

  A. conserved   B. theorized   C. realized   D. persisted

143. Large community meals might have served to <u>lubricate</u> social connections and alleviated tensions. （2018 年真题）

  A. facilitate   B. intimidate   C. terminate   D. mediate

144. Catalase activity reduced glutathione and vitamin E levels were decreased <u>exclusively</u> in subjects with active disease. （2018 年真题）

  A. definitely   B. truly   C. simply   D. solely

145. Ocular anomalies were frequently observed in this cohort of <u>offspring</u> born after in vitro fertilization. （2018 年真题）

  A. fetuses   B. descendants   C. seeds   D. orphans

146. Childhood poverty should be regarded as the single greatest public health <u>menace</u> facing our children. （2018 年真题）

  A. breach   B. grief   C. threat   D. abuse

147. A distant dream would be to <u>deliberately</u> set off quakes to release tectonic stress in a controlled way. （2018 年真题）

  A. definitely   B. desperately

  C. intentionally   D. identically

148. Big challenges still await companies <u>converting</u> carbon dioxide to petrol. （2018 年真题）

  A. applying   B. relating

  C. relaying   D. transforming

149. Concerns have recently been voiced that the drugs elicit unexpected cognitive side effects, such as memory loss, fuzzy thinking and learning difficulties.（2018 年真题）

A．ensue   B．encounter   C．impede   D．induce

150. A leaf before the eye shuts out Mount Tai, which means having one's view of the important overshadowed by the trivial.（2018 年真题）

A．insignificant   B．insufficient   C．substantial   D．unexpected

答案及解析

1. 【答案】B

【解析】offset 意为"补偿，抵消"；四个选项含义如下：take in ①吞入，吸入，例如：Fish can take in oxygen through their gills. 鱼能用鳃吸入氧气。②欺骗，例如：I was taken in by his story. 我被他的故事给骗了。③留宿，例如：The old man took in these homeless people. 这个老人收留了这些无家可归的人。make up ①弥补，例如：Saying sorry to me couldn't make up my damage. 对我说对不起不能弥补对我的伤害。②形成，构成，例如：Female students make up only one third of the student numbers in this university. 女学生仅占这所大学学生人数的三分之一。③编造，例如：The student made up an excuse for being late. 这个学生为迟到编造了一个借口。cut down 削减，例如：This company had to cut down its expenses in this project. 这家公司不得不削减这个项目的开支。bring about 导致，例如：What brought about the change in his attitude? 什么使得他改变了态度？

题干译文：可以很乐观地相信这些进步弥补了农业的大幅度减产。

2. 【答案】A

【解析】plot 意为"绘制，标出，策划"；四个选项含义为：mark 标注，注明；allocate 分派，分配；erase 抹去；pose 摆姿势。

题干译文：为了研究这个区域内病情的分布，在地图上标明情况很有用。

3. 【答案】A

【解析】elevation 的含义是"海拔"。四个选项含义为：altitude 高度，海拔；aptitude 才能，能力；latitude 纬度；longitude 经度。

题干译文：随着海拔升高，大气温度会降低。

4. 【答案】C

【解析】arbitrary 的含义是"任意的，专制的，武断的"。assertive 的含义是"断定的，过分自信的"，例如：He is an assertive boy, always insisting on his own rights and opinions. 他是个过分自信的男孩，总是坚持自己的权利和观点。decisive 的含义是"决定性的"；tasteful 的含义是"高雅的，雅致的"。根据句意可以知道 arbitrary 的含义不是"武断专制的"，而是"不加选择的，随意的"，故只有 C 符合句意。

题干译文：我不了解时尚，所以我对衣服的选择很随意。

5. 【答案】C

【解析】根据句意所提供的信息"不肯承认错误"可以判断画线词的含义为"倔强的，固执的"。四个选项含义如下：obsessive 着迷的，迷恋的，例如：an obsessive attention to details 十分注重细节。furious 狂怒的，暴怒的，固定搭配是 be furious with sb. at sth.，例如：He was furious with himself for the failure in the exam. 他生自己的气，怪自己考试不及格。stubborn 固执的，倔强的，例如：He is as stubborn as a donkey. 他倔得像头驴。rebellious 反抗的，叛逆的。

题干译文：这个孩子很倔强，不肯承认错误。

6. 【答案】B

【解析】题干画线词 indomitable 的含义为"不屈不挠的"，display 的含义为"呈现"，embody 的含义为"体现"。unsubdued 的含义为"不屈服的"；determined 的含义为"坚决的"；industrious 的含义是"勤勉刻苦的"。通过题干中的 athlete（运动员）可以推断出画线词的大概含义，只有 B 项符合句意。

题干译文：运动员所展现的不屈不挠的精神体现了这个国家的新风貌。

7. 【答案】D

【解析】根据画线部分的主要词汇 depth 可以知道 in-depth 的含义为"深入的"。specific 的含义是"明确的，具体的"，例如：specific instructions 明确的指示。shallow 的含义为"浅薄的"，不符合句意。profound 的含义为"深切的，深刻的，严重的"，例如：have a profound effect on 对……产生深远影响；profound insights 深刻的见解；profound disability 严重残疾。thorough 的含义为"深入的，细致的，彻底的"，例如：a thorough investigation 全面调查；a thorough cleaning 大扫除。只有 D 项与题干画线部分意思最接近。

题干译文：双方就如何进一步加强合作深入交换了意见。

8. 【答案】A

【解析】题干中画线词 insulate 的含义为"绝缘，隔热"。这里 insulate sb. / sth. from / against 含义是"免受……的（不良影响）"。四个选项含义为：isolate from 使隔离，使孤立，例如：He was isolated from other prisoners. 他被与其他犯人隔离开。secede 脱离，退出；be absent from 缺席，不在，例如：be absent from school 缺课。distinguish from 区分，区别，例如：He can distinguish a genuine antique from a reproduction. 他能区分真古董和仿制品。由此可知 A 项最适合。

题干译文：孩子应注意避免受到不良经验的影响。

9. 【答案】C

【解析】in the light of 的含义为"根据，按照"。四个选项含义为：throw light on 解释，阐明，例如：As the time went by, all the unsettled questions were thrown light on in the end. 随着时间的推移，所有未解决的问题都最终得到了解释。in line with 和……站成一排，与……相似或符合，例如：Your plan is in line with my ideas. 你的计划与我的想法一致。in accordance with 依照，例如：In accordance with his father's wish he gave the money to the school. 依照他父亲的愿望，他把钱捐给了学校。in terms of 就……而言，例如：In terms of learning strategies, I don't think this teaching method is beneficial to students. 就学习策略而言，我认为这个教学方法对学生不利。

题干译文：根据目前的状况，我必须重新审视我的计划了。

10. 【答案】D

【解析】题干画线词 aggressive 的含义是"侵略的，进取的"。根据题干的信息，aggressive 的含义应该是褒义的。四个选项含义为：invasive 侵略的，在医学上含义为"侵袭的"，例如：invasive cancer 扩散性肿瘤。belligerent 好斗的，挑衅的；progressive 进步的，逐步的，例如：a progressive muscular disease 逐渐严重的肌肉病症。enterprising 有进取心的，与画线词意思相同。

题干译文：在当今激烈的就业市场，人们尤其是年轻人要有进取心、要勤奋。

11. 【答案】A

【解析】题干画线词 assimilate 的含义为"吸收，消化"。四个选项含义为：digest 的含义是"消化，吸收，理解"，与题干画线词意义相同；incorporate 的含义为"包含，纳入"，例如：The new design incorporates all the latest fashionable elements. 这个新设计包含所有最新的时尚元素。imitate 模仿；compile 编纂。

题干译文：理解这篇有关计算技术的报告很费时，因为我不是这个专业的。

12. 【答案】A

【解析】题干画线词组 be responsible for 的含义为"对……负责"。四个选项含义为：answer for 的含义为"对……负责"，例如：Everyone should answer for his or her action. 每个人都应该对自己的行为负责。account for 的含义有：①解释，说明，例如：He didn't account for his absence. 他没有解释缺席的原因。②占……时间、空间，例如：Girls account for two thirds of students in this college. 这所大学女生占三分之二。charge for 索价，例如：We won't charge you for delivery. 我们为你免费送货。compensate for 赔偿，补偿，例如：Nothing can compensate for my loss. 什么也不能补偿我的损失。

题干译文：作为社会一分子，人人应该对社会负责，为社会做贡献。

13. 【答案】B

【解析】画线词 resourceful 含义为"足智多谋的，机智的"；四个选项含义为：imaginary 虚构的，不真实的。imaginative 有创造性的，与画线词意义相近；plentiful 丰富的；versatile 多面手的，多才多艺的。

题干译文：令我惊奇的是，这个年轻人非常机智，可以找到很多方式用肢体语言表达他的情感。

14. 【答案】A

【解析】画线词组的含义为"并发症"。complication 的含义就是"并发症"；其他三项的含义为：complexity 复杂性；knottiness 困难，难题，纠纷；hindrance 障碍。

题干译文：为了降低怀孕的并发症，要求你在确定自己怀孕后改变生活方式。

15. 【答案】B

【解析】题干画线词 impetus 的含义是"推动力，促进"。四个选项含义为：impetuous 是形容词，含义为"冲动的，轻率的"，例如：She regretted her impetuous decision. 她后悔做出轻率的决定。impulse 为名词，含义为"推动"，例如：On impulse, I bought the expensive antique. 我一心血来潮就买下了这个昂贵的古董。hindrance 障碍；impasse 僵局，例如：They reached an impasse in the negotiations. 他们在谈判过程中陷入僵局。

题干译文：这个条约给两国间贸易以及各自工业发展提供了推动力。

16. 【答案】C

【解析】题干画线词 hideous 是形容词，含义是"骇人听闻的，可怕的"。torment 含义是"痛苦，折磨"，surrender oneself 含义是"自首，投降"。四个选项含义为：painful（身心）痛苦的；inhumane 残忍的，不人道的；horrid 可怕的，恐怖的；brutal 残忍的。只有 C 项与画线词义接近。

题干译文：当敌人抓到他的时候，他受尽折磨，但他根本就没屈服。

17. 【答案】D

【解析】题干中的画线词组 at stake 的含义可以通过语境信息推断出来，即"危险中"。on hand 的含义为"现有的"，相当于 available，例如：Medical service is on hand. 提供医疗服务。in circulation ①流通中，例如：A number of forged banknotes are in circulation. 大量假币在流通中。②社交，交际，例如：After a month in hospital, she is back in circulation. 住了一个月的医院后，她又活跃起来了。under consideration 的含义为"考虑中"，例如：The proposal is currently under consideration. 这个提议目前正在考虑中。at risk 含义为"在危险中"，与画线词组意思相同。

题干译文：在紧急情况下商业部门可以关门，但医院不可以，因为性命攸关。

18. 【答案】A

【解析】题干画线词 substitute 含义为"替代品"，常与介词 for 连用。题干中，the eve of Spring Festival 含义为"除夕"。四个选项含义为：alternative 选择物，替代品；allusion 提及，暗示，例如：His writings are full of classical allusions. 他的作品里有许多典故。alteration 变更，改造；altercation 争论，口角。

题干译文：我们从来就没想过其他事物是否可以成为除夕饺子的替代品，并且一样好吃。

19. 【答案】C

【解析】题干画线词组的含义为"被控告"，be dismissed 被开除，sales representative 销售代表。四个选项含义为：be accustomed to 相当于 be used to doing，即"习惯于"，例如：I am accustomed to taking a walk after supper. 我习惯于晚饭后散步。adhere to 坚持，遵循，例如：She adheres to teaching methods she learned over 20 years ago. 她还在遵循 20 年前她所学到的教学方法。be charged with 被控告，例如：He was charged with murder. 他被控谋杀。stick to 坚持，例如：

He promised to help us, but he didn't stick to his word. 他答应帮助我们，但他失言了。

题干译文：这个销售代理被开除了，因为他被控欺骗顾客。

20. 【答案】B

【解析】题干画线词 appalling 含义为"骇人听闻的，可怕的"。in person 含义为"亲手，亲自"，extenuate 含义为"减轻，使人原谅"，例如：Because of extenuating circumstances, the court acquitted him of the crime. 因考虑到情有可原，法庭判他无罪。各选项含义为：appealing 与画线词形似，但含义为：①吸引人的，有感染力的；②可怜的，恳求的。dreadful 可怕的，与画线词含义相同；imprudent 轻率的，鲁莽的；displeasing 不愉快的。

题干译文：这个中年男子亲手杀害了他的妻子和孩子，这种骇人听闻的行为罪不可恕。

21. 【答案】B

【解析】题干画线词组 compatible with 的含义为"与……一致"。四个选项含义如下：be suitable for 适合，例如：No one in the applicants is suitable for the job. 申请者中无人适合这个工作。be consistent with 与……一致，例如：The results are entirely consistent with our earlier research. 结果与我们先前的研究完全一致。be in harmony with 融洽，和睦，例如：People should be in harmony with the environment. 人们要与环境相和谐。be in favor of ①赞同，例如：He was in favor of the proposal. 他赞同这个提议。②看中，选择，例如：He abandoned teaching in favor of a career as a musician. 他弃教从事音乐。

题干译文：别再相信这个发言人了，因为他的行为与他的观念从来就不一致。

22. 【答案】A

【解析】题干画线词组 be vulnerable to sth. 意为"易受……伤害"，例如：In case of food poisoning, young children are easily vulnerable. 在食物中毒的问题上，年龄小的孩子容易受到危害。juvenile 意为"青少年"。各选项含义为：be susceptible to 容易受……的影响。be favorable to 对……有利、有帮助，例如：The terms of this agreement are favorable to both sides. 协议中的条款对双方都有利。be relevant to 与……紧密相关，例如：The evidence they found is relevant to the case. 他们找到的证据与这个案件相关。be capable of 有能力做。

题干译文：青少年更容易受消极影响和外部压力的影响，包括同龄人的压力。

23. 【答案】C

【解析】题干中 subject sb. to 的含义是"使经受"，例如：The essay subjected him to criticism. 这篇论文让他受到批评。vicious 恶毒的；insidious 阴险的；hazardous 危险的；notorious 声名狼藉的。故 C 正确。

题干译文：工作中有让你接触有害化学物质的东西吗？

24. 【答案】B

【解析】题干画线词 alleviate 的含义为"减轻，缓解"。四个选项含义如下：expel 驱散，消除；diminish 减少；endure 忍耐；chop 砍，剁。B 项符合画线词的含义。

题干译文：姜也可以通过促进血液循环帮助减轻感冒的痛苦。

25. 【答案】D

【解析】题干画线词 deadly 的含义为"致命的"，victim 的含义为"受害者"，orphan 的含义为"孤儿"。四个选项含义如下：brutal 残忍的；terrible 可怕的；horrible 恐怖的；lethal 致命的。

题干译文：上千人成为受害者，许多孩子在这场致命的地震中成为孤儿。

26. 【答案】A

【解析】题干画线词组 on the sly 含义为"秘密地，偷偷地"，例如：He has to visit his children on the sly. 他必须偷偷地去看他的孩子。选项中只有 A 项 secretly 符合这个词组的含义。其他三项：punctiliously 谨小慎微地；dilatorily 慢吞吞地，迟缓地；cunningly 狡猾地。

题干译文：在觉得没人看到的时候，她打开了橱柜，偷偷地拿出了一些糖果。

27. 【答案】A

【解析】题干画线词组 on occasion 的含义为"偶尔，有时"。四个选项含义为：at times 偶尔；at a time 每次，一次，例如：take three pills at a time 一次服三粒药片。at all times 始终（无论什么时候），例如：You should have a cool head at all times. 无论什么时候你都应该保持清醒的头脑。at one time 曾经，一度，例如：She was my best friend at one time. 她曾经是我最好的朋友。

题干译文：我们在几年前就没再保持深厚的友谊，尽管我们偶尔互相拜访。

28. 【答案】B

【解析】题干画线词含义为"富有的"。各选项含义如下：powerful 强大的；affluent 丰富的，富裕的；promising 有希望的，有前途的；almighty 全能的。可知只有选项 B 符合画线词含义。

题干译文：英国人属于欧洲富有国家之一，和其他国家相比，他们享有很高的生活水平。

29. 【答案】C

【解析】题干画线词组 without question 含义为"毫无疑问"。各选项含义如下：out of the question 不可能，例如：Another trip abroad this year is out of the question. 今年再次出国旅行是不可能的。apparently 显然，相当于 obviously；undoubtedly 的含义即为"毋庸置疑地"；naturally 自然地。

题干译文：毫无疑问，这里人们的生活在过去的二十年间发生了翻天覆地的变化。

30. 【答案】B

【解析】题干画线词 indignant 的含义为"愤怒的"，常与介词 at 或者 about 连用，例如：They were indignant at the way they had been treated. 他们对自己受到的待遇很愤怒。各选项含义如下：imprudent 轻率的，鲁莽的；wrathful 愤怒的；tenacious 顽强的；impatient 不耐烦的。

题干译文：工人们对不公待遇和老板漠然的态度很愤恨。

31. 【答案】C

【解析】题干画线单词 indisposition 的含义为"小病，微恙"。各选项含义如下：aliment

滋养品；situation 状况；ailment 疾病（尤指微恙）；incompetence 无能力。

题干译文：他不想老是问起她的健康情况，因为她对自己的病好像不是很在乎。

32. 【答案】D

【解析】题干画线词 wholesome 的含义为"有益健康的"。各选项含义如下：decent
端庄的，得体的；wholesale 批发的，大规模的；moral 有道德的；salubrious
的含义即为"有益健康的"。

题干译文：提供给社会和大众安全、有益健康的食品是政府十分重要的责任。

33. 【答案】C

【解析】题干画线词 absurd 的含义为"荒谬的"。四个选项含义为：unreasonable 不合
情合理的；immoral 不道德的；ridiculous 荒谬的；abnormal 不正常的。

题干译文：做同样的工作，女性的工资要比男性的低，太荒谬了。

34. 【答案】B

【解析】题干画线单词 upright 的含义为"正直的"。四个选项含义为：vertical 垂直的；
honest 诚实的，正直的；modest 谦虚的；incorruptible 清廉的。

题干译文：这个出租车司机很正直，从来不多要钱。

35. 【答案】D

【解析】题干画线单词 earnestly 的含义为"认真地"；各选项含义如下：cautiously 谨慎地；
severely 严重地；accurately 精确地；seriously 认真地，符合题干画线词含义。

题干译文：安全官员很认真地质疑是否合成材料使用越多，火灾的隐患就会越大。

36. 【答案】B

【解析】题干画线单词 jeopardize 的含义为"危害"，例如：If you are impolite to your
boss, it may jeopardize your chance of success. 如果你对老板不礼貌，也许会危
及你成功的机会。四个选项含义为：benefit 对……有利；endanger 危及，危害；
hinder 阻碍；disturb 扰乱。只有 B 项符合题干画线单词的含义。

题干译文：参议员认为支持这项措施将会危及改选。

37. 【答案】A

【解析】题干画线词 ambiguous 的含义为"模棱两可的，模糊不清的"。各选项含义如下：
obscure 朦胧的，模糊的，与题干画线词含义相同。ambitious 有野心的，雄心
勃勃的；indifferent 漠然的；explicit 清楚的。

题干译文：我们对他在如何彻底解决这个问题上模棱两可的态度很是生气。

38. 【答案】B

【解析】题干画线单词 disseminate 的含义为"传播，散布"，例如：disseminate
rumors 散布谣言；disseminate culture 传播文化。题干 envoy 的含义为"特使，
外交使节"。四个选项含义为：disclose 揭露，暴露；spread 传播；analyze 分
析；deliver 递送。

题干译文：在汉代，皇室派遣特使前往西方国家传播中国文化。

39. 【答案】D

【解析】题干画线词 anguish 的含义为"痛苦"。各选项含义如下：surprise 惊奇；

stress 压力；dilemma 进退两难的困境；misery 痛苦。由此可知 D 符合画线词含义。

题干译文：我永远不会忘记当他父母得知他死亡的消息时，脸上极其痛苦的表情。

40. 【答案】B

【解析】题干画线词 resourceful 的含义为"机智的"，四个选项含义为：versatile 多才多艺的。diligent 勤劳的，勤勉的；capable 有能力的；perfect 完美的，只有选项 clever 符合题干画线词含义。

题干译文：妻子们总是认为她们的丈夫一定是足智多谋、多才多艺的。

41. 【答案】A

【解析】题干画线单词 incidence 的含义为"发病率"，malaria 意思为"疟疾"，tropical 意思为"热带的"，句型 there is no denial that 意为"不可否认的是……"。各选项含义如下：morbidity 发病率，与画线单词含义相同；precedent 先例；mobility 活动性，灵活性；proficiency 熟练，精通程度。

题干译文：不可否认，在热带地区，疟疾的发病率很高。

42. 【答案】B

【解析】题干画线词组 in sequence 含义为"依次，顺次"；四个选项含义为：at length 详细地，相当于 in details；in order 依次，与题干画线词组含义相同；in advance 提前；in earnest 认真地。

题干译文：我们想让你依次报告那天早上发生的所有事情，不得延误。

43. 【答案】C

【解析】题干画线单词 expedient 的含义为"有利的"。各选项含义如下：beneficent 仁慈的，慈善的；contributive 贡献的，资助的；advantageous 有利的，为正确答案；profitable 有利可图的。

题干译文：大多数演讲者发现对公众发表演讲的时候使用笔记提示是有利的。

44. 【答案】D

【解析】题干画线单词 anonymous 的含义为"匿名的"。四个选项的含义为：undisturbed 不受干扰的；unnoticed 不被注意的；unrecorded 不被记录的；unnamed 匿名的，与题干画线单词含义相同。

题干译文：一些人打电话报警的时候更愿意匿名。

45. 【答案】A

【解析】题干画线单词 immature 的含义为"不成熟的"。各选项的含义如下：puerile 未成熟的，孩子气的，幼稚的，与画线单词词义相同。sophisticated 久经世故的；crude 天然的，未加工的；worldly 世间的。

题干译文：小孩子可能在某一年龄显示出相对早熟的行为模式，并且在后面的年龄段显现出相对不成熟的行为模式。

46. 【答案】B

【解析】题干画线单词 allegiance 的含义为"忠贞，效忠"，与介词 to 连用，固定搭配为：to pledge / swear allegiance to sb. 宣誓 / 发誓效忠某人。四个选项的含义为：truthfulness 真实，坦率；loyalty 忠诚，与介词 to 连用，例如：remain loyal to the principles 信守原则；faith 信仰，信任，与介词 in 连用；endurance 忍耐力。

题干译文：战前，战士们发誓效忠祖国。

47. 【答案】D

【解析】题干画线单词 instantaneous 的含义为"瞬间的，刹那的"。各选项含义如下：instance 实例，情况；spontaneous 自发的，自然产生的；homogenous 同质的；immediate 立即的，即刻的。

题干译文：如果你喝醉了，不要驾车，因为在致命的车祸中死亡就发生在一瞬间。

48. 【答案】A

【解析】题干画线单词 compulsive 的含义为"难控制的"。workaholic 的含义是"工作狂"，unrelenting 的含义是"不宽恕的，不缓和、不松懈的"。各选项含义如下：compulsory 必须做的，如 compulsory courses 必修课；obstructive 妨碍的；constructive 有建设性的；impulsive 冲动的。

题干译文：工作狂总是在任何时候都有难以抑制、不松懈想要工作的需求。

49. 【答案】B

【解析】题干画线单词 exterminate 的含义为"消除"，mosquitoes 意为"蚊子"，flies 意为"苍蝇"。各选项含义为：erase 擦除，抹去；eliminate 消除，符合画线单词含义；demolish 毁坏，推翻；ruin 毁坏。

题干译文：我们尽力消除热带地区的蚊子和苍蝇。

50. 【答案】C

【解析】题干画线词组 exempt from 的含义为"使……免除"，eyesight 意为"视力"，military service 指的是"服兵役"。各选项含义为：prevent from 防止；deprive from 剥夺，使丧失；free from 免于；hinder from 阻碍，例如：A former injury was hindering him from playing his best. 旧伤使他无法发挥出最好水平。

题干译文：你视力不佳，可以免兵役。

51. 【答案】B

【解析】画线词 dominate 的含义是"支配"。boost 的含义是"促进"；govern 的含义是"统治，掌管"；clarify 的含义是"澄清"；pioneer 的含义是"做先驱，开辟"。只有 B 项接近画线词的含义。physiology 的含义是"生理学"，body mass 的含义是"体重"。

题干译文：19 世纪的生理学是以食物能量转化为体重和身体活动的研究为主导的。

52. 【答案】C

【解析】画线词 sensible 的含义是"明智的，合情理的"。realistic 的含义是"现实的"；sensitive 虽然形似画线词，但其含义是"敏感的"；reasonable 的含义是"合情合理的"；sensational 的含义是"轰动的，耸人听闻的"。此题值得注意的是形似画线词的选项很可能不是答案。

题干译文：当然，在采取任何行动前听听别人的意见是明智的。

53. 【答案】D

【解析】画线词 veneration 的含义是"崇敬"。recognition 的含义是"承认"；sincerity 的含义是"真诚"；heritage 的含义是"遗产"；honor 的含义是"荣誉，荣幸"。只有选项 D 与画线词意思接近。ancestor 的含义是"祖先"。

题干译文：中国人极其尊敬他们的祖先。

54. 【答案】D

【解析】画线词 requisite 的含义是"必要的"，例如：He hasn't got the requisite qualifications for this job. 他不具备这项工作所需的资格。perfect 的含义是"极好的，优秀的"；exquisite 与画线词形似，但其含义是"精致的"，例如：Her skirt has very exquisite lace. 她的裙子有非常精致的花边。unique 的含义是"独特的，唯一的"；necessary 与画线词词义相近。managerial 的含义是"管理的"。

题干译文：我努力培养成为管理者所需的必要技能。

55. 【答案】B

【解析】画线词 index 的含义是"指标"；instance 的含义是"事例"；indicator 的含义是"指示"；appearance 的含义是"外表"；option 的含义是"选择"。maintenance 的含义是"保养，维护"。hasten 的含义是"催促"。

题干译文：如果锻炼是身体维护活动和生理年龄的一项指标，那么缺乏足够锻炼可能会导致或者加速衰老。

56. 【答案】A

【解析】画线词 strenuous 的含义是"费力的"，例如：He made strenuous attempts to stop her. 他为阻止她做出了极大的努力。arduous 的含义是"费力的，辛勤的"，例如：Although the work was arduous, he finished it in a short time. 虽然这项工作很费力，他仍然很快就做完了。demanding 的含义是"要求高的"，例如：Teaching is a demanding profession. 教学工作是个要求很高的职业。potent 的含义是"有效力的"；continuous 的含义是"连续不断的"。

题干译文：医生建议 Ken 避免强度大的运动。

57. 【答案】D

【解析】画线词 accountable 的含义是"负有责任的"，例如：I am not accountable to you for my actions. 我没有义务要对你说明我的行动。reliable 的含义是"可靠的"；flexible 的含义是"灵活的，有弹性的"；responsible 通常与介词 for 连用，与画线词近义。

题干译文：这个医院应该有必要就提供的服务质量进行说明。

58. 【答案】C

【解析】画线词 appraise 的含义是"评价，估价"。esteem 的含义是"尊敬"；appreciate 的含义是"感激，欣赏"；evaluate 与画线词近义，意思是"评价"；approve 的含义是"赞成"，通常与介词 of 连用，例如：Her father didn't approve of her marriage to the poor guy. 她父亲不同意她嫁给一个穷小子。

题干译文：绿色和平组织被邀请参加评估这样的经营活动的环境成本。

59. 【答案】B

【解析】 画线词 bleak 的含义是"阴郁的，严寒的，黯淡的"，例如：The future of this firm will be very bleak indeed if we keep losing money. 要是我们继续亏本的话，这家公司的前途会非常黯淡。chilly 的含义是"寒冷的，冷淡的"，例如：chilly welcome 冷淡的迎接；dismal 的含义是"阴沉的，凄凉的"，例如：take a dismal view of economy 对经济不抱乐观态度。promising 的含义是"有希望的，有前途的"；fanatic 的含义是"狂热的"，例如：be fanatic about pop music 痴迷于流行音乐。根据题干语境提示，可以得知 bleak 的含义是"渺茫的"。故 B 正确。

题干译文：公司仍旧希望找到买家，但未来看上去希望渺茫。

60. 【答案】D

【解析】画线词组 bear upon 的含义是"与……有关，影响"；ensure 的含义是"保证，确保"；ruin 的含义是"毁坏"；achieve 的含义是"达成"；influence 的含义是"影响"。vital 的含义是"至关重要的，生死攸关的，有活力的"，例如：The heart is a vital organ. 心脏是维持生命必需的器官。

题干译文：这些是关系到每个人幸福的重要决定。

61. 【答案】B

【解析】画线词 impair 的含义是"损害"。inhibit 的含义是"禁止，抑制"；injure 的含义是"受伤"；induce 的含义是"引诱，导致"，例如：Too much food probably induces sleepiness. 吃得太多可能会引起困意。intervene 的含义是"干涉，干预"。

题干译文：吃药可能会增强记忆，也可能会损害记忆。

62. 【答案】A

【解析】画线词 drawback 的含义是"缺点"；defect 的含义是"缺陷"；assistance 的含义是"帮助"；culprit 的含义是"犯人"；triumph 的含义是"胜利"。

题干译文：这个就是新医疗计划中的严重缺陷吗？

63. 【答案】C

【解析】画线词 exasperate 的含义是"恼怒"。frustrate 的含义是"挫败"；perplex 的含义是"困惑，糊涂"；irritate 的含义是"激怒"；cripple 的含义是"使……跛"。

题干译文：他们正在问的这些问题激怒了这个医生。

64. 【答案】D

【解析】画线词 callous 的含义是"麻木的，无情的"。involuntary 的含义是"非自愿的"；apparent 的含义是"明显的"；deliberate 的含义是"故意的"；indifferent 的含义是"冷漠的"；disregard 的含义是"漠视，忽视"。

题干译文：我们惊讶于这个医生对医学人文层面的无情漠视。

65. 【答案】B

【解析】画线词 panting 的含义是"喘息"。rocking 的含义是"摇动的"；gasping 的含义是"气喘的"；vibrating 的含义是"震动的"；resonating 的含义是"共鸣的，共振的"。akin to 的含义是"类似，近于"，例如：Pity is often akin to love. 怜悯经常类似于爱。

题干译文：多年以来，生物学家已经得知黑猩猩甚至一些猴子能够发出类似于人笑声的气喘声。

66. 【答案】A

【解析】画线词 jolly 的含义是"愉快的"。rejoicing 的含义是"高兴的"；reconciling 的含义是"和解，妥协"；refreshing 的含义是"有精神的"；resenting 的含义是"仇恨，生气"。此题根据 relaxed 的含义，可以得知 jolly 的含义与 relaxed 相近。

题干译文：晚会上每个人都很放松，心情愉快。

67. 【答案】D

【解析】画线词 judicious 的含义是"明智的，审慎的"。四个选项是形近词，要注意辨析。impudent 的含义是"鲁莽的"；imprudent 的含义是"轻率的"；purulent 的含义是"化脓的，脓性的"；prudent 的含义是"审慎的"。antibiotics 的含义是"抗生素"。

题干译文：谨慎地使用抗生素可以治愈细菌感染。

68. 【答案】D

【解析】画线词 hamper 的含义是"妨碍"。endanger 的含义是"使遭受危险"；endure 的含义是"忍耐，持续"；encounter 的含义是"意外遭遇"；encumber 的含义是"阻碍"，例如：The girl's long skirt encumbered her while running. 这女孩子的长裙在她跑的时候阻碍她的行动。

题干译文：他试着跑，但他的断腿阻碍了他。

69. 【答案】D

【解析】画线词 colossal 的含义是"巨大的"。consecutive 的含义是"连续的"；conductive 的含义是"传导性的"；considerate 的含义是"体贴周到的"；considerable 的含义是"相当大的"。

题干译文：整个假期太浪费钱了。

70. 【答案】C

【解析】画线词 controversial 的含义是"有争议的"。inevitable 的含义是"必然的，不可避免的"；applicable 的含义是"可适用的"；disputable 的含义是"有争议的"；incredible 的含义是"不可思议的"。

题干译文：修正有缺陷基因的想法在科学领域不是特别有争议。

71. 【答案】C

【解析】本题考查语义和词汇辨析。画线词 awkwardly 意为"笨拙地"。embarrassingly 意为"尴尬地"，reluctantly 意为"不情愿地"，clumsily 意为"笨拙地"，

dizzily 意为"眩晕地"。故 C 为正确选项。

题干译文：她很笨拙地摔倒了，腿摔折了。

72. 【答案】D

【解析】本题考查固定搭配。anything but 意为"不是……"，与 by no means 同义。more or less 意为"或多或少"，by and large 意为"总的说来"，more often than not 意为"多半"。故选 D。

题干译文：在大多数历史记录中，药学绝对算不上科学。

73. 【答案】B

【解析】本题考查语义。只有 fascinate 表示"吸引"。illuminate 意为"照亮"，alienate 意为"异化"，hallucinate 意为"出现幻觉"。故选 B。

题干译文：学生被医生举例的方式所吸引。

74. 【答案】C

【解析】本题考查语义与词汇辨析。tangible 意为"实际的，有形的，确凿的"，与 substantial 含义相同。intelligible 意为"可理解的"，infinitive 意为"无限的，不定式的"，deficient 意为"不足的"。故选 C。

题干译文：我们需要以数据统计、产品或是金钱回报等有形的方式来证明我们辛勤的工作。

75. 【答案】A

【解析】本题考查近义词辨析。sustain 意为"坚持，维持"，与 maintain 同义。reserve 意为"保留"，conceive 意为"察觉"，empower 意为"授权"。故本题选 A。

题干译文：限制某些食物种类或是承诺不切实际效果的饮食很难长时间维持，或者说长时间坚持会对健康不利。

76. 【答案】A

【解析】discipline 意为"纪律，学科"，与 specialties 意思相同。principle 意为"原则"，rationale 意为"基本原理"，doctrine 意为"教义"。故 A 为正确答案。

题干译文：临床药学的传统学科中处处可见分子学的影响。

77. 【答案】C

【解析】somatic 意为"身体的"，与 physical 含义相同。juvenile 意为"未成年的"，potent 意为"强有力的"，mature 意为"成熟的"，故选 C。

题干译文：一个人往往通过身体体征意识到青春期的开始。

78. 【答案】D

【解析】feasible 意为"可能的，可实行的"，与 viable 同义。rational 意为"合理的，理性的"，reciprocal 意为"互惠的，相应的"，versatile 意为"多才多艺的"，故本题选 D。

题干译文：他的手术应该能成功，因为看上去是可行的。

79. 【答案】B

【解析】intensely 意为"强烈地"，与 vitally 近义。irresistibly 意为"无法抵抗地"，potentially 意为"潜在地，可能地"，intriguingly 意为"有魅力地"。故本题选 B。

题干译文：这些有关质量、特殊护理和经验的益处的问题是极其重要的。

80. 【答案】B

【解析】strategy 意为"策略，技巧"，与 technique 近义。tend 意为"趋向"，notion 意为"理念"，breakthrough 意为"突破"。故本题应选 B。

题干译文：这份指南给出了最佳自我护理的策略和最新医疗发展的信息。

81. 【答案】B

【解析】画线词 a tingle of 的含义是"一丝丝，一阵阵"，这里指的是一阵激动。A 项 glimpse 的含义是"匆匆一瞥"，因而不能和 excitement 连用；C 项 panic 的含义是"恐慌"；D 项 pack 的含义是"包装，一包"，这两个词都不能和 excitement 连用；B 项 gust 表示"一阵（风）"。

题干译文：她是个疯狂的歌迷，见到迈克尔·杰克逊的时候她感到很激动。

82. 【答案】C

【解析】画线词 transcend 的含义是"超越"；A 项 discipline 的含义是"训练"；B 项 complain 的含义是"抱怨"，常与 about 连用；C 项 conquer 的含义是"克服，征服"；D 项 defy 的含义是"藐视，公然对抗"。

题干译文：母亲对弟弟的偏心使她心生怨恨，无法释怀。

83. 【答案】A

【解析】画线单词 trifle with 是"玩弄，轻视"的含义，与 belittle 同义。exaggerate 意为"夸张"；ponder 意为"思考"；eliminate 意为"删除，清除"。故本题选 A。

题干译文：任何人都不能小看这种恐惧，也不能向它妥协。

84. 【答案】B

【解析】画线单词 in light of 意思是"从……方面，考虑到……"，与 in view of 同义。in place of 意为"反而，然而"，与 instead of 同义；in spite of 意为"尽管"；in search of 意为"寻找"。故本题选 B。

题干译文：考虑到他的良好记录，警察接受了他的辩护。

85. 【答案】D

【解析】画线单词 terminate 意思是"终止，停止"，与 suspend"延迟，停止"同义。accuse 意为"控诉"；punish 意为"惩罚"；dismiss 意为"解散"。故选 D。

题干译文：市政府官员说，在应聘申请中有撒谎嫌疑的人会被终止聘用。

86. 【答案】B

【解析】画线单词 be blamed for 意思是"承担……责任"，与 be ascribed to 意思相近。be attached to 意为"附属于"；be composed of 意为"由……组成"；be related to 意为"与……有关"。故本题选 B。

题干译文：2009 年 4 月墨西哥城外猪流感的爆发造成一百多人死亡。

87. 【答案】A

【解析】画线单词 discharge 意思是"释放，散发"，与 put out 同义。pass off 意为"消失"；pull out 意为"拔出，拉出"；send out 意为"派出"。故本题选 A。

题干译文：森林起火燃烧时，会释放成百上千种化合物，包括一氧化碳。

88. 【答案】A

【解析】画线单词 from scratch 的意思是"从头做起，从零做起"，与 from the beginning 同义。from now on 意为"从现在起"；from time to time 意为"时不时，经常"；from the bottom 意为"从底部"。故本题选 A。

题干译文：不幸的是，修建中的桥在地震中坍塌了，他们不得不从头开始。

89. 【答案】D

【解析】画线单词 promise 的意思是"承诺，使很有可能"，与 ensure 含义相同。administer 意为"管理"；nurture 意为"培育"；inspire 意为"鼓励"。故选 D。

题干译文：双胞胎姐妹让英国科学家在白血病研究上有了突破，能使治疗方案效果更好，副作用更少。

90. 【答案】A

【解析】画线单词 disruption 的意思是"破坏"，与 disturbance 含义相近。distraction 意为"分散"；intersection 意为"横断，交叉"；interpretation 意为"解释"。故本题选 A。

题干译文：激进的环境保护主义者谴责杀虫剂中的污染物和合成化学物质破坏了人体荷尔蒙。

91. 【答案】C

【解析】画线词 defect 的含义是"缺陷，缺点"。选项 A 为"赤字"，选项 B 为"误差"，选项 C 为"缺点，缺陷"，选项 D 为"差异，矛盾"。

题干译文：圣诞节期间的购物者应该知道打折销售的产品可能是残次品。

92. 【答案】D

【解析】画线词组 take on 的含义是"承担"。选项 A 为"轻视"，选项 B 为"逃避"，选项 C 为"要求"，选项 D 为"承担"。

题干译文：这个培训项目的目的就是要提高孩子们的责任心以及乐于迎接挑战的勇气。

93. 【答案】B

【解析】画线词 tax 在题干中的含义是"使……承担过重"。选项 A 为"改善"，选项 B 为"使烦恼，负担"，选项 C 为"检查"，选项 D 为"征税"。

题干译文："9.11"事件后，奥运会使得东道国的安保服务承担更大的压力。

94. 【答案】C

【解析】画线词的含义是"惊厥，痉挛，震动，动乱"。此题可根据题干信息得出答案。

题干译文：小丑的表演很搞笑，观众无论大人还是小孩都在大笑。

95. 【答案】A

【解析】画线词的含义是"抵押贷款"，因而答案为 A。

题干译文：我们向中国银行申请抵押借款，并被通知今年年底还清。

96. 【答案】D

【解析】画线词的含义是"完全的，绝对的"。题干中 hypocrisy 的含义是"伪善"。

题干译文：提倡者高度重视体育精神，而反对者则贬低它，声称这完全就是伪善与自我欺骗。

97.【答案】A

【解析】画线词的含义是"不安的，激动的，焦虑的"。选项 A 为"恼怒的，生气的"，选项 B 为"顺从的"；选项 C 为"盖戳的，铭刻的"；选项 D 为"探测"。

题干译文：每当响尾蛇躁动时，它就开始摇摆尾巴并发出很大的响声。

98.【答案】B

【解析】画线词的含义是"洞察力"，选项 A 为"归纳，感应"；选项 B 为"感觉，洞察力"；选项 C 为"解释"；选项 D 为"渗透"。

题干译文：这个侦探对罪犯的伎俩有着不寻常的洞察力，清楚如何抓捕他们。

99.【答案】A

【解析】画线词的含义是"演讲"（传递信息给听众）。

题干译文：我弟弟一遍遍地练习演讲，直到他的发言和对时间的掌控都很完美为止。

100.【答案】C

【解析】画线词的含义是"不合理地"。选项 A 为"不合时宜地，过早地"；选项 B 为"意外地"；选项 C 为"不合理地"；选项 D 为"异常地，不依惯例地"。

题干译文：近几周房价和股价开始从不合理的惊人高位回落。

101.【答案】D

【解析】画线词 indispensable 的含义是"必不可少的"。选项 A 为"不可抗拒的"，选项 B 为"珍视的"，选项 C 为"不可分割的"，选项 D 为"必备的"。

题干译文：所有诺贝尔文学奖获得者的成功都是长期积累的过程，坚持不懈的努力是不可或缺的。

102.【答案】A

【解析】画线词 impart 的含义是"赋予"，选项 A 为"授予，放置"，选项 B 为"展示"，选项 C 为"强加，施加"，选项 D 为"放射，发出"。

题干译文：女王的到来使伦敦白金汉宫的接待酒会多了一份高雅。

103.【答案】B

【解析】画线词 manifest 作为形容词的含义是"明显的，显然的"，与 apparent 同义。选项 A 为"加强的"，选项 C 为"代表性的"，选项 D 为"阴险的，隐伏的"。

题干译文：医生清楚甲状腺功能不全在生长期儿童身上非常明显，表现为身心发展迟缓。

104.【答案】C

【解析】画线词 accommodate oneself to 的含义是"适应"，A 选项与 to 连用，含义为"屈服，让步"，选项 B 的含义是"扩大"，选项 D 的含义是"投向"。

题干译文：眼睛能自动调节适应不同距离，这一机制被应用在自动照相机技术上，并带来一个革命性的技术飞跃。

105.【答案】B

【解析】画线词 exacerbate 的含义是"使加剧，恶化"，与选项 B 同义。选项 A 为"根除"，选项 C 为"征服，击败"，选项 D 为"避免，防止"。

题干译文：不同宗教信仰者之间的区别是常见的，然而正是宗教迫害的压力加剧了冲突，造成了联盟的分崩离析。

106.【答案】B

【解析】画线词 obliterate 的含义是"抹去，擦去"。选项 A 为"复制"，选项 C 为"代替"，选项 D 为"编纂"，只有 B 表示"除去，消除"。

题干译文：毕加索特别贫穷的时候，他可能曾经尝试在帆布上抹掉原始作品重新作画。

107.【答案】A

【解析】画线词 deplore 的含义是"谴责，强烈反对"，与选项 A 近义。选项 B 的含义是"鄙视，轻视"，选项 C 的含义是"推翻，拆除"；选项 D 的含义是"腐烂"。

题干译文：为了保护动物，环境保护者反对核工厂修建项目。

108.【答案】A

【解析】画线词 fidelity 的含义是"忠诚"，与选项 A 同义。选项 B 为"道德"，选项 C 为"品质，特色"，选项 D 为"稳定"。

题干译文：尤其是政治人物，需要严格遵守道德忠贞的标准。

109.【答案】C

【解析】画线词 negligent 的含义是"疏忽的，粗心大意的"，与选项 C 同义。选项 A 为"暴怒的"，选项 B 为"热心的"，选项 D 为"残暴的"。

题干译文：病人抱怨医生疏忽大意，给他的检查不够全面。

110.【答案】A

【解析】画线词 wrath 的含义是"盛怒"，与选项 A 同义。选项 B 的含义是"混乱"，选项 C 为"绝望"，选项 D 为"苦恼，痛苦"。

题干译文：她整个早晨都在心平气和地处理所有投诉。

111.【答案】A

【解析】画线词 prompt 的含义是"激起，促使"。选项 A 为"促使"，选项 B 为"延长"，选项 C 为"迷惑"，选项 D 为"承诺"。

题干译文：英国每年有 1000 多个病人因等不及器官捐赠而死亡，这促使科学家去考虑其他制造器官的方式。

112.【答案】A

【解析】画线词 stigma 的含义是"耻辱，污名"。选项 A 为"耻辱"，选项 B 为"歧视"，选项 C 为"骚扰"，选项 D 为"隔离"。

题干译文：治疗方案的改进改变了艾滋病人的前景，但是对艾滋病仍有严重的歧视。

113.【答案】C

【解析】画线词 lassitude 的含义是"无精打采"。选项 A 为"消耗"，选项 B 为"脱水"，选项 C 为"筋疲力尽"，选项 D 为"残废"。

题干译文：船只失事的幸存者在因为体力透支而导致无力坚持的时候最终获救。

114.【答案】D

【解析】画线词 illegible 的含义是"难以辨认的，不清楚的"。选项 A 为"负面的"，选项 B 为"令人疑惑的"，选项 C 为"雄辩的"，选项 D 为"不清楚的"。

题干译文：科学家发明了立体扫描技术来阅读原本无法辨认的木雕石头，这是一种可以应用在其他领域的方式，比如医疗。

115.【答案】C

【解析】画线词 scrutinize 的含义是"仔细研究"。选项 A 为"期望"，选项 B 为"澄清"，选项 C 为"检查"，选项 D 为"证实，核对"。

题干译文：顶尖的运动员会和教练仔细研究成功和失败，并从中吸取教训，但他们从不会远离自己长期的目标。

116.【答案】D

【解析】画线词 imperative 的含义是"表示权威的"。选项 A 为 challenging"挑战的"，选项 B 为"庄严的"，选项 C 为"有敌意的"，选项 D 为"苛刻的，苛求的"。

题干译文：毋庸置疑的语气显示了他的傲慢自大和刚愎自用。

117.【答案】C

【解析】画线词 eclipse 的含义是"使丧失重要性，使失色"。选项 A 为"擦掉"，选项 B 为"激发"，选项 C 为"使有阴影"，选项 D 为"搁置"。

题干译文：美国和欧盟关于经济合作的讨论可能因为近期日益增多的贸易摩擦而前途叵测。

118.【答案】A

【解析】画线词 foster 的含义是"培育，培养"。选项 A 为"培育"，选项 B 为"消除"，选项 C 为"同化，吸收"，选项 D 为"刺穿，戳穿"。

题干译文：价格快速的增长促使大家相信，未来也会呈更大幅度的增长，高价促进需求，而非压制需求。

119.【答案】C

【解析】画线词 unprecedented 的含义是"前所未有的"。选项 A 为"难以预料的"，选项 B 为"非传统的"，选项 C 为"无法媲美的"，选项 D 是"无法预料的"。

题干译文：摄像技术近期的一些发展允许动物在以前难以接近的地方，以前所未有的详细方式被研究。

120.【答案】B

【解析】画线词 manipulate 的含义是"操纵，应付"。选项 A 为"估计"，选项 B 为"处理"，选项 C 为"改正，校正"，选项 D 为"期望"。

题干译文：一个经验丰富的谈判专家在处理棘手问题时应该很有技巧。

121.【答案】D

【解析】画线词 scrutiny"彻底检查"；A. sanction"准许，批准"；B. restriction"限制"；C. census"统计，调查"；D. examination"检查"。

题干译文：无论怎样，注射死刑都要经过联邦政府审查。

122.【答案】B

【解析】画线词 potent"有力的"；A. inexpensive"廉价的"；B. powerful"强有力的"；C. conventional"传统的"；D. lethal"致命的"。

题干译文：不起眼的西红柿可能成为抗击前列腺癌的利器。

123. 【答案】D

【解析】画线词组 at odds with "与……不一致"；A. in tune with "与……一致"；B. in favor of "赞成，支持，有利于"；C. for the sake of "为了……利益"；D. in disagreement with "与……不一致"。

题干译文：男性对于他们应该照料多少的看法与女性截然不同。

124. 【答案】A

【解析】画线词 eminent "著名的"；A. renowned "著名的"；B. notorious "臭名昭著的"；C. popular "受欢迎的"；D. mysterious "神秘的"。

题干译文：黄山以其自然风光著名，值得一去。

125. 【答案】C

【解析】画线词 diversity "多样性"；A. severity "严重性"；B. reliability "可靠性"；C. variety "种类"；D. specificity "特性"。

题干译文：肥胖是多种因素造成的持续性状态。

126. 【答案】A

【解析】画线词 lapse "过失，小错，疏忽"；A. error "错误"；B. sin "罪恶"；C. guilt "罪行"；D. offense "冒犯"。

题干译文：他通常行为举止端正，这次无礼仅仅是一个过失。

127. 【答案】D

【解析】画线词 jaundice "黄疸，偏见"；A. grievance "委屈，冤情"；B. sympathy "同情"；C. jealousy "嫉妒"；D. indignation "愤怒，愤慨"。

题干译文：你能感受到她评论中的偏见吗？

128. 【答案】B

【解析】画线词组 to little avail 的意思是"没什么用，不奏效"。by no means "绝不"；in vain "徒劳无功"；of no account "没有考虑到"；at stake "处于危险中"。

题干译文：1912 年，德国医生尝试使用甲状腺细胞来治疗甲状腺功能低下的孩子，但丝毫不奏效。

129. 【答案】C

【解析】画线词 lavishly 的意思是"非常浪费地，奢华地"。fearlessly "无畏地"；conspicuously "显著地，明显地"；wastefully "浪费地"；ferociously "厉害地，激烈地"。

题干译文：在很多人看来，他挥霍无度。

130. 【答案】A

【解析】画线词 progression 的意思是"进展"。要注意，"疾病的进展"言下之意是疾病恶化了。deterioration "恶化"；accumulation "积累"；expansion "扩展"；promotion "提升"。

题干译文：现在，没有医疗手段可以阻止风湿性二尖瓣狭窄的恶化。

131. 【答案】B

【解析】画线单词 drowsy 的意思是"打瞌睡的，想睡觉的"，与 sleepy 含义相近，故本题选 B。

题干译文：如果你服用的药物让你昏昏欲睡，就向经理汇报。

132.【答案】D

【解析】画线单词 prevalent 的意思是"流行的，普遍存在的"。crucial "至关重要的"，virulent "有毒的"，colossal "庞大的"，widespread "普遍的"，本题正确答案为 D。

题干译文：糖尿病是世界上最普遍和最具潜在危险的疾病之一。

133.【答案】C

【解析】a multitude of 的意思是"大量的，很多的"，与 plenty of 含义相近。

题干译文：同样，烟灰和烟雾中含有大量的致癌物质。

134.【答案】C

【解析】画线单词 elucidate 的意思是"阐明，解释"。implicate "暗示"，imply "暗示，暗含"，illuminate "阐明，启示"，initiate "发起，开始"。正确答案为 C。

题干译文：关于雌激素效应的许多问题仍有待阐明，各种调查正在通过持续的实验室研究和临床研究来寻求答案。

135.【答案】D

【解析】画线单词 substitute 的意思是"代替，替代"。accomplishment "成就"，refreshment "提神，恢复精神"，complement "补充"，replacement "代替"。正确答案为 D。

题干译文：网络聊天是以咖啡会友的暗淡无力的替代品。

136.【答案】A

【解析】画线单词 overly 的意思是"过度地，极端地"。extremely "极端地"，exclusively "仅仅"，exactly "精确地"，explicitly "清楚地"。本题正确答案为 A。

题干译文：患者住院时间长了，往往会形成过度依赖，不再愿意自己照顾自己。

137.【答案】C

【解析】画线单词 aggravate 的意思是"使恶化"。ameliorate "改善"，aggregate "合计"，deteriorate "恶化"，duplicate "复制"。正确答案为 C。

题干译文：试图限制市中心的停车场进一步加剧了交通堵塞问题。

138.【答案】C

【解析】画线单词 contaminate 的意思是"污染"。inflame "使恶化"，inflict "使遭受打击"，infect "传染，感染"，infiltrate "浸润"。本题正确答案为 C。

题干译文：据报道，细菌污染了美国国内 80% 的零售生鸡。

139.【答案】A

【解析】画线单词 inhibit 的意思是"抑制，遏制"。curb "控制"，induce "诱导"，lessen "减少"，impel "促使"。curb 与 inhibit 含义最相近，因此最佳答案为 A。

题干译文：研究人员最近发布了美国枪支暴力数据，并认为合法持枪的规定并不能阻止暴力犯罪。

140.【答案】C

【解析】画线单词 stereotype 的意思是"刻板印象"。specification"尺寸，规格"，sensation"感觉，知觉"，convention"传统，规约"，conservation"保护，保守"。根据题意，这里强调的是"长久以来形成的固定看法"，与 conventions 的含义最相近，因此最佳答案为 C。

题干译文：无论我们对固定印象如何不安，许多研究仍然显示中西教育差异明显。

141.【答案】B

【解析】competent"合格的，胜任的"，与 capable 含义相同。

题干译文：真正称职的医生，能坐下来，感受他人的"秘密"，表现出对病人的个人兴趣和充分理解。

142.【答案】C

【解析】perceive"认为，认知"。conserve"保留"，theorize"理论化"，realize"意识到"，persist"坚持己见"。本题最佳答案为 realized。

题干译文：医生通常认为治疗是由病人发起的。

143.【答案】A

【解析】lubricate"润滑"。facilitate"帮助，促进"，intimidate"威吓"，terminate"终结"，mediate"调解"。本题 mediate 为混淆选项，调解往往指有矛盾时才调解，而 lubricate 在这里明显是褒义，表达将社区关系向更好的方向发展的只有 facilitate。

题干译文：大型社区聚餐或许能作为社会联系的润滑剂，缓解紧张关系。

144.【答案】D

【解析】exclusively"独一无二地"，与 solely 含义相同。simply 也有"only"的含义，但没有排外性，更多地强调"少"的意义。

题干译文：过氧化氢酶活性降低了谷胱甘肽，维生素 E 水平仅在具有活动性疾病的受试者中降低。

145.【答案】B

【解析】offspring"后代，子孙"。fetus"胚胎"，descendant"后代，继承者"，seed"种子"，orphan"孤儿"。根据题意，正确答案为 B。

题干译文：体外受精繁衍出的后代序列中经常出现眼部异常。

146.【答案】C

【解析】menace"威胁"，与 threat 同义。breach"违背"，grief"痛苦"，abuse"滥用"。

题干译文：童年贫困应被视为儿童面临的最大的公共健康威胁。

147.【答案】C

【解析】deliberately"故意地，有意地"，与 intentionally 含义相同。definitely"确定地"，desperately"绝望地"，identically"相同地"。

题干译文：一个未来的理想是特意引发地震，以可控的方式释放地球构造应力。

148.【答案】D

【解析】convert "转化，转变"，与 transform 的含义相同。apply "应用"，relate "联系"，relay "接力"。

题干译文：巨大的挑战仍然横亘在企业将二氧化碳转化成汽油的道路上。

149.【答案】D

【解析】elicit "引起，诱发"，与 induce 的含义相同。ensue "随之而来"，encounter "遭遇，碰到"，impede "妨碍"。

题干译文：最近有人担心这些药物会引起对认知方面意料之外的副作用，如记忆力减退、思维模糊和学习障碍。

150.【答案】A

【解析】trivial "琐碎的，不重要的"。insignificant "不重要的"，insufficient "不充足的"，substantial "实质的，重要的"，unexpected "意料之外的"。根据题意，正确答案为 A。

题干译文：一叶障目，不见泰山，意思是人们对重要事情的看法被琐碎的事情所蒙蔽。

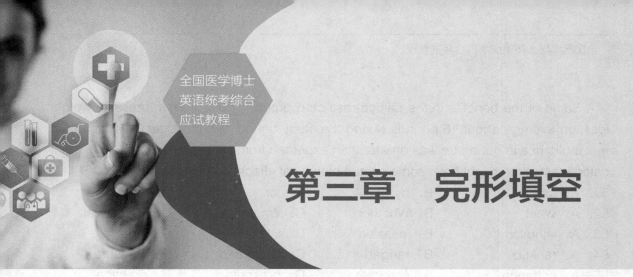

第三章　完形填空

一、考试大纲的要求

根据考试大纲的要求，这部分考题主要侧重测试考生在篇章中理解、运用语言知识的综合能力。此部分的篇章约为 200 个词的短文，短文中有 10 处空白。要求考生在理解全文大意和上下文的基础上，从每题的四个备选项中选出一个最佳答案，使得所填内容符合语法、句型结构以及上下文的逻辑关系。此部分共 10 道小题，每题 1 分，共计 10 分，考试时间约为 10 分钟。通过这一考试要求的表述，我们可以得出这样的结论：完形填空的特点在于它的综合性，考查考生的阅读能力、语法分析能力、词汇掌握熟练程度，因而具有相当的难度。

二、真题演练与解析

 2020 年真题

Scientists have long known a fairly reliable way to extend the life span in lab animals: reduce the amount of calories they eat by 10 to 40 percent.

This strategy, known __51__ caloric restriction, has been shown to increase the life span of various organisms and reduce their rate of cancer and other age-related ailments. __52__ it can do the same in people has been an open question. But an intriguing new study suggests that in young and middle-aged adults, chronically restricting calorie __53__ can affect their health.

In this study, researchers looked at 143 healthy men and women who __54__ in age from 21 to 50. They were instructed to __55__ caloric restriction for two years. They could eat the foods they wanted __56__ they cut back on the total amount of food that they ate to reduce the calories they consumed by 25 percent. Many did not __57__ that goal. But the group saw many of their metabolic health markers improve __58__ they were already in the normal range.

Some of the benefits in the calorie-restricted group __59__ from impressive weight loss, on average about 16 pounds during the study period. But the extent to which their metabolic health got better was greater than expected from weight loss alone, __60__ that caloric restriction might have some unique biological effects on disease pathways.

51. A. as   B. by   C. for   D. to
52. A. What   B. Whether   C. Whatever   D. Whichever
53. A. injection   B. invasion   C. intake   D. input
54. A. ranked   B. ranged   C. fluctuated   D. measured
55. A. enhance   B. entertain   C. preserve   D. practice
56. A. as well as   B. as soon as   C. so long as   D. so far as
57. A. attest   B. affirm   C. assert   D. achieve
58. A. as if   B. so that   C. in case   D. even though
59. A. traced   B. evolved   C. stemmed   D. stimulated
60. A. suggest   B. suggests   C. suggested   D. suggesting

答案与解析

51. 【答案】A
【解析】考查介词。known as... 是固定搭配，意思是"被称为"。该句的意思是"这个策略，被称为热量限制"。

52. 【答案】B
【解析】考查逻辑。前一句说到，这个被称为热量限制的方法，可增加各种生物的寿命，减少罹患癌症和其他与年龄相关的疾病的风险。该句需要一个 wh- 词来引导主语从句，it 指代上文"减少罹患癌症和其他与年龄相关的疾病的风险"，这件事目前在 various organisms 上有效，但对人类是否有效还不得而知。因此这里选择 whether 符合句意。

53. 【答案】C
【解析】考查词义。injection "注射"，invasion "侵略"，intake "摄入"，input "输入"。这里讲的是热量摄入，故 intake 是正确答案。

54. 【答案】B
【解析】考查固定搭配。range...from 是固定搭配，意思是"从……到……"。该句意思是"研究者调查了 143 个健康男性和女性，年龄从 21 岁到 50 岁不等"。

55. 【答案】D
【解析】考查词义。enhance "强化，加强"，entertain "娱乐；招待"，preserve "保留"，practice"实施；练习"。这里想表达受试者按要求实行两年的热量摄入限制。practice 是最佳答案。

56. 【答案】C
【解析】考查逻辑关系。这里讲如何执行热量限制的方案：想吃什么都可以，只要减少 25% 的热量摄入。空格后内容为前面内容的条件。as well as "并且；还"，as soon as "一……就……"，so long as "只要"，so far as "到目前为止"。本题正确答案为 C。

57. 【答案】D

【解析】考查词义。attest "证实"，affirm "确认"，assert "肯定"，achieve "达到"。上一句讲到实施热量限制时的方案和目标，本句顺承下来则是讲是否能达到该目标。因此 D 为正确答案。

58. 【答案】D

【解析】考查逻辑关系。as if "仿佛，似乎"，so that "以便于"，in case "万一"，even though "即使"。上一句讲到：很多人不能达成目标，但仍然能看到自己的新陈代谢指标有所改善，即使指标已经处于正常范围内。

59. 【答案】C

【解析】考查句意。热量摄入控制的益处源于减重。stem from "起源于"，表示因果关系。

60. 【答案】D

【解析】考查非谓语动词。四个选项为 suggest 的不同形式，如果句子缺少谓语动词，则可以考虑 suggest（一般现在时）、suggests（一般现在时第三人称单数）、suggested（一般过去时）；如果有谓语动词，则考虑 suggesting，即非谓语形式。该句主干为 the extent was greater than...，主干完整，所以只能选择 suggesting。

2019 年真题

"Looking at someone's eyes helps us understand whether a person is feeling sad, angry, fearful, or surprised. As adults, we then make decisions about how to respond and what to do next. __51__, we know much less about eye patterns in children — so, understanding those patterns can help us learn more about the __52__ of social learning," Michalska said.

To examine these questions, Michalska and the team of researchers showed 82 children, 9 to 13 years old, and images of two women's faces on a computer screen. The computer was equipped with an eye tracking device that allowed them to measure __53__ on the screen children were looking, and for how long. The participants were __54__ shown each of the two women a total of four times. Next, one of the images was paired with a loud scream and a fearful expression, and __55__ one was not. At the end, children saw both faces again without any sound or scream.

"We examined participants' eye contact when the face was not expressing any emotions, to __56__ if children make more eye contact with someone who is associated with something bad or __57__, even when they are not expressing fear at that moment. We also looked at whether children's anxiety scores were __58__ to how long children made eye contact."

The following three conclusions can be drawn from the study:

1. All children spent more time looking at the eyes of a face that was paired with the loud scream than the face that was not paired with the scream, __59__ they pay attention to potential threats even in the absence of outward cues.

2. Children who were more anxious avoided eye contact during all three phases of the experiment, for both kinds of faces. This had consequences for how afraid they were __60__ the faces.

3. The more children avoided eye contact, the more afraid they were of the faces.

The conclusions suggest that children spend more time looking at the eyes of a face when previously paired with something frightening suggesting they pay more attention to potentially threatening information as a way to learn more about the situation and plan what to do next. However, anxious children tend to avoid making eye contact, which leads to greater fear experience.

51. A. But   B. and   C. Therefore   D. So
52. A. impact   B. benefit   C. development   D. anxiety
53. A. what   B. where   C. why   D. the place
54. A. constantly   B. originally   C. always   D. presumably
55. A. another   B. other   C. the other   D. others
56. A. question   B. object   C. determine   D. express
57. A. threat   B. threaten   C. threatening   D. threatened
58. A. related   B. decided   C. relation   D. decision
59. A. suggest   B. suggested   C. to suggest   D. suggesting
60. A. to   B. of   C. at   D. about

答案与解析

51. 【答案】A
    【解析】文章主题是眼神交流时，面部表情对孩子心理状态的影响。空格前讲的是 adults（成年人）在眼神交流后会决定如何应对。空格后讲到对 children（儿童）的眼神交流模式还知之甚少，空格前后在语义上形成转折和对比关系，因此填入 but 最合适。

52. 【答案】C
    【解析】承接前文：因为对儿童眼神交流模式知之不多，因此多做研究有助于更多地了解孩子的社会学习（social learning）发展。因此 development 是正确答案。

53. 【答案】B
    【解析】考查连接词。measure（测量）为动词，后面跟宾语从句，从句中的谓语为

were looking，因此连接词应该是副词性关联词 where。如果用 what 连接，谓语应该是 were looking at。

54. 【答案】B

【解析】考查副词。该句的大意为：他们＿＿会被展示两个女人的照片，一共展示 4 次。constantly "持续地"，和 always 意思相近。presumably "可能地，预想地"，originally "原本，最初"。可知选项 B 符合句子含义。

55. 【答案】C

【解析】考查固定搭配。前文提到 two，故后文应为 one...the other。注意 another 表示三者以上的范围。

56. 【答案】C

【解析】考查句意和动词。空格前讲到 "当面部表情没有表达出任何情绪时，我们会查看参与者的眼神交流"，并以此来确定孩子们是否会与跟坏事关联的人有更多的眼神接触。question "质疑"，object "反对"，determine "确定"，express "表达"。根据题意，正确答案为 C。

57. 【答案】C

【解析】考查动词形式。这里有一个并列结构 bad or ＿＿＿＿。根据并列结构的语义要求，空格处应填入的单词词性和语义与 bad 相近，因此 threatening 是正确答案。

58. 【答案】A

【解析】考查固定搭配。be related to "与……有关联"，句子大意为：我们也会观察孩子们的焦虑程度是否与更多的眼神交流有关联。

59. 【答案】D

【解析】考查非谓语动词。该句有完整的主谓宾结构，逗号后需要非谓语动词来承担伴随状语的功能，故 suggesting 是正确答案。

60. 【答案】B

【解析】考查介词。be afraid of "惧怕……" 是固定搭配。

2018 年真题

The same benefits and drawbacks are found when using CT scanning to detect lung cancer—the three-dimensional imaging improves detection of disease but creates hundreds of images that increase a radiologist's workload, which, ___51___, can result in missed positive scans.

Researchers at University of Chicago Pritizker School of Medicine presented ___52___ data on a CAD (computer-aided diagnosis) program they've designed that helps radiologist spot lung cancer ___53___ CT scanning. Their study was ___54___ by the NIH and the university.

In the study, CAD was applied to 32 low-dose CT scanning with a total of 50 lung nodules, 38 of which were biopsy-confirmed lung cancer that were not found during initial clinical exam. __55__ the 38 missed cancers, 15 were the result of interpretation error (identifying an image but __56__ it as non cancerous) and 23 __57__ observational error (not identifying the cancerous image).

CAD found 32 of the 38 previously missed cancers (84% sensitivity), with false-positive __58__ of 1.6 per section.

Although CAD improved detection of lung cancer, it won't replace radiologists, said Sgmuel G. Armato, PhD, lead author of the study. "The computer is not perfect," Armato said. "It will miss some cancers and call some things cancer that __59__. The radiologists can identify normal anatomy that the computer may __60__ something suspicious. It's a spell-checker of sorts, or a second opinion."

51. A. in common   B. in turn   C. in one   D. in all
52. A. preliminary   B. considerate   C. deliberate   D. ordinary
53. A. being used   B. to use   C. using   D. use
54. A. investigated   B. originated   C. founded   D. funded
55. A. From   B. Amid   C. Of   D. In
56. A. disseminating   B. degenerating   C. dismissing   D. deceiving
57. A. were mistaken for   B. were attributed to
    C. resulted in   D. gave way to
58. A. mortalities   B. incidences   C. images   D. rates
59. A. don't   B. won't   C. aren't   D. wasn't
60. A. stand for   B. search for   C. account for   D. mistake for

答案及解析

51. 【答案】B
【解析】本题考查上下文关系。第一段讲到用 CT 扫描的优劣势。优势为 3D 成像可以帮助筛查疾病，但同时因为成百上千张影像增加了放射科医生的工作量，这相应也会导致漏筛。in turn 是正确答案。

52. 【答案】A
【解析】本题考查句意。preliminary "初期的"，considerate "体贴的"，deliberate "故意的"，ordinary "普通的"。根据上下文的语义，初期数据是符合题意的搭配。

53. 【答案】C
【解析】本题考查非谓语动词。这里用现在分词的主动形式做方式状语，help sb. do sth. using...。这里非谓语动词的逻辑主语为 radiologist，是主动关系。

54. 【答案】D
【解析】本题考查动词。该项目受到了 NIH 的资助，而不是"调查""起源"或是"建立"。

55. 【答案】D
【解析】通过介词考查逻辑关系。本段第一句讲到，在该研究中，将 CAD 应用于 32

个低剂量 CT 扫描，总共 50 个肺结节，其中 38 个是经初步临床检查未发现的活检证实的肺癌。空格处紧跟其后，是在这 38 个漏掉的癌症病例中……，因此用 in 最合适。

56. 【答案】C

【解析】本题考查动词的含义。disseminating "传播"，degenerating "恶化，退化"，dismissing "打发"，deceiving "欺骗"。根据句意，本题选择 dismissing 最合适，意思是 "……但却当成非癌而搁置了"。

57. 【答案】B

【解析】本题考查逻辑关系。38 个漏诊的案例中，15 个是阐释错误，23 个归因于观察失误。这里需要表示因果关系的词组，只有 B 和 C 符合题意，且前面是结果，observational error 是原因，只有 B 是正确的。

58. 【答案】D

【解析】本题考查名词辨析。本句的大意为 "CAD 在 38 个以前漏诊的癌症中发现了 32 个（84% 的敏感性），假阳性率为每节 1.6 个"。表示 "概率"。

59. 【答案】C

【解析】本题考查句子结构。这里是个省略句，完整的表达应该是：It will miss some cancers and call some things cancer that are not cancers. 因此本题正确答案为 C。

60. 【答案】D

【解析】本题考查句意和词组。原句 The radiologists can identify normal anatomy that the computer may __60__ something suspicious 大意是：放射科医生能将电脑误诊的疑似病例通过正常的解剖手段识别出来。因此本题正确答案为 mistake for，形成前后的对照。

三、考查内容及相应的应试技巧

（一）考查内容

下面就完形填空所涉及的考查内容进行简单讲述。

1. 阅读能力是考查的难点和重点

完形填空是以篇章的形式设置考题，因而值得考生注意的是，此部分考查内容首要就是测试考生的阅读能力。具体地说，这种考查内容主要涉及考生对阅读文章整体脉络、文章上下文逻辑关系的把握。考生在阅读完形填空的篇章时，要注意每一个自然段落的主旨大意，不要仅仅局限于空白处所在的句子。每个段落的主旨大意联系起来就是文章内容的脉络。

2. 词汇、语法是考查的基础

对于词汇的考查，形式和内容类似于词汇部分的 Section A，考查内容涉及形近词的辨认能力、对同义词或近义词的识别能力、对短语或词组的熟悉程度、对短语或词组搭配的掌握。

完形填空考查内容不仅涉及以上要点，而且还涉及语法的应用，主要包括以下一些内容：动词题（时态、语态、非谓语动词）、从句、特殊句型、虚拟语气、倒装等。因而考生要对这些语法项目的内容有所了解，并能灵活运用。

（二）应试技巧

1. 完形填空的解题步骤

第一，通读完形篇章，把握文章脉络

考生不要在不了解篇章大意的情况下，匆忙解题，这会有可能出现由于文章大意掌握不准确，或偏差，连续出现解题错误的情况。所以，考生首先应该将文章快速通读一遍，了解大意，确定每个段落的主旨内容。

第二，进行选择，分析判断

如果是根据上下文解题，就要抓住解题信息。当在句内无法解题时，可以参看上下文多一点的信息，或者暂时跳过该题，不要在一道题上耽误过多时间，因为有时候前面题的答案就在后面的篇章里出现。

第三，再次通读全文，检查结果

做完所有题目后，还要通读一遍全文，从语义、逻辑结构、语法、搭配等方面考虑得出的答案是否合理。

2. 解题策略以及应注意的问题

第一，充分利用篇章知识

通过分析上面的真题，可以很清楚地发现上下文信息对于解题帮助很大。出题人在设置题目的时候，也是要考虑到篇章中是否存在解题信息。基于这两点，考生要把文章发展的脉络、线索作为解题的主要手段，切忌只看到题目出现的某一句。通常没有出现考题的内容对解题很有帮助，不要忽略。

第二，注重表示逻辑关系的衔接词

文章的各种逻辑关系，如列举、结果、让步、对比、目的、条件、转折等，需要通过各种衔接词加以体现和表达。没有这些逻辑词，文章就显得语义模糊不清，不能形成篇章。因而考生要重视这些逻辑词，它们可帮助考生理解文章发展的脉络。

第三，注意答案就在文中

在有些情况下，某一题的答案就隐藏在篇章中，因而考生在理解上下文的时候，要做个敏感的有心人，随时根据自己的发现调整选项的选择。

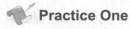 四、完形填空专项练习及最新真题解析

Practice One

If we accept that we cannot prevent science and technology from changing our world, we can at least try to __1__ that the changes they make are in the right directions. In a democratic society, this means that the public needs to have a basic understanding of science, __2__ it can make informed decisions and not __3__ them in the hands of experts. At the moment, the public has a rather ambivalent attitude __4__ science. It has come to expect the steady increase in the standard of __5__ that new developments in science and technology have brought to continue, but it also distrusts science because it doesn't understand it. This distrust is evident in the cartoon __6__ of the mad scientist working in his laboratory to produce a Frankenstein. It is also an important __7__ behind support for the Green parties.

What can be done to __8__ this interest and give the public the scientific background it needs to make informed decisions on subjects like acid rain, the greenhouse effect, nuclear weapons, and genetic engineering? Clearly, the basis must lie in what is taught in schools. But in schools science is often __9__ in a dry and uninteresting manner. Children learn it by rote to pass examinations, and they don't see its __10__ to the world around them. Moreover, science is often taught in terms of equations. Although equations are a concise and accurate way of describing mathematical ideas, they frighten most people.

1. A. assess   B. discern   C. ensure   D. anticipate
2. A. because   B. so that   C. despite that D. though
3. A. clutch   B. leave   C. fabricate   D. nurture
4. A. about   B. with   C. upon   D. toward
5. A. living   B. life   C. survival   D. lives
6. A. literature   B. person   C. art   D. figure
7. A. role   B. concept   C. element   D. index
8. A. constrain   B. harness   C. foster   D. extinguish
9. A. presented   B. conducted   C. portrayed   D. utilized
10. A. meaning   B. contribution   C. application   D. relevance

短文概要

对科学基本的了解和认知。

答案及解析

1. 【答案】C
    【解析】本题考查句意和动词辨析。题干大意为：我们至少要努力确保科技带来的变化方向是正确的。A 项 assess "评定，估价"；B 项 discern "识别；了解"；C 项 ensure "确保，保证"；D 项 anticipate "预期，预计"。

2. 【答案】B
    【解析】本题考查逻辑关系。题干大意为：在民主社会，这就意味着公众需要对科学有一个基本的了解，以便它做出的明智决策能为公众所知情。A 项 because "因为"；B 项 so that "以便，所以"；C 项 despite that "尽管，不管"；D 项 though "虽然，尽管"。

3. 【答案】B

【解析】本题考查动词词组。题干大意为：……而不是在专家的掌握之中。leave...in the hands of "把……掌控在某人手中"。

4. 【答案】D

【解析】本题考查介词。题干大意为：目前，公众对于科学的态度相当矛盾。attitude toward 是固定搭配，表示"对……的态度"。

5. 【答案】A。

【解析】本题考查固定搭配。题干大意为：一方面公众期望科技新发展继续稳定提高生活水平……根据句意可知本处是指"生活水平"的提高，其正确表达法是 the standard of living。故选 A。

6. 【答案】D

【解析】本题考查名词词义。题干大意为：这种不信任在疯狂科学家的卡通人物身上体现得尤为明显，他创造了一个科学怪人。

7. 【答案】C

【解析】本题考查名词词义，题干大意为：它也是人们支持绿色组织的一个重要因素。A 项 role "角色"；B 项 concept "观念"；C 项 element "元素"；D 项 index "指标"。

8. 【答案】B

【解析】本题考查动词词义。题干大意为：怎样利用这个兴趣给公众补充科学背景知识。A 项 constrain "束缚"；B 项 harness "治理；利用；驾驭"；C 项 foster "培养，养育"；D 项 extinguish "熄灭，扑灭"。

9. 【答案】A

【解析】本题考查动词词义。题干大意为：在学校，科学常常以枯燥乏味的形式出现。A 项 present "介绍，呈现"；B 项 conduct "管理，引导"；C 项 portray "描绘，扮演"；D 项 utilize "利用"。

10. 【答案】D

【解析】本题考查名词词义。题干大意为：孩子们为了通过考试只会死记硬背，他们看不到科学与世界的相关性。A 项 meaning "意义，含义"；B 项 contribution "贡献"；C 项 application "申请"；D 项 relevance "相关性"。

Practice Two

The problem of caring for the weak and sick members of society has existed from the very earliest times. But the idea is a new one in the history of man.

The Greek, for instance, had __1__ public institutions for the sick. Some of their doctors maintained surgeries where they could carry on their work, but they were very small, and only one patient could be treated __2__. The Romans, in times of war, established infirmaries, __3__ were used to treat sick and injured soldiers. Later on, infirmaries were founded in the larger cities and were __4__ out of public funds.

__5__, the Roman influence was responsible for the establishment of hospitals. As Christianity grew, the care of the sick became the duty of the Church. During the Middle Ages monasteries and convents provided most of the hospitals monks and nuns were the nurses.

The custom of making pilgrimages to religious shrines also helped advance the __6__ of hospitals. These pilgrimages were often long, and the travelers had to stop overnight at small inns along the road. These inns were called hospitalia, or guest houses, from the Latin word "hospes", meaning "a guest". The inns connected with the monasteries __7__ themselves to caring for travelers who were ill or lame or weary. In this way the name "hospital" became connected with __8__ for the afflicted.

Since living conditions during the Middle Ages were not very comfortable or hygienic, the hospitals of those days were __9__ clean or orderly. In fact, many a hospital would put two or more patients in the same bed!

During the seventeenth century, there was a general improvement in living conditions. People began to feel that it was the duty of the state to care for its ailing citizens. But it wasn't __10__ the eighteenth century that public hospitals became general in the larger towns of England. Soon, the idea of public hospitals began to spread and they appeared all over Europe.

1. A. a few   B. no   C. many   D. few
2. A. at a time   B. at no time   C. once and again D. once for all
3. A. they   B. that   C. in which   D. which
4. A. supplied   B. recruited   C. built   D. supported
5. A. In the same way B. In a big way   C. In a way   D. In the way
6. A. history   B. idea   C. condition   D. equipment
7. A. devoting   B. that devoted   C. devoted   D. for devoting
8. A. housing   B. hospitality   C. casing   D. friendship
9. A. far from being   B. far to being
   C. so far as to be   D. so much from being
10. A. in   B. by   C. up to   D. until

短文概要

医院发展的历史。

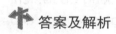答案及解析

1. 【答案】B

【解析】本题考查句意。根据后文可知，Greek 是没有公共医疗机构的，于是有些医生自行建立了一些小的手术室，故 B 项正确。

2. 【答案】A

【解析】本题考查句意和词组。此处句意为：手术室非常小，一次只能为一个病人做手术。故 at a time "一次" 是正确答案。at no time "任何时候都不"；once and again "再次"；没有 once for all 这个词组。

3. 【答案】D

【解析】本题考查定语从句。根据所填词前面的逗号可知，此处为非限制性定语从句，因此 which 是正确的，指代上文的 infirmaries。

4. 【答案】D

【解析】本题考查句意和动词。此处指这些医务室是由公共资金支持赞助的，因此 support 是正确答案。supply "供应"；recruit "招聘"；build "建立"。

5. 【答案】C

【解析】本题考查词组。in a way "在某种程度上"；in the same way "同样地"；in the way "挡道"；in a big way "彻底地，大规模地"。

6. 【答案】B

【解析】本题考查句意和搭配。根据下文可知朝圣的风俗使许多 inns 出现，从而演变成为 hospital，故此处应是帮助提出了 "医院" 的概念。同时，四个选项中只有 idea 可与 advance "提出" 搭配，故本题正确答案为 B。

7. 【答案】C

【解析】本题考查句意和动词。devote oneself to 表示 "投身于……"。

8. 【答案】C

【解析】本题考查句意和名词。casing "包装，保护性的外套"。housing "提供住宅"；hospitality "好客，盛情"；friendship "友谊"。

9. 【答案】A

【解析】本题考查词组。句意：因为中世纪生活条件既不舒适也不卫生，所以那时的医院既不干净也无秩序。far from "没有"；so far as "就……而论，在……的范围内"。

10. 【答案】D

【解析】本题考查固定搭配。句意：直到 18 世纪，在英国一些较大的城镇，公立医院才变得普遍起来。not until "直到……才"。

Practice Three

Women appear to be more vulnerable than men ___1___ many ___2___ consequences of alcohol use. A recent *NIAAA Alcohol Alert* reports that women achieve higher concentrations of alcohol in the blood and become more ___3___ than men after drinking equivalent amounts of alcohol. They are more ___4___ than men to alcohol-related organ damage and to trauma resulting ___5___ traffic crashes and interpersonal violence. This *Alcohol Alert* examines gender differences in alcohol's effects and considers some factors that may place women at risk for alcohol-related problems.

Women's drinking is most common between ages 26 and 34 and among women who are ___6___ or separated. Binge drinking (i.e., consumption of five or more drinks per occasion on 5 or more days in the past month) is most common among women ages 18 to 25. Among racial groups, women's drinking is more prevalent among whites, although black women are more likely to drink heavily.

Household surveys indicate that alcohol use is more ___7___ among men than women in the United States. In one survey, 34 percent of women reported ___8___ at least 12 standard drinks during the previous year compared with 56 percent of men. Among drinkers surveyed, 10 percent of women and 22 percent of men consumed two or more drinks per day on average. Men are also more likely than women to become alcohol ___9___. Men have greater rates of alcohol-use disorders than women. A new study of emotional and alcohol- ___10___ responses to stress has found that when men become upset, they are more likely than women to want alcohol.

1. A. for   B. in   C. to   D. at
2. A. positive   B. adverse   C. side   D. significant
3. A. sober   B. drunk   C. robust   D. impaired
4. A. susceptible   B. adaptable   C. accustomed   D. related
5. A. in   B. from   C. of   D. as
6. A. unmarried   B. housebound   C. divorced   D. hospitable
7. A. prevalent   B. unpopular   C. ordinary   D. preferable
8. A. digested   B. digesting   C. consumed   D. consuming
9. A. dependent   B. independent C. predominant D. disorders
10. A. sensitive   B. insensitive C. craving   D. crazy

短文概要

本文论述男女饮酒后的影响差异。

答案及解析

1. 【答案】C
   【解析】此题解题的关键在于"动词＋介词搭配"。be vulnerable to sth. 表示"更易受……影响"。故答案为C。

2. 【答案】B
   【解析】此题解题的关键在于上下文信息。A项 positive "积极的"；B项 adverse "相反的，不利的"；C项 side "旁边"，side effect "副作用"；D项 significant "重要的"。根据下文内容提到喝酒的不利结果，本段逻辑关系为总分，例证关系。此句含义：女性看上去要比男性更容易受饮酒不利结果的影响。因而答案为B。

3. 【答案】D
   【解析】A 项 sober "清醒的"；B 项 drunk "喝醉的"；C 项 robust "强有力的"；D 项 impaired "受损的"。仅参考此句不能解题，下文提到女性容易患上器官损伤等疾病，因而此处与上下文逻辑关系最吻合的就是 D 项。此句含义：据报告称，与男性相比，饮用同等量酒后，女性血液中的酒精浓度更高，身体更容易受损。

4. 【答案】A
   【解析】解题关键在于固定搭配。A 项 be susceptible to sth. "对……敏感"，与 be vulnerable to 同义；B 项 be adaptable to "适宜于……，适用于……"；C 项 be accustomed to "习惯于……"；D 项 be related to "和……有关"。根据介词 to 后面的名词可知，此处含义为 "患病"，因而 A 项为答案。

5. 【答案】B
   【解析】此题考点为 "动词 + 介词搭配"。result in 含义为 "导致……发生"，例如：Carelessness resulted in the accident. 粗心导致这个事故的发生。result from 意为 "由于"，表示原因，例如：The accident resulted from his carelessness. 事故的发生是因为他的粗心。此处表示原因，因而为 from，选 B。

6. 【答案】C
   【解析】此题解题的关键在于和空白处并列的 separated，因而空白处应该为 separated 的近义词，故答案为 C。

7. 【答案】A
   【解析】根据空白处下一句的数据可以判断此题空白处的词义，故答案为 prevalent，意为 "普遍的，流行的"。D 项 preferable 表示 "更适合，更可取"，与介词 to 连用，例如：Anything is preferable to the tense atmosphere at home. 什么都比家里的紧张气氛要好。

8. 【答案】D
   【解析】根据句意此处含义应该为 "饮酒"，故 A、B 可以排除。digest 的含义为 "消化，吸收"。根据语法知识，report 为谓语动词，故 consume 应该是表示主动的非谓语动词，答案即为 D。此句含义：在一项调查中，与 56% 的男士相比，有 34% 的女士报告说在去年至少饮用了 12 标准杯的酒。

9. 【答案】A
   【解析】根据下文的含义，男士在遇到情感问题或压力的时候，要比女性更想饮酒。所以此空白处的含义应该为 "对酒精的依赖"，答案为 A。B 项 independent "独立的"；C 项 predominant "处于主导地位的"；D 项 disorders 为名词，指的是 "紊乱，失调"。

10. 【答案】C
    【解析】根据句意可以得出答案，句意参考第 9 题。A 项 sensitive "敏感的"；B 项 insensitive "不敏感的"；C 项 craving "渴望的"；D 项 crazy "疯狂的"。

Practice Four

Elderly people respond best to a calm and __1__ environment. This is not always easy to provide as their behaviour can sometimes be __2__. If they get excited or upset they may become more confused and more difficult to look after. Although sometimes it can be extremely difficult, it is best to be patient and not get upset yourself. You should always encourage old people to do as much as possible for themselves but be ready to __3__ a helping hand when necessary.

__4__ memory makes it difficult for the person to recall all the basic kinds of information we take for granted. The obvious way to help in this situation is to supply the information that is missing and help them __5__ what is going on. You must use every opportunity to provide information but remember to keep it simple and __6__.

"Good morning, Mum. This is Fiona, your daughter. It is eight o'clock, so if you get up now, we can have breakfast downstairs."

When the elderly person makes confused statements, such as, about going out to his or her old employment or visiting a dead relative, correct him or her in a __7__ matter-of-fact fashion: "You don't work in the office any more. You are retired now. Will you come and help me with the dishes?"

We rely heavily on the information provided by signposts, clocks, calendars and newspapers. These assist us to organise and direct our behavior. __8__ old people need these aids __9__ to __10__ their poor memory. Encourage them to use reminder boards or diaries for important coming events and label the contents of different cupboards and drawers. Many other aids such as information cards, old photos, scrap books, addresses or shopping lists could help in individual cases.

1. A. excited   B. hasty   C. unhurried   D. nervous
2. A. ridiculous   B. childlike   C. unacceptable   D. irritating
3. A. carry   B. offer   C. lend   D. provide
4. A. Implicit   B. Failing   C. Sensory   D. Semantic
5. A. make sense of   B. make sense
   C. see sense   D. knock some sense into
6. A. complicated   B. implicit
   C. straightforward   D. ambiguous
7. A. calm   B. impatient   C. fussy   D. furious
8. A. Excited   B. Irritated   C. Disappointed   D. Confused
9. A. all the time   B. at times   C. in no time   D. at a time
10. A. remind of   B. compensate for
    C. prevent from   D. derive from

短文概要

本文讨论如何照料老人，尤其是该如何帮助记忆力不好的老年人。

答案及解析

1. 【答案】C

    【解析】A 项 excited "兴奋的"；B 项 hasty "匆忙的"；C 项 unhurried "不慌不忙的，从容的"；D 项 nervous "紧张的"。此题解题关键在于 calm，空白处应该为 calm 的近义词，故答案为 C。

2. 【答案】D

    【解析】此题解题的关键在于后面具体的表述。我们可以得知如果老年人很激动或者紧张不安，他们就会变得很困惑，也很难照料。因而空白处所在句子的含义为：因为他们的行为有时候很恼人，所以这并不容易。A 项 ridiculous "荒谬可笑的"；B 项 childlike "幼稚的"；C 项 unacceptable "不可接受的"；D 项 irritating "恼人的"。

3. 【答案】C

    【解析】此题考点为固定搭配 be ready to lend a helping hand，表示"乐于助人"。

4. 【答案】B

    【解析】A 项 implicit "含蓄的，不直接言明的"；B 项 failing "失败的"；C 项 sensory "感官的"，sensory memory 表示"感官记忆"；D 项 semantic "语义的"，semantic memory 表示"语义记忆"。此句含义：对于一个记忆力下降的人来说，要想回想起我们认为理所当然的基本信息是很困难的。根据句意，B 项正确。

5. 【答案】A

    【解析】A 项 make sense of "理解，弄懂"，例如：I can't make sense of the novel. 我读不懂这本小说。B 项 make sense 有两种含义。①有道理，有意义，例如：Your explanation doesn't make sense. 你的解释不通。②明智的，例如：It makes sense to buy the most up-to-date version. 买最新版本是明智的。C 项 see sense 搭配不存在。D 项 knock some sense into sb. "强使某人理智行事"。此句含义：在这种状况下最直接的办法就是提供已经消失的信息并且帮助他们明白正在发生的事情。

6. 【答案】C

    【解析】A 项 complicated "复杂的"；B 项 implicit "含蓄的"；C 项 straightforward "直截了当的"；D 项 ambiguous "模棱两可的"。根据此句中的 simple 可以推断空白处为 simple 的近义词，故 C 项为答案。此句含义：你一定要利用每一次机会提供信息，但是记得让信息简单且直白。

7. 【答案】A

    【解析】根据后面引语里面的话，可以推断：更正的方式应该是温和且实事求是的。A

项 calm "冷静的"，为答案；B 项 impatient "不耐心的"；C 项 fussy "急躁的"；D 项 furious "发怒的"。此句含义：当老年人出现困惑的时候（因为记忆不好了），要用温和、实事求是的方式纠正他们。

8. 【答案】D

【解析】四个备选单词的含义比较简单，关键看语境含义："我们通常很依赖路标、时钟、日历和报纸提供给我们的信息。这些帮助我们安排、指导我们的行为。"根据这句话的含义我们知道这些都是提醒的作用。那么对于老人来说，尤其是对于记忆力不好的老人来说他们尤其需要这些帮助。根据推断，答案为 confused，表示 "困惑的"。

9. 【答案】A

【解析】A 项 all the time "总是，一贯"；B 项 at times "有时，间或"；C 项 in no time "立即"；D 项 at a time "每次，一次"。

10. 【答案】B

【解析】remind sb. of "使某人想起"，例如：The picture reminds me of France. 这张图片让我想起了法国。B 项 compensate for "弥补"；C 项 prevent from "防止"；D 项 derive from "源自，来源于"。此句含义：使用这些提示可以帮助老年人弥补他们很差的记忆。

Practice Five

Fear is often a(n) ___1___ emotion. When you become frightened, many physical changes occur within your body. Your heartbeat and ___2___ quicken; your pupils expand to admit more light; large quantities of energy-producing adrenaline（肾上激素）are poured into your bloodstream. ___3___ a fire or accident, fear can ___4___ life-saving flight. Similarly, when a danger is psychological rather than physical, fear can force you to take self-protective measures. It is only when fear is disproportional to the danger ___5___ that it becomes a problem.

Some people are simply more vulnerable ___6___ fear than others. A visit to the newborn nursery of any large hospital will demonstrate that, from the moment of their births, a few fortunate infants respond calmly to sudden fear-producing situations such as a loudly slammed door. Yet a neighbour in the next bed may cry out with profound fright. From birth, he or she is more ___7___ learn fearful responses because he or she has inherited a tendency to be more ___8___.

Further, psychologists know that our early experiences and relationships strongly ___9___ and determine our later fears. A young man named Bill, for example, grew up with a father who regarded each adversity as a ___10___ obstacle to be overcome with imagination and courage. Using his father as a model, Bill came to welcome adventure and to trust his own ability to solve problem.

1. A. useful   B. unbeneficial   C. strong   D. mixed
2. A. steps   B. pace   C. responses   D. breath
3. A. Suffering from   B. Confronted with
     C. In relation to   D. In the face of
4. A. avoid   B. hinder   C. delay   D. fuel
5. A. at hand   B. in hand   C. to hand   D. by hand
6. A. in   B. to   C. at   D. on
7. A. tend to   B. attendant upon   C. prone to   D. subjected to
8. A. sensory   B. sensible   C. sensational   D. sensitive
9. A. affect   B. hinder   C. avoid   D. shape
10. A. temporary   B. permanent   C. unconquered   D. formidable

短文概要

本文讨论恐惧的好处以及早期经历对人以后恐惧心理的影响。

答案及解析

1. 【答案】A

   【解析】解此题需要参看下面的信息来确定哪个形容词适合在这里形容恐惧。你害怕的时候，会出现许多身体变化。后面的内容就要具体看出现哪些变化，而且要看出这些变化是积极的还是消极的。因而这道题需要解决所有其他题目之后再决定。此句属于主题句。整个段落都在讲述恐惧的好处，故答案为 A。

2. 【答案】C

   【解析】根据具体的身体变化可以推断空白处的答案。"你的心跳加快，瞳孔放大以接受更多的光，大量用来产生能量的肾上腺激素进入血流。"如果仅仅看本句，可以排除 A 和 B。这时需要继续往下看相关信息。"当遇到火灾或事故的时候，恐惧有助于逃命。"看到这里就可以判断此题 C 项 response 反应加快要比 breath 呼吸加快更恰当。

3. 【答案】B

   【解析】在做出正确选项前，可以推断此处的含义为"遇到火灾或事故"。可以排除 C 项 in relation to "和……有关"。A 项 suffer from "遭受"；D 项 in the face of "面对"。二者虽然含义与此句吻合，但是这两个词组的主语通常为人，因而在这里不合语法。故答案为 B。

4. 【答案】D

   【解析】此题解题的关键在于 similarly，意为"同样地"，即用后面的已知信息推知前面的含义。"同样，当危险是心理上的而不是身体上的时，恐惧可以迫使你启用自我保护的措施。"因而可以推断前面的未知信息是有助于或者促进逃命的含义。答案为 fuel，原意为"提供燃料"。

5. 【答案】**A**

   【解析】此题考点为形近词组辨析。A 项 at hand 意为 "在手边，在附近，即将到来"；B 项 in hand "在手头，在进行中"；C 项 to hand "在手边，随时可以得到"，例如：I'm afraid I don't have the latest figures to hand. 恐怕我手头没有最新的数据。D 项 by hand "用手，亲手"。此句为强调句，含义为：只有当恐惧与即将到来的危险不成比例的时候，它才成为一个问题。

6. 【答案】**B**

   【解析】此题为固定搭配，be vulnerable to "易受……影响"，此句含义：一些人比其他人更容易受恐惧的影响。

7. 【答案】**C**

   【解析】本段举例新生儿。A 项 tend to "倾向于"，意思吻合但不合语法，这个词组为动词短语，不与 be 动词连用。B 项 be attendant upon "随之而来的"，例如：We had all the usual problems attendant upon starting a new business. 我们遇到了创业时通常会出现的所有问题。C 项 be prone to "易于……，有做……的倾向"。D 项 be subjected to "使服从"。此句含义：从出生开始，他或她就更易学习恐惧的反应，因为他或她与生俱来有一种对事物更敏感的趋势。故答案为 C。

8. 【答案】**D**

   【解析】此题考点为形近词辨析。A 项 sensory "感官的"；B 项 sensible "明智的"；C 项 sensational "轰动性的，极好的"；D 项 sensitive "敏感的"。句意参看第 7 题。

9. 【答案】**D**

   【解析】此题解题关键在于后面的例子，由例子的含义可以推断出主题句的大意。D 项 shape 表示 "形成"，与 determine 近义，故 D 为答案。

10. 【答案】**A**

    【解析】事例告诉我们这个叫 Bill 的年轻人由他父亲抚养长大，他的父亲把每一个挫折视为暂时的困难，并且相信智慧和勇气可以战胜困难。根据这句话的含义，他父亲坚定地认为困难不是不可战胜的。A 项 temporary "暂时的"；B 项 permanent "永久的"；C 项 unconquered "不可战胜的"；D 项 formidable "令人可怕的"。只有 A 符合他父亲对困难的态度。

Practice Six

Statuses are marvelous human __1__ that enable us to get along with one another and to determine where we "fit" in society. As we __2__ our everyday lives, we mentally attempt to place people __3__ their statuses. For example, we must judge whether the person in the library is a reader or a librarian, whether the telephone caller is a friend or a salesman, whether the unfamiliar person on our property is a thief or a meter reader, and so on.

The statuses we __4__ often vary with the people we encounter, and change throughout life. Most of us can, at very high speed, assume the statuses that various situations require. Much of social interaction consists of ___5___ and selecting among appropriate statuses and allowing other people to assume their statuses in relation to us. This means that we fit our actions to those of other people based on a ___6___ mental process of ___7___ and interpretation. Although some of us find the task more difficult than others, most of us perform it rather ___8___.

A status has been compared to ready-made clothes. Within certain limits, the buyer can choose style and fabric. But an American is not free to choose the costume（服装）of a Chinese peasant or that of a Hindu prince. We must choose from among the clothing presented by our society. Furthermore, our choice is limited to a size that will fit, as well as by our pocketbook（钱包）. Having made a choice within these limits we can have certain ___9___ made, but ___10___ minor adjustments, we tend to be limited to what the stores have on their racks. Statuses too come ready-made, and the range of choice among them is limited.

1. A. discoveries   B. inventions   C. creations   D. innovation
2. A. go about   B. go by   C. go down   D. go through
3. A. in relation to   B. in line with   C. in the light of   D. on account of
4. A. resume   B. assume   C. consume   D. distinguish
5. A. recognizing   B. realizing   C. identifying   D. interpreting
6. A. instant   B. temporary   C. permanent   D. constant
7. A. trials   B. praise   C. appraisal   D. consideration
8. A. effortlessly   B. unendurably   C. knottily   D. smoothly
9. A. alternations   B. alterations   C. alternatives   D. decisions
10. A. far from   B. in terms of   C. apart from   D. in view of

短文概要

本文就人类的身份进行讨论。

答案及解析

1. **【答案】B**

   【解析】 A 项 discovery "发现"，常表示"原来存在，后来被发现的事物"；B 项 invention "发明"；C 项 creation "创造"；D 项 innovation 作为不可数名词，含义为"创新，改革"，作为可数名词含义为"新思想，新方法"。此句含义：身份地位是人类的发明创造，它使我们能够彼此相处，并且决定了我们在社会中适合的位置。故 B 为答案。

2. **【答案】A**

   【解析】 此题为形近词组辨析。A 项 go about "着手做某事"，例如：How can I go about a part-time job? 我怎样才能找到一份兼职呢？ B 项 go by 有两个含义。

①（时间）逝去，过去，例如：Things will get easier as time goes by. 随着时间的推移，事情会越来越简单。②遵循（某事物），例如：That is the rule you have to go by. 这个规则你必须遵守。C 项 go down "下沉，下跌"，例如：The price of oil is going down. 油价正在下跌。D 项 go through 有三个含义。①仔细察看，例如：I used to start the day by going through e-mails. 过去我常常是从查看邮件开始我新的一天。②经历，遭受，例如：He went through a tough period during the war. 战争期间他经历了很困难的时期。③用完，耗尽，例如：The child went through the whole loaf of bread after school. 放学后这个孩子吃光了整条面包。此句含义：当我们开始一天的生活时，我们会试图从情感上根据地位将人们划分归类。故答案为 A。

3. 【答案】C

【解析】A 项 in relation to "和……有关"；B 项 in line with "符合"；C 项 in the light of "根据，依照"；D 项 on account of "由于，因为"，例如：She retired earlier on account of poor health. 她因为身体不好提早退休了。原句含义参见第 2 题。

4. 【答案】B

【解析】A 项 resume "恢复"；B 项 assume "假定"；C 项 consume "消费"；D 项 distinguish "分辨"。原文大意为：我们假定的身份地位因我们遇到的人而有所不同，并且在一生中都会发生变化。

5. 【答案】C

【解析】A 项 recognize "认出"；B 项 realize "认识到……"；C 项 identify "鉴别，确定"；D 项 interpret "解释，说明"。此句含义：社会交往包含在适合的身份地位中确定、选择并且允许其他的人认定他们和我们有关的身份地位。C 项符合句意。

6. 【答案】D

【解析】此题较难。A 项 instant "立即的，快速的"；B 项 temporary "临时的"；C 项 permanent "永久的"；D 项 constant "持续的"。此句含义：这就意味着我们要根据时刻进行的解释和评价使我们的行为符合其他人的行为。这一过程不是一朝一夕，应该是持久的。这也符合本段第 1 句话告诉我们的：变化调整要伴随一生。（The statuses we assume often vary with the people we encounter, and change throughout life.）

7. 【答案】C

【解析】A 项 trial "试验"；B 项 praise "表扬"；C 项 appraisal "评价，评估"；D 项 consideration "考虑"。只有 C 符合本句含义。原文含义参看第 6 题。

8. 【答案】A

【解析】此题解题关键在于 although 这个连词，这就告诉我们空白处应该为 difficult 的反义词。A 项 effortlessly "不费力气地"；B 项 unendurably "无法忍受地，不能持久地"；C 项 knottily "棘手地，困难多地"；D 项 smoothly "平稳地"。

9. 【答案】B

【解析】此段落用一个比喻做进一步的阐述。A 项 alternation "交替，轮流"；B 项 alteration "改变"；C 项 alternative "选择"；D 项 decision "决定"。此题关键在于 but 后面的 minor adjustments（微调）。因而答案为 B。

10. 【答案】C

【解析】A 项 far from "远离，远非"；B 项 in terms of "根据，按照"；C 项 apart from "除……之外"；D 项 in view of "考虑到，由于"。此句含义：除了做一点微调，我们总是局限于货架上现有的货品。只有 C 项符合此句的逻辑关系。

Practice **Seven**

Most children with healthy appetites are ready to eat almost anything that is offered them and a child rarely dislikes food __1__ it is badly cooked. The __2__ a meal is cooked and served is most important and an __3__ served meal will often improve a child's appetite. Never ask a child whether he likes or dislikes a food and never __4__ likes and dislikes in front of him or allow anybody else to do so. If the father says he hates fat meat or the mother __5__ vegetables in the child's hearing he is __6__ to copy this procedure. Take it for granted that he likes everything and he probably will. Nothing healthful should be __7__ from the meal because of a __8__ dislike. At meal time it is a good idea to give a child a small __9__ and let him come back for a second helping rather than give him as much as he is likely to eat all at once. Do not talk too much to the child during meal time, but let him get on with his food; and do not allow him to leave the table immediately after a meal or he will soon learn to swallow his food so he can hurry back to his toys. Under __10__ circumstances must a child be coaxed or forced to eat.

1. A. if   B. until   C. that   D. unless
2. A. procedure   B. process   C. way   D. method
3. A. adequately   B. attractively   C. urgently   D. eagerly
4. A. remark   B. tell   C. discuss   D. argue
5. A. opposes   B. denies   C. refuses   D. offends
6. A. willing   B. possible   C. obliged   D. likely
7. A. omitted   B. allowed   C. served   D. prevented
8. A. supposed   B. proved   C. considered   D. related
9. A. part   B. portion   C. section   D. quotient
10. A. some   B. any   C. such   D. no

短文概要

本文讲述如何促进孩子的食欲以及一些教育方面的禁忌。

🔺 答案及解析

1. 【答案】D

   【解析】解此题的关键在于此句的含义及逻辑关系。"许多胃口好的孩子总是能够把食物几乎都吃掉。他们几乎不会讨厌食物，除非食物做得太难吃了。"根据句意和逻辑关系，只有 unless 这个含有否定含义的连词最合适。

2. 【答案】C

   【解析】A 项 procedure "程序，手续"；B 项 process "过程"；C 项 way "方式"；D 项 method "方法"。此句含义为：烹饪方式和色泽很关键，菜色很好的食物会促进孩子的食欲。根据这个含义，此题空白处应该为 C，意为"做菜和上菜的方式"。

3. 【答案】B

   【解析】A 项 adequately "充足地"；B 项 attractively "诱人地，吸引人地"；C 项 urgently "迫切地"；D 项 eagerly "热心地"。根据第 2 题的大概含义，应该是菜色好的饭菜会促进孩子的食欲，所以 attractively 符合句意。

4. 【答案】C

   【解析】A 项 remark "评论"，与介词 on 或者 upon 连用，例如：remark on the subject 对于话题的评论。D 项 argue "争论"，与介词 for 或者 against 连用。此句含义：永远不要问孩子是否喜欢还是不喜欢某种食物，也不要在孩子面前讨论喜欢吃的和不喜欢吃的，也不让别人这样做。只有 C 项既符合句意又符合语法。

5. 【答案】C

   【解析】A 项 oppose "反对，对抗"，例如：oppose war and violence 反对战争、暴力；B 项 deny "否认"；D 项 offend "冒犯，违反"。此题空白处单词应该是 hate 的近义词，本句大概含义为：如果孩子听到父亲说他不喜欢吃肥肉或者母亲不吃蔬菜，他也可能会这样。C 项 refuses 为答案。

6. 【答案】D

   【解析】此题表示孩子也有可能像父母那样。表示可能性的说法只有 D 项 be likely to do sth.。A 项 be willing to do "自愿做某事"；B 项 possible，句型为 it is possible for sb. to do sth.；C 项 be obliged to do sth. "不得不，必须做"，例如：I felt obliged to leave after such an unpleasant quarrel. 发生了这样不愉快的争吵之后，我觉得有必要离开。

7. 【答案】A

   【解析】此题解题的关键在于主语 nothing healthful。根据对文章主旨含义的掌握可以判断，有营养的食物不应该认为不喜欢就不去吃，主语为否定词，因而 A 为正确答案。

8. 【答案】A

   【解析】参照此句的大意：有营养的食物不应该认为不喜欢就不去吃。只有 A 符合句意。

9. **【答案】B**

　　【解析】此句大意：就餐时，给孩子一小份比较好，让他能再要一次（食物），而不是一次就给他可能吃完的量。根据句中的 as much as he is likely to eat all 以及 come back for a second helping 可以推断前面为一小份。A 项 part "部分，部件"；B 项 portion "（食物）一份"；C 项 section "部门"；D 项 quotient "份额"。故 B 为答案。

10. **【答案】D**

　　【解析】此句话为倒装句。根据全文对于孩子吃饭的观念，可以判断这里的含义大概为：不要哄骗或者强迫孩子吃饭。因而空白处应该为否定词，under no circumstance 这里的含义就是"在任何情况下都不要……"。

Practice Eight

In ___1___ children, every parent watches eagerly the child's ___2___ of each new skill — the first spoken words, the first independent steps, or the beginning of reading and writing. It is often ___3___ to hurry the child beyond his natural learning rate, but this can set up dangerous feelings of failure and states of worry in the child. This might happen at any stage. A baby might be forced to use a toilet too early; a young child might be encouraged to learn to read before he knows the meaning of the words he reads. On the other hand, though, if a child is left alone too much, or without any learning opportunities, he loses his natural ___4___ for life and his desire to find out new things for himself.

Parents vary greatly in their degree of strictness towards their children. Some may be especially strict in money matters. Others sever over time of coming home at night or punctuality for meals. ___5___, the controls imposed represent the needs of the parents and the values of the community as much as the child's own happiness.

As regards the development of moral standards in the growing child, ___6___ is very important in ___7___ teaching. To forbid a thing one day and excuse it the next is no foundation for morality. Also, parents should realize that "example is better than ___8___". If they are not sincere and do not practise what they preach（说教）, their children may grow ___9___, and emotionally insecure when they grow old enough to think for themselves, and realize they have been to some extent fooled.

A sudden awareness of a marked difference between their parents' ___10___ and their morals can be a dangerous disappointment.

1. A. bringing about　　B. bringing up　　C. bringing down　　D. bringing in
2. A. acquisition　　　　B. attainment　　　C. achievement　　　D. performance
3. A. forcing　　　　　　B. persuading　　　C. allowing　　　　　D. tempting
4. A. potential　　　　　B. talent　　　　　C. enthusiasm　　　　D. capability

5.　A. First of all　　　　B. In detail　　　　C. Above all　　　　D. In general
6.　A. patience　　　　　B. consistency　　　C. consideration　　D. strictness
7.　A. maternal　　　　　B. paternal　　　　　C. parental　　　　　D. school
8.　A. blame　　　　　　B. precept　　　　　　C. action　　　　　　D. revile
9.　A. timid　　　　　　　B. naughty　　　　　　C. confused　　　　D. disappointed
10.　A. principles　　　　B. principals　　　　C. morale　　　　　　D. instructions

短文概要

本文论述父母应该如何教育孩子，以及在教育过程中父母的一些错误行为。

答案及解析

1.　【答案】B
　　【解析】A 项 bring about "引起，导致"，例如：What brought about the change in his attitude? 什么改变了他的态度？B 项 bring up "抚养，提出（讨论等）"；C 项 bring down "减少，打败"；D 项 bring in "提出（新法案等）"。这句话是指在抚养孩子的过程中，因而答案为 B。

2.　【答案】A
　　【解析】A 项 acquisition "（知识、技能等）获得，得到"；B 项 attainment "成就，造诣，达到，获得（success in achieving sth.）"；C 项 achievement "成就"；D 项 performance "表演，表现"。此句含义：父母们总是很热切地观察自己的孩子学会每一个新技能。所以答案为 A。

3.　【答案】D
　　【解析】此句解题的关键在于上下文的逻辑关系。根据第 2 题可以知道在抚养孩子的过程中，父母们都急切地观察孩子学会每一个新技能。此题所在句子继续告诉我们：这也就使得家长急切地希望孩子能超越自然学习的频率而超前学习，但是这就导致孩子心理上危险的失败感和担忧。与上下文父母急切的心情和做法一致的选项只有 tempt to do sth.，表示"诱使，对做什么事情动了心"。

4.　【答案】C
　　【解析】前文提到由于父母急切的心情，使得孩子会超前学习的情况。on the other hand 表示"另一方面"。"如果一个孩子不被关注，或者没有学习机会，他就失去了自己学习新知识的愿望。"此空白处应该为 desire 的近义词。A 项 potential "潜能"；B 项 talent "才能，天赋"；C 项 enthusiasm "热情"；D 项 capability "能力"。只有 C 项表示一种愿望和想法，因而为正确答案。

5.　【答案】D
　　【解析】A 与 C 选项为近义词组，表示"首先，首要的是"；B 项 in detail "详尽地"；D 项 in general 表示总结性，意思是"概括地说，总的来说"。此句话是基于上述父母对孩子的限制和严格管教做出的总结性论述，因而 D 为答案。

6. 【答案】B

　　【解析】as regards "关于，至于"。此句含义为：就儿童成长过程中道德标准的形成而言，某事是至关重要的。此题解题的关键在于下面的具体论述。下一句话提到：不要某一天禁止一件事，而第二天就原谅了，毫无道德基础。这也就说明：在教育孩子的时候，要前后保持一致。四个备选单词中只有 B 项 consistency 表示"一致性，连贯性"，为正确选项。

7. 【答案】C

　　【解析】通篇在讲述父母应该如何教育孩子。A 项 maternal "母亲的"；B 项 paternal "父亲的"；C 项 parental "父母的"。文章没有提到学校教育该如何进行，因而 D 项与文章无关。

8. 【答案】B

　　【解析】此题解题的关键也在于下一句话。这句话大意为：榜样比____更好。下一句提到如果父母不真诚，并不按照他们说教的去做，他们的孩子____。从这句话可以判断题目真正的含义为"身教胜于言教"。B 项 precept 为"规则"，与"言教"近义，是正确选项。D 项 revile 意为"辱骂，斥责"。

9. 【答案】C

　　【解析】前句中提到父母要注意"身教胜于言传"。如果父母不这样去做，说一套做一套，孩子就会____。从字里行间可以推断孩子可能会不知所措，很困惑。A 项 timid "胆小的，怯懦的"；B 项 naughty "淘气的"；C 项 confused "困惑不解的"；D 项 disappointed "失望的"。故答案为 C。

10. 【答案】A

　　【解析】此题解题的关键在于后面的单词 morals（道德标准），空白处需要一个与之近义的单词。principle 含义为"原则"；principal 为名词时，含义为"校长"，为形容词时，含义为"主要的"；morale 含义为"士气"；instruction 含义为"指示，指导"。A 项与 morals 近义。

Practice Nine

Reading involves looking at graphic symbols and formulating mentally the sounds and ideas they represent. Concepts of reading have changed __1__ over the centuries. During the 1950's and 1960's especially, increased attention has been devoted to defining and describing the reading process. Although specialists agree that reading involves a complex organization of higher mental functions, they disagree on the exact nature of the process. Some experts, who regard language primarily as a code using symbols to represent sounds, view reading as simply the decoding of symbols into the sounds they stand __2__.

These authorities __3__ that meaning, being concerned with thinking, must be taught independently of the decoding process. Others maintain that reading is __4__ related to thinking, and that a child who pronounces sounds without __5__ their meaning is not truly reading. The reader, according to some, is not just a person with a theoretical ability to read but one who actually reads.

Many adults, although they have the ability to read, have never read a book in its entirety. By some expert they would not be __6__ as readers. Clearly, the philosophy, objectives, methods and materials of reading will depend on the definition one use. By the most __7__ and satisfactory definition, reading is the ability to __8__ the sound-symbols code of the language, to interpret meaning for various __9__, at various rates, and at various levels of difficulty, and to do so widely and enthusiastically. __10__ reading is the interpretation of ideas through the use of symbols representing sounds and ideas.

1.　A. substantively　　B. substantially　　C. substitutively　　D. subjectively
2.　A. by　　　　　　　B. to　　　　　　　C. off　　　　　　　D. for
3.　A. content　　　　　B. contend　　　　　C. contempt　　　　D. contact
4.　A. inexplicably　　　B. inexpressibly　　　C. inextricably　　　D. inexpediently
5.　A. interpreting　　　B. saying　　　　　　C. explaining　　　　D. reading
6.　A. regarded　　　　B. granted　　　　　C. classified　　　　D. graded
7.　A. inclusive　　　　B. inclinable　　　　C. conclusive　　　　D. complicated
8.　A. break up　　　　B. elaborate　　　　C. define　　　　　　D. unlock
9.　A. purposes　　　　B. degrees　　　　　C. stages　　　　　　D. steps
10. A. By the way　　　　　　　　　　　　B. In short
　　C. So far　　　　　　　　　　　　　　D. On the other hand

短文概要

本文讨论阅读的含义。

答案及解析

1.　【答案】B
　　【解析】文章首句提出此短文的话题：阅读包括看图解符号以及明确地叙述它们所呈现的声音和观点。A 项 substantively "实质上"；B 项 substantially "非常，大量"；C 项 substitutively "替代地"；D 项 subjectively "主观地"。此空白处需要一个程度副词修饰动词 change，因而 B 为正确选项。

2.　【答案】D
　　【解析】A 项 stand by "袖手旁观"，例如：How could you stand by and do nothing for the poor girl? 你怎么能袖手旁观，不为这个可怜的女孩儿做点儿什么呢？B 和 C 选项的词组不存在。stand for "代表"，例如：WTO stands for World Trade Organization. WTO 代表世界贸易组织。此句含义：一些专家把语言看作用符号代表声音的编码，这些人把阅读简单地看成把符号解码成它们所代表的声音。

3. 【答案】B

【解析】A 项 content "满足，满意"；B 项 contend "主张"；C 项 contempt "轻蔑"；D 项 contact "接触，联系"。此处的含义为：这些权威们认为……因而 B 项为正确选项。并且下面一句话中，others 与 these authorities 相对应，而 maintain（主张）则与 contend 对应，为答案复现。

4. 【答案】A

【解析】A 项 inexplicably "费解地，无法解释地"；B 项 inexpressibly "不能表达地"；C 项 inextricably "无法分开地"；D 项 inexpediently "不适宜地"。此句含义为：另一些专家认为，阅读和思维有着一种无法解释的关系。

5. 【答案】A

【解析】此句含义：（那些专家）还认为一个孩子只发音但没有明白含义，就没有真正地阅读。interpret 的含义为 "用语言解释，说明"。

6. 【答案】C

【解析】此段落首句告诉我们：尽管许多成年人有能力阅读，但他们从没完整地阅读。A 项 be regarded as "被看作……"。B 项 granted，固定搭配通常为 take sth. for granted "认为……理所应当"；C 项 be classified as "被划分为……，被界定为……"。D 项 be graded as "被划分等级"。此句的含义为：根据某类专家的观点，他们不能界定为阅读者。下一句中的 definition 也给出了此题解题的关键词。

7. 【答案】C

【解析】解此题的关键在于 satisfactory，意为 "令人满意的"，空白处应该为 satisfactory 的近义词。此句含义为：根据最确实的、最满意的定义，阅读……A 项 inclusive "包含的，包括的"；B 项 inclinable "倾向于……的"；C 项 conclusive "最后的，确实的"；D 项 complicated "复杂的"。

8. 【答案】D

【解析】此句为阅读的定义：阅读就是为了解释说明各种目的的含义，解开语言声音符号密码的能力。A 项 break up "破裂，中断"；B 项 elaborate "精心制作，详尽阐述"；C 项 define "下定义"；D 项 unlock "解开"。故 D 项符合句意。

9. 【答案】A

【解析】此句含义参看第 8 题，为了各种目的。正确选项为 A。

10. 【答案】B

【解析】根据此句话可以推断出这句话为总结性的语句。A 项 by the way "顺便说一下"；B 项 in short "简而言之"；C 项 so far "迄今为止"；D 项 on the other hand "另一方面"。只有 B 项为总结性的短语。

Practice Ten

Culture shock might be called a(n) __1__ disease of people who have been suddenly transplanted abroad. Like most ailments, it has its own symptoms cure.

Culture shock is precipitated by the anxiety that results from losing all our familiar signs and __2__ of social intercourse. Those signs or cues include the thousand and one ways in which we __3__ ourselves to the situation of daily life: when to shake hands and what to say when we meet people, when and how to give tips, how to __4__ purchases, when to accept and when to refuse invitations, when to take statements seriously and when not. These cues, which may be words, gestures, facial expressions, customs, or norms, are __5__ by all of us in the course of growing up and are as much a part of our culture as the language we speak or the beliefs we accept. All of us depend on our peace of mind and our efficiency on hundreds of these cues, most of which we do not carry on the level of conscious awareness.

Now when an individual enters a strange culture, all or most of these familiar cues are __6__. He or she is like a fish out of water. No matter how broad-minded or full of goodwill you may be, a series of props have been knocked from under you, followed by feeling of frustration and __7__. People react to the frustration in much the same way. First they __8__ the environment which causes the discomfort. "The ways of the __9__ country are bad because they make us feel bad." When foreigners in a strange land get together to __10__ about the host country and its people, you can be sure they are suffering from culture shock.

1. A. acute   B. chronic   C. infectious   D. occupational
2. A. symbols   B. signals   C. indications   D. clues
3. A. familiarize   B. orient   C. convert   D. contribute
4. A. do   B. accomplish   C. complete   D. make
5. A. required   B. inquired   C. acquired   D. acknowledged
6. A. adjusted   B. modified   C. rejected   D. removed
7. A. nervousness   B. anxiety   C. excitement   D. grief
8. A. remove   B. refuse   C. reject   D. leave
9. A. guest   B. target   C. host   D. master
10. A. grouse   B. be appraised   C. comment   D. be unsatisfied

短文概要

本文简述文化冲击的成因以及表现。

答案及解析

1. 【答案】D

【解析】空白处需要一个形容词修饰 disease（疾病）。A 项 acute disease "急性病"；B 项 chronic disease "慢性病"；C 项 infectious disease "传染性疾病"；D 项 occupational disease "职业病"。正确选项由后面的定语从句界定：文化冲突可以称作一种职业病，突然移居国外的人常患此病。根据句意，正确选项为 D。

2. 【答案】A

【解析】解此题的关键在于前面的单词 signs，空白处应该为这个单词的近义词。symbol "符号，标志"; signal "信号"; indication "指示"; clue "线索"。此句含义：文化冲突是由在社会交往中，我们所有熟悉的标志和符号的消失引起的。

3. 【答案】B

【解析】此题解题的关键在于后面的介词搭配 to。A 项 familiarize oneself / sb. with sth. "使熟悉，了解"，例如：I need time to familiarize myself with our office procedures. 我需要时间熟悉办公程序。B 项 orient sb. to / towards to sth. "使适应，确定方向"，例如：New students should orient themselves to everything in the new school soon. 新生应该尽快适应新学校的一切。C 项 convert sth. (from sth.) into sth. "使转变"，例如：The hotel is going to be converted into a nursing home. 这家旅馆将要变成一所养老院。D 项 contribute to "为……做贡献"。此句含义：那些符号包括使我们适应日常生活各种状况的 1001 种方式。根据句意，正确选项为 B。

4. 【答案】D

【解析】此题考点为固定搭配，含义为"买东西"，只有 D 项 make 可以与 purchases 搭配。

5. 【答案】C

【解析】此题考点为形近词辨析。require "要求"; inquire "询问"; acquire "获得"; acknowledge "承认"。此句含义：这些提示，也许是文字、手势、面部表情、习俗或者规则，都是在成长的过程中获得的。C 项 acquire 与句意吻合。in the course of "在……过程中"。

6. 【答案】D

【解析】此题解题需要了解本句和下一句的含义。"当一个人进入一个陌生的文化中，所有或者大多数熟悉的提示都不见了。他或她就像是离开水的鱼。" A 项 adjust "调整"; B 项 modify "更改"; C 项 reject "拒绝，抛弃"; D 项 remove "移动，消除"。D 项符合句意。

7. 【答案】B

【解析】此题解题的关键在于 frustration（沮丧），空白处应该为这个词的近义词。原文大意是：无论心胸多么宽阔，多么善意，你都可能遇到一系列的问题，随之而来的就是沮丧和不安。

8. 【答案】C

【解析】根据原文大意，首先人们会排斥让他们感到不适的环境。因而空白处的含义为"拒绝接受，排斥"。只有 C 项符合此意。

9. 【答案】C

【解析】此题为答案复现，在最后一句话中出现了答案 host。这里 host country 的含义为"东道国"。

10. 【答案】A

【解析】此题解题的关键在于"动词＋介词搭配"，grouse about "埋怨，发牢骚";

appraise "评价，评估"，为及物动词，不需要与介词连用；comment 与介词 on 或者 upon 连用，含义为 "表达意见"；unsatisfied 为形容词，固定搭配为 be unsatisfied with，意为 "对……不满意"。

Practice Eleven

One aspect of American culture is a great belief in independence and ___1___. Children are encouraged to be independent. Many children are given ___2___ Americans call a "weekly allowance" and are ___3___ to have part-time jobs at young age: for boys, newspaper routes, and for girls, baby-sitting. Parents often encourage their children to open bank accounts, and some high school and college students have their own credit cards.

Although American families stress independence, America is also a youth-oriented nation, and a great deal of public attention is paid to children. In many American families, husband and wife will ___4___ up their own plans to go to a vacation ___5___ in order to please their children by choosing amusement parks like Disney World and Disneyland. The toy industry in America is large and ___6___ rapidly. Americans buy expensive toys for their children. For an American family, Christmas, Easter, and a child's birthday are ___7___ events. All of these holidays ___8___ on the children. Many American couples form friendships based upon their children's friendships. For instance, two couples often become friends because their children are friends. Television shows on Saturday morning are ___9___ to children, and a lot of advertising is aimed ___10___ children.

1. A. self-respect   B. self-defence   C. self-discipline   D. self-reliance
2. A. what   B. which   C. that   D. when
3. A. forced   B. inspired   C. considered   D. forbidden
4. A. keep   B. turn   C. give   D. put
5. A. spot   B. district   C. zone   D. park
6. A. enlarging   B. increasing   C. growing   D. enhancing
7. A. major   B. critical   C. familiar   D. domestic
8. A. depend   B. fall   C. concentrate   D. center
9. A. turned   B. devoted   C. adapted   D. adjusted
10. A. to   B. for   C. at   D. on

短文概要

本文讲述美国文化中的独立特性以及父母对孩子的重视。

答案及解析

1.　【答案】D

【解析】此题解题的关键在于 independence 的近义词。self-respect "自尊"；self-defence "自我防卫"；self-discipline "自律"；self-reliance "自力更生"。

2. 【答案】A

　　【解析】此题考点为语法知识中的名词从句。从句中缺少宾语，因而正确选项为 A。weekly allowance 指的是 "零花钱"。

3. 【答案】B

　　【解析】根据上文含义，美国父母希望自己的孩子独立。因而这里应该是父母鼓励孩子在小时候就做兼职。与 "鼓励" 近义的选项为 inspire，意为 "激励，鼓励"。

4. 【答案】C

　　【解析】此段首句告诉我们美国家庭重视独立，但是美国同时也是一个关注孩子的国家。因而此句话应该是父母为了取悦孩子放弃自己的度假计划，答案为 give up，意为 "放弃"。keep up "跟上，保持"；turn up "出现"；put up "表现，推荐，提升"。

5. 【答案】A

　　【解析】此题为固定搭配，vacation spot "旅游胜地"。

6. 【答案】C

　　【解析】此句含义：由于美国家庭十分重视孩子，因而美国的玩具业也很庞大，发展迅速。只有 C 项表示 "发展"。enlarge "扩大"；enhance "提高，增强"。

7. 【答案】A

　　【解析】此句含义：对于美国家庭来说，圣诞节、复活节和孩子的生日都是重大活动。critical "关键的"；domestic "国内的"。

8. 【答案】D

　　【解析】depend on "依靠，依赖"；concentrate on "集中于"；center on "以……为中心"。

9. 【答案】B

　　【解析】此句含义：电视节目和大量广告都以孩子为目标。turn to "转向"；be devoted to "致力于"；adapt to "使适合于"；adjust to "调整以适合于"。

10. 【答案】C

　　【解析】aim at 表示 "以……为目标"，是固定搭配。

Practice Twelve

In the last fifty years, modern medical research has made a number of important ___1___ in heart surgery. For example, in 1954, Henry Swan, an American, established cryosurgery — surgery in which the tissue to be cut up is frozen — as a standard procedure. In that landmark operation, Swan ___2___ the patient's body temperature and slowed down the patient's circulation. This ___3___ the surgeon to perform the operation in a dry area. This technique was successful ever since.

Another major advance was the development of open heart surgery. C. Walter Lillehie first accomplished this in 1954. Although open heart surgery is still a __4__ operation, recently surgeons perform it __5__ greater and greater success. A discovery that __6__ to the success of heart surgery was the use in 1963 of an artificial heart to circulate blood during the operation. This gave the patient greater safety and the doctor, Michael De Baker, more working time. Perhaps the most famous and most promising action in heart surgery was made in 1967 by Christian Barnard, a South African. He attempted to __7__ healthy human heart into a person who had a __8__ heart. Although the patient only lived for a short while after the operation, Barnard continued his transplants in other patients __9__ he hoped to perfect the transplanting operation. We all hope that this important advance in heart surgery can be __10__ in the future.

1. A. moves   B. changes   C. advances   D. programs
2. A. maintained   B. leveled   C. measured   D. lowered
3. A. encouraged   B. acquired   C. required   D. urged
4. A. fatal   B. dangerous   C. rare   D. pilot
5. A. with   B. by   C. for   D. in
6. A. contributed   B. attributed   C. distributed   D. committed
7. A. transmit   B. employ   C. transform   D. transplant
8. A. faulty   B. defective   C. weak   D. fragile
9. A. although   B. even if   C. because   D. when
10. A. fostered   B. perfected   C. promised   D. forwarded

短文概要

本文介绍在心脏手术方面的进展。

答案及解析

1. 【答案】C
    【解析】根据下文可知：近 50 年来，现代医学研究在心脏手术方面取得了许多重要的进步。advance 为"进步"的含义。

2. 【答案】D
    【解析】根据前文可知，cryosurgery 是一种在手术中被切开的细胞组织，是冷冻的。因而此部分的含义是：要降低病人的体温，使病人的血液循环减缓。所以 lower 正确。

3. 【答案】C
    【解析】此句含义为：这就要求外科医生要在比较干燥的环境下进行手术。require"要求做……"。

4. 【答案】B

【解析】本句前文提到另一个开心脏手术的进步。根据此句话中的 although 所提示的逻辑关系，再加上后面的 success，因而可以判断这样的手术风险大。A 项 fatal "致命的，致死的"；B 项 dangerous "危险的"。

5. 【答案】A

【解析】此题为介词搭配。with success 相当于 successfully。

6. 【答案】A

【解析】此题考点为固定搭配，contribute to 含义为 "贡献于"，此句含义为：促成心脏手术的发现是 1963 年在手术中使用人造心脏形成血液循环。

7. 【答案】D

【解析】根据上下文可以推断，这个医生试图将一个健康人的心脏移植到有心脏病的病人身上。符合这一含义的只有 D 项 transplant "移植（器官）"。并且在下文出现答案选项，属于答案复现。

8. 【答案】B

【解析】根据第 7 题得知空白处应该为有心脏病缺陷的病人。A 项 faulty "有错误的"；B 项 defective "有缺陷的，有毛病的"；C 项 weak "虚弱的"；D 项 fragile "易碎的，脆弱的"。故答案为 B。

9. 【答案】C

【解析】此题测试考生对原文语句逻辑关系的理解。"尽管那个进行心脏移植手术的病人术后只存活了一小会儿，但这个医生继续在其他病人身上进行移植，因为他希望能完善移植手术。"空白处应该为因果关系，故 C 为正确答案。

10. 【答案】B

【解析】第 9 题提到这个医生的不懈努力，因而在这句话中 "我们也希望心脏手术这一重大进步能在今后更加完善"。B 符合句意。

Practice Thirteen

Planning is a very important activity in our lives yet really sophisticated. It can give pleasure, even excitement, __1__ cause quite severe headaches. The more significant the task __2__ is, the more careful the planning requires. Getting to school or to work on time is a task requiring little or no planning, and it is almost a __3__. A month's touring holiday abroad, or better __4__, getting married, it would be a different matter altogether. If the holiday involves a church wedding, with fifty guests, a reception, a honeymoon in Venice, and __5__ to a new home, this requires even more planning to make sure that it is successful. Planning is our way of trying to ensure success and __6__ avoiding costly failures we cannot afford. It is equally essential and fundamental to mankind as a whole, to individual nations, to families and single people; the __7__ may vary, but the degree of importance does not. In essence, a nation planning its resources and needs does not differ from the familiar weekly shopping or monthly household budget. __8__ are designed to ensure an adequate supply of essentials, at a rate of spending within the limits of __9__ , and if properly carried out, will __10__ shortages, wastage and over-expenditure.

1. A. on the end   B. or   C. least   D. more or less
2. A. arrangement   B. aside   C. ahead   D. above
3. A. assignment   B. burden   C. endeavor   D. routine
4. A. more   B. otherwise   C. still   D. moreover
5. A. attending   B. gripping   C. returning   D. staying
6. A. of   B. for   C. with   D. between
7. A. scale   B. scope   C. extent   D. range
8. A. Some   B. All   C. Both   D. Many
9. A. production   B. wage   C. income   D. property
10. A. avoid   B. keep   C. solve   D. cause

短文概要

规划的定义和重要性。

答案及解析

1. 【答案】B
   【解析】本题考查句子结构。or 表示选择。这里前后两个单词 excitement 和 headache 的意思是相反的，表示选择的话只能用 or。on the end 没有这种搭配；least "最小的，最少的"；more or less "或多或少"，放在文中语义不对。

2. 【答案】C
   【解析】本题考查句意和形容词。ahead "在前面，提前"。该句的意思是：要使将来的任务有意义，就需要用更多的心思来做规划。

3. 【答案】D
   【解析】本题考查句意和形容词。routine "日常工作，日常的事情"。该句的意思是：去上学或者工作不需要做什么规划，这几乎是我们每天都做的事情。assignment "分配，安排"；burden "负担"；endeavor "努力"。

4. 【答案】C
   【解析】本题考查逻辑关系。该句的意思是：如果你幸运的话，你就会在国外度过一个月的假期，或者更好的情况，你结婚了。more "更加"，只能放在被修辞词的前面。otherwise "否则"；moreover "甚至，并且"。

5. 【答案】C
   【解析】本题考查句意和动词。return "返回"，后面用 to 加上地方，表示"回到某地"，这里指"回到家"。attend "出席"；grip "紧握"；stay "停留"。

6. 【答案】A

【解析】本题考查并列结构。and 前后的成分要一致，前面用的是 of 词组，and 后也应用 of，做 our way of 的并列成分。

7. 【答案】A

【解析】本题考查句意和名词辨析。scale "规模"；scope "范围，眼界"；extent "程度，长度"；range "幅度"。这里的意思是：尽管规模不同，但是重要性的程度却是一样的。

8. 【答案】C

【解析】本题考查不定代词。both "两者都"，这里指代国家预算和家庭预算。

9. 【答案】C

【解析】本题考查名词辨析。income "收入"，这里指一个家庭所有的收入来源，范围比其他三个词广。意思是：以收入限制范围内的速度花钱。production "生产"；wage "工资"；property "财产"（包括不动产）。一个家庭的花销一般是根据收入情况来决定的。

10. 【答案】A

【解析】本题考查句意和动词。avoid "避免"。该句的意思是：如果计划实施顺利，将会避免资金不足、浪费，以及过度消费的情况。

Practice Fourteen

Visual impairment carries with __1__ ability to travel through one's physical and social environment until adequate orientation and mobility skills have been established. Because observational skills are more limited, self-control within the immediate surroundings is limited. The visually impaired person is less able to anticipate __2__ situations or obstacles to avoid.

Orientation refers to the __3__ map one has of one's surroundings and to the relationship between self and that environment. It is best generated by moving through the environment and __4__ together relationships, object by object, in an organized approach. With __5__ visual feedback to reinforce this map, a visually impaired person must rely on memory for key landmarks and other clues, which enable visually impaired persons to __6__ their position in Space.

Mobility is the ability to travel safely and efficiently from one point to another within one's physical and social environment. Good orientation skills are necessary to good mobility skills. Once visually impaired students learn to travel safely as pedestrians（行人）they also need to learn to use public transportation to become as __7__ as possible.

To meet the __8__ demands of the visually impaired person, there is a sequence of instruction that begins during the preschool years and may continue after high school. Many visually impaired children lack adequate concepts regarding time and space or objects and events in their environment. During the early years much attention is focused on the development of some fundamental __9__, such as inside or outside, in front of or behind, fast or slow, which are essential to safe, __10__ travel through familiar and unfamiliar settings.

1. A. complex   B. vital   C. restricted   D. remarkable
2. A. varying   B. difficult   C. hazardous   D. distressful
3. A. mental   B. visual   C. graphic   D. demographic
4. A. putting   B. getting   C. reinforcing   D. piecing
5. A. few   B. little   C. much   D. inadequate
6. A. testify   B. affirm   C. identify   D. certify
7. A. flexible   B. independent   C. frequent   D. skillful
8. A. expanding   B. extending   C. continual   D. desperate
9. A. behaviors   B. concepts   C. awareness   D. memory
10. A. comfortable   B. effective   C. efficient   D. efficacious

短文概要

本文介绍了视觉障碍的两个关键因素——定位和移动，以及如何帮助视觉障碍的人群。

答案及解析

1. 【答案】C
   【解析】此题考点为上下文。第 1 句话是视觉障碍的定义，故应该是能力不足或有限，选项 C 正确。

2. 【答案】C
   【解析】此题考点为上下文。此题解题关键可以参考 or 所连接的并列名词 obstacles。这句话的含义是：因为有视觉障碍的人的观察技能比较有限，所以他们在所处环境中的自控能力有限，因此不能预先估计危险状况或者应该避免的障碍。

3. 【答案】A
   【解析】此题考点是上下文。本段讲述定位，并且第 1 句话即为定义。根据本段的细节信息可知视觉障碍的人无法形成视觉图像，故只能依靠移动过程中对于所触及的物体或者地标进行记忆，形成大脑中的图像以保证确定自己的方位。故选项 A 最符合本段含义。graphic 的含义是"图表的"；demographic 的含义是"人口统计学的"。

4. 【答案】D
   【解析】此题考点为上下文。在移动中，把物体之间的关系按照有序的方式结合起来，这样形成最好的心理地图。piece 作为动词，其含义是"把碎片结合起来"，故为正确答案。

5. 【答案】B
   【解析】此题考点为上下文。视觉障碍的人应该是没有视觉反馈的，因而选项 B 符合句意。本句含义为：作为视觉障碍的人，他们不能对物体产生视觉反馈以加强

6. 【答案】B

【解析】此题考点为上下文，且需要形近词辨析。A 项 testify "证明，作证"；B 项 affirm "确定，断定"；C 项 identify "识别，鉴定"；D 项 certify "保证"。此处含义应该是 "通过记忆中的主要地标或者线索确定自己在空间中的位置"，故选项 B 符合句意。

7. 【答案】B

【解析】此题考点为上下文。这个段落介绍移动能力的定义以及对于视觉障碍的人来说移动能力的重要性。段落最后提到 "视觉障碍的人既要学会安全行走又要学会使用公共交通，这样做的目的应该是使得他们能够在社会上独立"，故选项 B 符合语义。句意：一旦视觉障碍的学生学会如何作为行人在路上安全行走，他们也需要学会使用公共交通，以便能够尽可能地独立。

8. 【答案】A

【解析】此题考点为固定搭配。A 项 expanding "扩展的，扩充的"；B 项 extending "伸展的"；C 项 continual "不断的"；D 项 desperate "绝望的，不顾一切的"。根据句意可知应该是满足视觉障碍人更多的需求，所以选项 A 符合句意。

9. 【答案】B

【解析】此题考点为原词再现。上一句提到：许多视觉障碍的孩子缺乏对时间、空间、物体或者环境中事件的概念。所以下一句提到在他们早期培训中，重点要集中在他们一些基本概念的建立上。根据这一逻辑关系，选项 B 为答案。

10. 【答案】C

【解析】此题考点为上下文。B 项 "有效的"，尤指能看得到效果和成效的；D 项 efficacious 的含义是 "灵验的，有效的"。最后一句提到这些基本的概念是他们在熟悉或不熟悉环境中安全行走的基础。除了 "安全的" 以外，符合句意的形容词只有 C。

Practice Fifteen

Without exposure to the cultural, intellectual, and moral traditions that are our heritage, we are excluded from a common world that __1__ generations. On the one hand, such exclusion tends to __2__ us to recreate everything, a needless and largely impossible task; on the other hand, it tends to make us __3__, to suggest that we are indeed the creators of the world and of all good ideas — __4__ in fact we are only a fragment of the history of man. __5__ entirely to ourselves, we could make only the slimmest contributions to wisdom.

While the humanities overlap the fine and liberal arts, they are also related of necessity to the science and to technology. Some of the __6__ of the humanities raise questions about what ends are worthy to be __7__, what ideals deserve __8__. But since it is futile to know what is worth doing without having any idea of how to get things done, effective study in the humanities requires respect for and attainment of factual knowledge and technological skill. __9__, it is pointless to know how to get things done without having any idea what is worth doing, so that informed study in applied science demands __10__ in the humanities.

1. A. crosses   B. passes down   C. survives   D. exists
2. A. warn   B. facilitate   C. compel   D. encourage
3. A. arrogant   B. exhausted   C. productive   D. reliable
4. A. since   B. when   C. whereas   D. which
5. A. Provided   B. Left   C. Reserved   D. Kept
6. A. arenas   B. communities   C. subjects   D. disciplines
7. A. followed   B. investigated   C. served   D. abandoned
8. A. identification B. maintenance   C. reverence   D. endeavor
9. A. Similarly   B. Contrarily   C. Virtually   D. Literally
10. A. concentration B. presupposition   C. revelation   D. reflection

短文概要

人文学科与应用科学的关系。

答案及解析

1. 【答案】B
   【解析】B。本题考查文意和动词。cross "交叉，横断"；pass down "传承"；survive "生存"；exist "存在"。B 符合文意。

2. 【答案】C
   【解析】本题考查文意和动词。warn "警告，提醒"；facilitate "促进，帮助"；compel "强迫，迫使"；encourage "鼓励，怂恿"。C 项符合文意。

3. 【答案】A
   【解析】A。本题考查文意和形容词。arrogant "自大的，傲慢的"；exhausted "疲惫的，耗尽的"；productive "能生产的，有生产力的"；reliable "可靠的，可信赖的"。根据句意，正确答案为 A。

4. 【答案】C
   【解析】C。本题考查上下文逻辑关系。空格前后的句子是转折关系。since 表示因果，when 表示时间，whereas 表示转折和对比，which 则表示 "哪一个"。故本题正确答案为 C。

5. 【答案】D
   【解析】D。本题考查动词的固定搭配。provide for sb. "为……提供"；leave to sb. "留给……，交托……"；reserve "预防，储备"；keep to oneself "不

6. 【答案】C

   【解析】C。本题考查文意和名词。arena "竞技场"；community "社区，团体"；subject "学科，科目"；discipline "纪律"。空格前提到 to the science and to technology，这些都属于 subjects。故本题正确答案为 C。

7. 【答案】A

   【解析】A。本题考查上下文语义和动词的惯用法。follow "听从，跟随"；investigate "研究，调查"；serve "服务"；abandon "放弃"。根据句意，正确答案为 A。

8. 【答案】B

   【解析】B。本题考查文意和名词。identification "鉴定，识别"；maintenance "维护，维修"；reverence "敬畏，尊敬"；endeavor "努力，尽力"。根据文意，正确答案为 B。

9. 【答案】A

   【解析】A。空格上句提到的 futile 意思是 "无用的，无效的"。空格所在的句子中 pointless 意为 "无意义的"，前后语义走向是一致的。similarly "同样地，类似地"；contrarily "相反地，反之"；virtually "事实上，几乎"；literally "逐字地，照字面意义地"。根据题意，正确答案为 A。

10. 【答案】D

    【解析】D。本题考查句意和名词。concentration "专注，集中"；presupposition "假定，预想"；revelation "启示，揭露"；reflection "深思，沉思"。根据题意，正确答案为 D。

Practice Sixteen

Vitamins are organic compounds necessary in small amounts in the diet for the normal growth and maintenance of life of animals, including man.

They do not provide energy, __1__ do they construct or build any part of the body. They are needed for __2__ foods into energy and body maintenance. There are thirteen or more of them, and if __3__ is missing a deficiency disease becomes __4__.

Vitamins are similar because they are made of the same elements — usually carbon, hydrogen, oxygen, and __5__ nitrogen. They are different __6__ their elements are arranged differently, and each vitamin __7__ one or more specific functions in the body.

__8__ enough vitamins is essential to life, although the body has no nutritional use for __9__ vitamins. Many people, __10__, believe in being on the "safe side" and thus take extra vitamins. However, a well-balanced diet will usually meet all the body's vitamin needs.

1. A. either   B. so   C. nor   D. never
2. A. shifting   B. transferring   C. altering   D. transforming
3. A. any   B. some   C. anything   D. something

4. A. serious　　　　B. apparent　　　　C. severe　　　　D. fatal

5. A. mostly　　　　B. partially　　　　C. sometimes　　　　D. rarely

6. A. in that　　　　B. so that　　　　C. such that　　　　D. except that

7. A. undertakes　　　　B. holds　　　　C. plays　　　　D. performs

8. A. Supplying　　　　B. Getting　　　　C. Providing　　　　D. Furnishing

9. A. exceptional　　　　B. exceeding　　　　C. excess　　　　D. external

10. A. nevertheless　　　　B. therefore　　　　C. moreover　　　　D. meanwhile

短文概要

维生素的重要性。

答案及解析

1. 【答案】C

   【解析】选项必须既能引导倒装句，又能与前面的否定相呼应。either 表示"也"，可以用在否定句中，但一般放在句尾；so 可以引导倒装句，但它用在肯定句中，表示"也"；nor 也可以引导倒装句，并可用在否定句中，构成 not…nor…（既不……也不……）固定结构；never 也可以引导倒装句，表示否定，但它必须放在句首。故选 C。

2. 【答案】D

   【解析】由文意可知，空格填入的分词需和 into 搭配，并符合文意。transform 常与 into 搭配，强调的是"事物大的变革或质的改变"。在此从 food（食物）到 energy（能量）的转变是一种质的改变，因此 D 符合句意。shift 不与 into 搭配；transfer 多用于位置的改变，也不与 into 搭配；alter 强调部分或少量的变动，程度较轻。以上三个词都不能表示事物质的改变，故选 D。

3. 【答案】A

   【解析】空格所在句子是一个由 and 连接的并列句，前一个分句 There are thirteen or more of them 中的 them 指的是 vitamins，后一个分句是一个由 if 引导的条件状语从句，意为："如果……缺乏，（会出现）维生素缺乏症。"由于 if 引导的从句中谓语动词 is 是单数，因而只能由一个表示单数意义的不定代词作为备选项。首先排除 some，它一般用于肯定句，做主语时谓语动词用复数；其次 anything 与 something 泛指任何事或某些事，放入句中不符合句意；any 放入后相当于 any of them，即"任何维生素"。注意 any 一般用于否定或疑问句中，做主语时，谓语动词常用单数，故选 A。

4. 【答案】B

   【解析】根据上下文，这里需要填入一个准确描述疾病症状的词。serious、severe 和 fatal 这几个词都表示程度严重，甚至危及生命。但上下文没有暗示缺乏一种维生素会导致严重的后果，因此这三个词都不可作为备选项。apparent 只是简单地描述了疾病的症状，为正确选项，故选 B。

5. 【答案】C

【解析】本句破折号后举例说明维生素的组成成分：碳、氢、氧和_____氮，and 表明各成分之间为并列关系，选项应与 usually 相呼应。usually 是频率副词，选项也应是频率副词。mostly 和 partially 不是频率副词，而是强调事物部分与整体的关系，rarely 是频率副词，但它含否定含义，若用于句中，之前的连词 and 应改为表示转折关系的 but。故选 C。

6. 【答案】A

【解析】上句提到维生素相似的原因，这句开始提到维生素也是有区别的，由于两个句子是平行的结构，本句的后半句也会解释为什么不同。因此空格处应填入表示因果关系并连接原因状语从句的短语。except that 不表示因果，so that 和 such that 后面接结果。只有 in that 后面接原因，并且空格前面的 different 与介词 in 连用，表示"在哪一方面不同"。故选 A。

7. 【答案】D

【解析】本题考查动词与 function 的搭配。四个选项中能与 function 搭配的只有 perform，即 perform a function（具有……的功能，发挥……的作用），其他选项的常用搭配有：undertake a mission/task/project "承担使命 / 任务 / 工程"；hold a share "持有股份"；play a role/part "扮演……角色"。故选 D。

8. 【答案】B

【解析】本题空格所在句子是让步状语从句的复合句，空格部分和 enough vitamins 构成动名词的复合结构做主句的主语。空格处填入的动名词的逻辑主语也就是后面 although 引导的让步状语从句中的主语，即：the body。动名词所表示的动作必须是 the body 发出来的，又能接 enough vitamins 做宾语。选项中，Supplying，Providing 和 Furnishing 均表示"提供，供应"，动作的发出者不是"身体"。句子表达的含义是身体需要获取维生素的营养，而不是"提供"，因此只有 Getting（获取，获得）符合。故选 B。

9. 【答案】C

【解析】本题空格所在部分是 although 引导的让步状语从句。have use for 是固定短语，意为"需要"，主要用于否定和疑问句中，因此根据所在从句的含义，判断出人体对什么维生素没有营养上的需要。首先排除 external 和 exceptional，因为不存在"外部的维生素"或"例外的维生素"；exceeding 用来指被修饰的成分超出了一般的限度，它不能直接修饰"维生素"；只有 excess 指"超过正常或所需数额的数量"，强调"摄入过多的维生素"符合逻辑。故选 C。

10. 【答案】A

【解析】由题意可知，空格处应填入一个逻辑连接词，上文提到，过量服用维生素对身体没有营养价值，接着作者指出很多人的心态：出于"安全"考虑，服用额外的维生素。从语义上看，两句之间存在转折关系，选择项应该是一个表示转折关系的词，因此 nevertheless 符合题意，故选 A。

2017 年真题

It was the kind of research that gave insight into how flu strains could mutate so quickly. The same branch of research concluded in 2005 that the 1918 flu started in birds before passing to humans. Parsing（分析）this animal-human __51__ could provide clues to __52__ the next potential superflu, which already has a name: H5N1, also known as avian flu or bird flu.

This potential killer also has a number: 59%. According to WHO, nearly three-fifths of the people who __53__ H5N1 since 2003 died from the virus, which was first reported __54__ humans in Hong Kong in 1997 before a more serious __55__ occurred in Southeast Asia between 2003 and 2004. Some researchers argue that those mortality numbers are exaggerated because WHO only __56__ cases in which victims are sick enough to go to the hospitals for treatment.

__57__, compare that to the worldwide mortality rate of the 1918 pandemic; it may have killed roughly 50 million people, but that was only 10% of the number of people infected, according to a 2006 estimate.

H5N1's saving grace — and the only reason we're not running around masked up in public right now — is that the strain doesn't jump from birds to humans, or from humans to humans, easily. There have been just over 600 cases (and 359 deaths) since 2003. But __58__ its lethality, and the chance it could turn into something far more transmissible, one might expect H5N1 research to be exploding, with labs __59__ the virus's molecular components to understand how it spreads between animals and __60__ to humans, and hoping to discover a vaccine that could head off a pandemic.

51. A. rejection   B. interface   C. complement   D. contamination
52. A. be stopped   B. stopping
    C. being stopped D. having stopped
53. A. mutated   B. effected   C. infected   D. contracted
54. A. in   B. on   C. with   D. from
55. A. trigger   B. launch   C. outbreak   D. outcome
56. A. counts   B. amounts to   C. accounts for   D. accumulates
57. A. Thereafter   B. Thereby   C. Furthermore   D. Still
58. A. given   B. regarding   C. in spite of   D. speaking of
59. A. parses   B. parsed   C. parsing   D. to parse
60. A. potently   B. absolutely
    C. potentially   D. epidemiologically

答案及解析

51. 【答案】B

【解析】本题考查上下文语义和名词含义。rejection"排异"；interface"接合点，交界"；complement"补充物"；contamination"污染，感染"。空白处前一句话讲到这种流感在鸟类中出现了很多起，才开始向人类传播。因此 parsing（分析）鸟类和人类的交叉感染是符合上下文语义走向的。

52. 【答案】B

【解析】本题考查固定搭配。a clue to doing sth. 的结构中，to 为介词，后面常常跟名词或者动名词形式，意思是"做某事的线索"。

53. 【答案】D

【解析】本题考查动词词义辨析。mutate"变异"；effect"引起"；infect"使感染"。infect 用于疾病感染人，而 contract 用于人感染疾病，文中是人感染疾病，故答案为 contract。

54. 【答案】A

【解析】本题考查介词。"在某个方面"介词常常用 in。on 表示"以……为主题"。

55. 【答案】C

【解析】本题考查语义。疾病"爆发"的表达方式为 outbreak。trigger"诱因"；launch"发起"；outcome"结果"。根据语义，C 为正确选项。

56. 【答案】A

【解析】本题考查语义和动词含义。account for"解释，说明"。count"把……算入"；amount to"达到"；accumulate"积累"。句意：有些研究者认为这些死亡数据有些夸大，因为 WHO 只会将严重到需要去医院就诊的病例算入。count 是最贴切的选项。

57. 【答案】D

【解析】本题考查逻辑关系。still 有让步的含义，意思是"尽管如此"。thereby 表示因果关系，furthermore 表示递进关系，thereafter 表示"之后"。该题上一句讲到有些研究者认为这些死亡数据有些夸大，因为 WHO 只会将严重到需要去医院就诊的病例算入。空格后则强调该数字仍然是惊人的。因此这里选择有让步含义的副词 still。

58. 【答案】A

【解析】本题考查逻辑关系。这里需要原因和条件，只有 given 能有此功能，意思是"鉴于，因为"，这里是连词。speaking of 的意思是"谈到，谈起"。

59. 【答案】C

【解析】本题考查 with 引导的介宾短语充当状语。with sth. doing sth. 结构，在本句中意思是"同时，实验室要探究病毒的分子构成"。

60. 【答案】C

【解析】本题考查句子含义和副词。这里表示可能对人类的传染，只有 potentially 表示"可能地，潜在地"。

2016 年真题

　　Humans are the only species known to have consciousness, awareness that we have brains and bodies __51__ adaptability, that we can affect the course our lives take, that we can make choices __52__ that vastly affect the quality of our lives—biologically, intellectually, environmentally, and spiritually. As humans, we have the ability to mold our __53__ beings to become what or who we wish to become. While some of us may, __54__, have genetic and biological imperatives that may require medication or training to overcome, or at least to modulate, the vast majority of us do, in fact, hold our emotional __55__ in our bank.

　　All that __56__, until the last decade, scientists believed that the human brain and its connections were formed during gestation and infancy and remained __57__ unchanged through childhood. They believed that humans had a given number of neurons in a specific brain structure, and __58__ the number might vary among people, once you were done with childhood development, you were set in this __59__. Your connections were already made, and the learning and growing period of your brain was over. In the last decade, however, researchers have found __60__ evidence that this is not so, and that something called neuroplasticity continues throughout our lives.

51. A. careful about　　B. capable of　　　C. accessible to　　D. susceptible to
52. A. in the event　　　B. in an attempt　　C. at the moment　　D. along the way
53. A. exclusive　　　　B. very　　　　　　C. just　　　　　　D. exact
54. A. indeed　　　　　B. however　　　　C. moreover　　　　D. therefore
55. A. demonstration　　B. dimension　　　C. destiny　　　　D. determination
56. A. has been said　　B. being said　　　C. was said　　　　D. is said
57. A. more or less　　　B. pretty much　　C. as ever　　　　D. if any
58. A. while　　　　　　B. despite　　　　C. nevertheless　　D. since
59. A. case　　　　　　B. mold　　　　　C. sense　　　　　D. condition
60. A. different　　　　B. similar　　　　C. insufficient　　D. significant

答案及解析

51. 【答案】B
　　【解析】文章第一句的大意是：人类是唯一有意识的物种：我们的大脑和肢体能够适应选择的生活轨迹……careful about "当心，注意"；capable of "能够"；accessible to "可接近的"；susceptible to "易受……影响的，对……敏感的"。根据题目含义，本题最佳答案为 B。

52. 【答案】D
　　【解析】根据选项可知，本题考查句意和词组。"...that we can make choices __52__ that vastly affect the quality of our lives..." 的大意是 "这种意识能让我们一直做

出对自己生活产生重大影响的决策"。in the event "在某个事件上"；in an attempt "尝试"；at the moment "当下"；along the way "一路上，沿途"。根据题意，D 为最佳选项。

53. 【答案】B

【解析】本题考查句意和形容词含义。该句的大意为"作为人类，我们都有将自己____的存在变成自己希望变成的样子"。exclusive "专用的，独有的"；very "极端的，正好的"；just "正直的，公正的"；exact "精确的"。根据题干意思判断，very 是最佳答案。

54. 【答案】A

【解析】本题考查逻辑关系。indeed "实际上"；however "然而"表示转折；moreover "并且"表示递进；therefore "因此"表示因果。该句句首 while 表示让步"虽然"，根据语法规则，however 在这里就不能再添加。该句大意是"尽管一些人____有需要药物或者训练才能克服的生理冲动，但绝大多数人可以将情绪____"；第一个空格处填入 indeed 表示强调某种事实，承认这种现象的存在，是最符合语义走向的。

55. 【答案】B

【解析】根据该句的大意为"……大多数人能将情绪控制好"。demonstration "展示"；dimension "体积，范围"；destiny "命运"；determination "决定，意志"。根据题意，选项 B（dimension）是最佳答案。

56. 【答案】B

【解析】本题考查非谓语动词和习惯用法。该句的主谓结构为 scientists believe，因此 all that 后的谓语动词应该相应变成非谓语结构。纵观四个选项，只有 B 符合要求。all that being said 是独立主格结构，充当状语，意思是"综上所述"。

57. 【答案】B

【解析】more or less "或多或少"；pretty much "十分，非常"；as ever "和以往一样"；if any "即使有的话也……"。该句的下文说到，科学家们认为一旦人脑成形，神经元便会保持稳定。由此信息便可知空格中应该为 pretty much unchanged，意思是"保持高度稳定"。

58. 【答案】A

【解析】本题考查逻辑关系。while 放在句首，表示让步，放在句中表示对比；despite "尽管"，表示让步，后面连接的是 that 从句；nevertheless "然而"，表示转折，放在句中时往往用标点隔开；since "因为，既然"，表示因果。"They believed that humans had a given number of neurons in a specific brain structure..." 讲到，科学家们相信在人类某个大脑结构中存在一定数量的神经元。and 后的句子中有两个信息缺失，需要我们找到语义线索来确定逻辑关系。vary "变化"，done with childhood development "完成儿童发展"，be set "定型"，由以上三个重点线索可知，这里的逻辑关系应该为"虽然……变化，但是一旦完成儿童发展，你就会……定型"。因此这里应该选择表示"尽管"的连词。

因引导句子，故 while 是正确答案。

59.【答案】B

【解析】该句的意思是"一旦完成儿童发展，大脑便会定型"。in the mold 是正确答案。
in this case"这种情况"；in this sense"在这个意义上"；in this mold"以这种形式"；in this condition"在这种条件下"。

60.【答案】D

【解析】本题考查语义走向和形容词。different"不同的"；similar"相似的"；insufficient "不充足的"；significant"重要的，有意义的"。文章的最后两句话大意是：你的神经元连接已经成型，大脑的学习和生长阶段已然结束。但是，在最近十年里，研究者们却发现了___的证据，证明情况并非如此，神经重构贯穿人类的一生。这里找到的证据应为"重要的，关键的"。此处并非谈论证据的"相似"或"不同"，而是强调证据对论点的支持力度。因此本题正确答案为 significant。

2015 年真题

A mother who is suffering from cancer can pass on the disease to her unborn child in extremely rare cases, __51__ a new case report published in *PNAS* this week.

According to researchers in Japan and at the Institute for Cancer Research in Sutton, UK, a Japanese mother had been diagnosed with leukemia a few weeks after giving birth, __52__ tumors were discovered in her daughter's cheek and lung when she was 11 months old. Genetic analysis showed that the baby's cancer cells had the same mutation as the cancer cells of the mother. But the cancer cells contained no DNA whatsoever from the father, __53__ would be expected if she had inherited the cancer from conception. That suggests the cancer cells made it into the unborn child's body across the placental barrier.

The *Guardian* claimed this to be the first __54__ case of cells crossing the placental barrier. But this is not the case — microchimerism, __55__ cells are exchanged between a mother and her unborn child, is thought to be quite common, with some cells thought to pass from fetus to mother in about 50 to 75 percent of cases and to go the other way about half __56__.

As the BBC pointed out, the greater __57__ in cancer transmission from mother to fetus had been how cancer cells that have slipped through the placental barrier could survive in the fetus without being killed by its immune system. The answer, in this case at least, lies in a second mutation of the cancer cells, which led to the __58__ of the specific features that would have allowed the fetal immune system to detect the cells as foreign. As a result, no attack against the invaders was launched.

__59__, according to the researchers there is little reason for concern of "cancer danger". Only 17 probable cases have been reported worldwide and the combined __60__ of cancer cells both passing the placental barrier and having the right mutation to evade the baby's immune system is extremely low.

51. A. suggests　　　　B. suggesting　　　C. having suggested　D. suggested
52. A. since　　　　　 B. although　　　　 C. whereas　　　　　D. when
53. A. what　　　　　 B. whom　　　　　　C. who　　　　　　　D. as
54. A. predicted　　　　B. notorious　　　　 C. proven　　　　　 D. detailed
55. A. where　　　　　 B. when　　　　　　 C. if　　　　　　　　D. whatever
56. A. as many　　　　 B. as much　　　　　C. as well　　　　　 D. as often
57. A. threat　　　　　 B. puzzle　　　　　　C. obstacle　　　　　D. dilemma
58. A. detection　　　　 B. deletion　　　　　 C. amplification　　　D. addition
59. A. Therefore　　　　B. Furthermore　　　 C. Nevertheless　　　 D. Conclusively
60. A. likelihood　　　　 B. function　　　　　 C. influence　　　　 D. flexibility

答案及解析

51. 【答案】A
　　【解析】本题考查动词时态。文章第一句为主题句：本周发布的一份新案例研究表明，患癌母亲在极为罕见的情况下，才会将疾病传染给未出生的婴儿。因为本题有非常明确的时间状语 this week，同时医学权威发布的结果应当为有一定代表性的结论，故选用动词的一般现在时。因此本题正确答案为 A。这与第二段中的 This suggests... 形成呼应。

52. 【答案】C
　　【解析】本题考查逻辑关系引导词。本句大意是：一位母亲在分娩几周后被诊断为白血病，而女儿在 11 个月大的时候，在其脸颊和肺部都发现了肿瘤。根据题意，两个分句之间有对比和转折的逻辑关系，因此本题正确答案为 C。

53. 【答案】D
　　【解析】本题考查从句引导词。本题的主句结构完整，意思是该女婴癌细胞中未发现父亲的 DNA，这就让大家认为她是在受孕过程中染上疾病的。这里需要一个引导词，能指代主句内容，同时还能引导从句，只有 as/which 才有此功能。因此本题正确答案为 D。

54. 【答案】C
　　【解析】本题考查句意和形容词。本句大意是：《卫报》称这是第一个得以证实的细胞穿透胎盘屏障的案例。上文用一个日本病人的案例对此进行了证明，因此本题正确答案为 C。

55. 【答案】A
　　【解析】本题考查逻辑关系和从句引导词。本句大意是：这不是微嵌合状态的病例，在该状态下，细胞在母体和胎儿之间发生交换，非常常见。50% 到 75% 的情况下，一些细胞从胚胎游向母体，50% 的情况下则是反向行之。此处从句表示该种情况发生的状态，用 where 最合适。因此本题正确答案为 A。

56. 【答案】D

【解析】本题考查副词。这里表示细胞从母亲到胎儿和胎儿到母亲两种方式的概率，能表示"概率，频率"的，只有 often。因此本题正确答案为 D。

57. 【答案】B

【解析】本题考查句意和名词。这里的大意为：这些越过胎盘障碍的癌细胞如何不会被免疫系统杀死，这是个令人费解的事情。因此本题正确答案为 B。

58. 【答案】B

【解析】本题考查句意与名词。对上面提出的 puzzle，答案是癌细胞进行了第二次变异，使检测异质细胞的免疫系统丧失功能。这里只能选择能表示"消失，磨灭"含义的词，才能符合文意。因此 deletion 是正确答案。

59. 【答案】C

【解析】本题考查逻辑关系。这里上文讲的是母体向胎儿传染癌症的情况，空格后则在舒缓对 cancer danger 的紧张情绪，这是明显的转折关系。因此本题正确答案为 C。

60. 【答案】A

【解析】本题考查句意和名词。这里进一步解释为何不用担心 cancer danger，因为全世界范围内只有 17 个可能性案例，能突破胎盘障碍的癌细胞同时能避免胎儿免疫系统筛查的免疫，两种方式结合起来的可能性实在很低。因此本题选 likelihood。

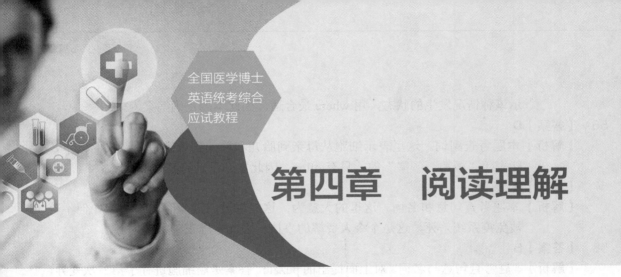

第四章　阅读理解

一、考试大纲的要求

　　该测试部分由 6 篇阅读短文组成，每篇短文约有 300 个单词，每篇文章后有 5 个问题，要求考生根据对文章的理解，在每个问题后的四个备选项中选出正确答案。此部分测试考生通过阅读英文书刊获取信息的能力（包括阅读速度和理解程度）。要求考生在阅读完一篇短文后，能理解其主题思想、主要内容和主要细节；能根据所读材料的内容进行推理判断，理解某些单词和短语在具体语境中的意义，理解句与句之间的内在逻辑关系；能领会作者的观点和思想感情，判断其对事物的态度。测试材料主要涉及医学科普、自然科普和人文等各种题材和体裁的文章。此部分共 30 题，每题 1 分，共计 30 分。考试时间约为 65 分钟。

二、真题演练与解析

　　首先，请各位考生严格按照考试的时间要求，在 65 分钟内实际演练下面的真题。通过演练，一方面，可正确且快速定位自己目前的水平，以便制订相应的复习策略；另一方面，可对医学博士英语统考的阅读部分测试有一个精准的把握，从而在复习过程中有的放矢，提高效率。

Passage One

In a society where all aspects of our lives are dictated by scientific advances in technology, science is the essence of our existence. Without the vast advances made by chemists, physicists, biologists, geologists, and other diligent scientists, our standards of living would decline, our flourishing, wealthy nation might come to an economic depression, and our people would suffer from diseases that could not be cured. As a society we ignorantly take advantage of the amenities provided by science, yet our lives would be altered interminably without them.

Health care, one of the aspects of our society that separates us from our archaic ancestors, is founded exclusively on scientific discoveries and advances. Without the vaccines created by doctors, diseases such as polio, measles, hepatitis, and the flu would pose a threat to our citizens, for although some of these diseases may not be deadly, their side effects can be a vast detriment to an individual affected with the disease.

Yet another aspect of science, discoveries of the world beyond us, has increased our knowledge and contributed to our culture. Such discoveries were once viewed as an impossible task, but the technology brought to life by NASA employees has accomplished this aspiration, and numerous others. In addition, science has developed perhaps the most awe-inspiring, vital invention in the history of the world, the computer. Without the presence of this machine, our world could exist, but the conveniences brought into life by the computer are unparalleled.

Despite the greatness of present-day innovators and scientists and their revelations, it is requisite to examine the amenities of science that our culture so blatantly disregards. For instance, the light bulb, electricity, the telephone, running water, and the automobile are present-day staples of our society; however, they were not present until scientists discovered them.

Because of the contributions of scientists, our world is ever metamorphosing, and this metamorphosis economically and personally comprises our society, whether our society is cognizant of this or not.

61. In the first paragraph the author implies that we _____.
    A. would not survive without science
    B. take the amenities of science for granted
    C. could have raised the standards of living with science
    D. would be free of disease because of scientific advances

62. The author uses health care and vaccines to illustrate _____.
    A. how science has been developed
    B. what science means to society
    C. what the nature of science is
    D. how disease affects society

63. Nothing, according to the author, can match the invention of the computer in terms of _____.
    A. power   B. novelty   C. benefits   D. complexity

64. The author seems to be unhappy about _____.
    A. people's ignorance of their culture
    B. people's ignoring the amenities of science

C. people's making no contributions to society

    D. people's misunderstanding of scientific advances

65. The author's tone in the passage is _____.

    A. critical   B. cognizant   C. appreciative   D. paradoxical

Passage Two

    Biotechnology is expected to bring important advances in medical diagnosis and therapy, in solving food problems, in energy saving, in environmentally compatible industrial and agricultural production, and in specially targeted environmental protection projects. Genetically altered microorganisms can break down a wide range of pollutants by being used, for example, in bio-filters and wastewater-treatment facilities, and in the clean-up of polluted sites. Genetically modified organisms can also alleviate environmental burdens by reducing the need for pesticides, fertilizers, and medications.

    Sustainability, as a strategic aim, involves optimizing the interactions between nature, society, and the economy, in accordance with ecological criteria. Political leaders and scientists alike face the challenge of recognizing interrelationships and interactions between ecological, economic, and social factors and taking account of these factors when seeking solution strategies. To meet this challenge, decision-makers require interdisciplinary approaches and strategies that cut across political lines. Environmental discussions must become more objective, and this includes, especially, debates about the risks of new technologies, which are often ideologically charged. In light of the complex issues involved in sustainable development, we need clearer standards for orienting and assessing our environmental policies. In this context I consider the current work on indicator models as a means to assess and monitor the success of sustainability strategies, to be of great significance.

    Sustainable development can succeed only if all areas of the political sector, of society, and of science accept the concept and work together to implement it. A common basic understanding of environmental ethics is needed to ensure that protection of the natural foundation of life becomes a major consideration in all political and individual action. A dialogue among representatives of all sectors of society is needed if appropriate environmental policies are to be devised and implemented.

66. Biotechnology _____.

    A. can help save energy and integrate industry and agriculture

    B. can rid humans of diseases and solve food problems

    C. can treat pollution and protect environment

    D. All of the above.

67. Wastewater can be treated _____.
    A. in genetic engineering
    B. by means of biotechnology
    C. in agriculture as well as in industry
    D. without the need for breaking down pollutants
68. When he says approaches and strategies that cut across political lines, the author means that they _____.
    A. involve economic issues   B. observe ecological criteria
    C. are politically significant   D. overcome political barriers
69. It can be inferred from the passage that the complexity of sustainable development _____.
    A. makes it necessary to improve the assessing standards
    B. renders environmental discussion possible
    C. charges new technologies risks
    D. requires simplification
70. The success of sustainable development lies in _____.
    A. its concept to be of great significance
    B. good social teamwork
    C. appropriate environmental policies
    D. the representatives of all sectors of society

Passage Three

Folk wisdom holds that the blind can hear better than people with sight. Scientists have a new reason to believe it.

Research now indicates that blind and sighted people display the same skill at locating a sound's origin when using both ears, but some blind people can <u>home</u> in on sounds more accurately than their sighted counterparts when all have one ear blocked. Canadian scientists describe the work in the Sept. 17 *Nature*.

Participants in the study were tested individually in a sound-insulated room. They faced 16 small, concealed loudspeakers arrayed in a semicircle a few feet away. With a headrest keeping their heads steady, the participants pointed to the perceived origins of the sounds.

The researchers tested eight blind people, who had been completely sightless from birth or since a very early age. They also tested three nearly blind persons, who had some residual vision at the periphery of their gaze; seven sighted people wearing blindfolds; and 29 sighted people without blindfolds. All participants were tested beforehand to ensure that their hearing was normal.

When restricted to one-ear, or monaural, listening, four of the eight blind people identified sound sources more accurately than did the sighted people, says study coauthor Michel Pare, a neuroscientist at the University of Montreal. The sighted people showed especially poor localization of sounds from the speakers on the side of the blocked ear.

In sighted people who can hear with both ears, "The brain learns to rely on binaural [stereo] cues. These data suggest that blind people haven't learned that and keep monaural cues as the dominant cues," says Eric I. Knudsen, a neurobiologist at Stanford University School of Medicine. "I find it surprising."

71. One thing is sure that participants in the study _____.
    A. had normal hearing   B. were born blind
    C. wore blindfolds   D. were divided into two groups

72. Under what conditions, according to Pare, did the blind testers perform better than their sighted counterparts?
    A. When both used one ear.
    B. When the speakers were concealed.
    C. When the sounds were tuned down.
    D. When both were restricted to blindfolds.

73. Knudsen explained the better hearing on the part of the blind in term of _____.
    A. cognitive psychology   B. visual images
    C. binaural cues   D. monaural cues

74. The Canadian scientists did their test to answer the question whether _____.
    A. the blind can hear as well as the sighted
    B. the blind have hearing capabilities
    C. blind people track sounds better
    D. folk wisdom is educational

75. What folk wisdom holds in the passage _____.
    A. has been scientifically tested in Canada and U.S., with different results produced
    B. has been scientifically verified
    C. merits further investigation
    D. is surprising to everyone

Passage Four

It used to be that a corporation's capital consisted of tangible assets such as buildings, machines, and finished goods. But, in the information economy, value has shifted rapidly from tangible to intangible assets, such as management skills and customer loyalty. But how do you measure intangible assets?

Karl Erik Sveiby began trying to answer that question as a magazine publisher in

Sweden and went to become Scandinavia's leading authority on knowledge-based businesses. In his latest book, *The New Organizational Wealth*, he offers insights into valuing and managing intangible assets.

Noting that Microsoft Corporation, the world's largest software firm, once traded at an average share price of $70 at a time when its book value was $7, Sveiby asks: "What is it about Microsoft that makes it worth 10 times the value of its recorded assets? What is the nature of that additional value that is perceived by the market but not recorded by the company?"

Sveiby's answer is intangible assets, which he defines as employee competence, internal structures (systems, patents, etc.), and external structures (customer and supplier relationships and the organization's image). Because of these factors, it follows that owners hold a kind of intangible equity in the company, in addition to tangible assets such as cash and accounts receivable.

Since knowledge is a key intangible asset, the ability to transfer knowledge from one employee to another, or from outside sources to employees, is a key business capacity, in Sveiby's view. The greater the transfer of knowledge, the more overall employee competence improves. The best method for transferring knowledge, says Sveiby, is through direct experience with a subject rather than simply listening to someone or reading about it.

Experience enables learning more than overt teaching because people acquire knowledge tacitly, by observation and listening in an unstructured environment. And, he adds, people will more readily learn from an activity if they enjoy it.

Once the flow of information within an organization is managed properly, the competence of the organization increases, and the relations with customers improve. But Sveiby also points out that knowledge and information are not the same thing. Information has no value until it becomes integrated knowledge and therefore useful.

76. In the information economy, it is a challenge _____.
    A. to place a high value on intangible assets
    B. to transfer tangible into intangible assets
    C. to change the concept of assets
    D. to quantify intangible assets

77. Microsoft Corporation, in Sveiby's view _____.
    A. is skillful at managing intangible assets
    B. creates most intangible assets in the world
    C. does not hold any tangible, but much intangible assets
    D. possesses much additional intangible assets recognized by the market

78. The transfer of knowledge which is a key intangible asset, according to Sveiby _____.
    A. has much to do with overall employee competence
    B. is best done through hands-on experience
    C. reflects business capacity
    D. All of the above.

79. Integrated knowledge, information _____.
    A. begins to spread within an organization
    B. will lose much of its value
    C. will remain useful forever
    D. is an intangible asset

80. Which of the following can be the best title for the passage?
    A. Knowledge as Capital.   B. Exploding Knowledge.
    C. The Power of Knowledge.   D. Information and Knowledge.

Passage Five

High-speed living has become a fact of life, and the frantic pace is taking its toll, according to science writer James Gleick. It's as if the old "Type A" behaviour of a few has expanded into the "hurry sickness" of the many.

"We do feel that we're more time-driven and time-obsessed and generally rushed than ever before," writes Gleick in *Faster: The Acceleration of Just About Everything*, a survey of fast-moving culture and its consequences. We may also be acting more hastily, losing control, and thinking superficially because we live faster.

Technology has conditioned us to expect instant results. Internet purchases arrive by next-day delivery and the microwave delivers a hot meal in minutes. Faxes, e-mails, and cell phones make it possible and increasingly obligatory — for people to work faster. Gleick cites numerous examples of fast-forward changes in our lives: stock trading and news cycles are shorter; sound bites of presidential candidates on network newscasts dropped from 40 seconds in 1968 to 10 seconds in 1988; and some fast-food restaurants have added express lanes.

High expectations for instant service make even the brief wait for an elevator seem interminable（漫长的）. "A good waiting time is in the neighborhood of 15 seconds. Sometime around 40 seconds, people start to get visibly upset," writes Gleick. We're dependent on systems that promise speed but often deliver frustration. Like rush-hour drivers fuming when a single accident halts the evening commute, people surfing the Internet squirm if a Web page is slow to load or when access itself is not instantaneous. And the concept of "customer service" can become an oxymoron（逆喻）for consumers waiting on hold for a telephone representative.

Uptempo living has turned people into multitaskers — eating while driving, writing an e-mail while talking on the phone, or skimming dozens of television programs on split screen. Gleick suggests that human beings may be capable of adjusting to these new levels of stimuli as high-speed culture challenges our brains "in a way they were not challenged in the past, except perhaps in times of war". We may gain the flexibility to do several things at once but lose some of our capacity to focus in depth on a single task.

81. With living pace getting quicker and quicker, the number of those of "Type A" behaviours is _____.
    A. on the rise   B. out of control
    C. on the decline   D. under investigation

82. High-speed living brings about the following consequences, exclusive of _____.
    A. superficial thinking   B. loss of control
    C. waste of time   D. more haste

83. The best conclusion can be drawn from the 3rd paragraph is that _____.
    A. technology is building a fast-moving culture
    B. we are living in the age of information
    C. economy is booming with technology
    D. the frantic pace is taking its toll

84. As the author implies, the faster we live _____.
    A. the less we do   B. the less patient we are
    C. the more time we save   D. the more efficient we have

85. Living faster and faster, the multitaskers tend _____.
    A. to scratch the surface of a thing
    B. to do things better at the same time
    C. to be flexible with their time schedules
    D. to have intense concentration on trivial things

Passage Six

Eating is related to emotional as well as physiologic needs. Sucking, which is the infant's means of gaining both food and emotional security, conditions the association of eating with well-being or with deprivation. If the child is breast-fed and has supportive body contact as well as good milk intake, if the child is allowed to suck for as long as he or she desires, and if both the child and mother enjoy the nursing experience and share their enjoyment, the child is more likely to thrive both physically and emotionally. On the other hand, if the mother is nervous and resents the child or cuts him or her off from the milk supply before either the child's hunger or sucking need is satisfied, or handles the child hostilely during the feeding, or props the baby with a bottle rather than holding the child, the child may develop physically but will begin to show signs of emotional disturbance at an early age. If, in addition, the infant is further abused by parental indifference or intolerance, he or she will carry scars of such emotional deprivation throughout life.

Eating habits are also conditioned by family and other psychosocial environments. If an individual's family eats large quantities of food, then he or she is inclined to eat large amounts. If an individual's family eats mainly vegetables, then he or she will be inclined to like vegetables. If mealtime is a happy and significant event, then the person will tend to think of eating in those terms. And if a family eats quickly, without caring what is being eaten and while fighting at the dinner table, then the person will most likely adopt the same eating pattern and be adversely affected by it. This conditioning to food can remain unchanged through a lifetime unless the individual is awakened to the fact of conditioning and to the possible need for altering his or her eating patterns in order to improve nutritional intake. Conditioning spills over into and is often reinforced by religious beliefs and other customs so that, for example, a Jew, whose religion forbids the eating of pork, might have guilt feelings if he or she ate pork. An older Roman Catholic might be conditioned to feel guilty if he or she eats meat on Friday, traditionally a fish day.

86. A well-breast-fed child _____.
   A. tends to associate foods with emotions
   B. is physiologically and emotionally satisfied
   C. cannot have physiologic and emotional problems
   D. is more likely to have his or her needs satisfied in the future

87. While sucking, the baby is actually _____.
   A. conscious of the impact of breast-feeding
   B. interacting with his or her mother
   C. creating a nursing environment
   D. impossible to be abused

88. A bottle-fed child _____.
   A. can be healthy physiologically, but not emotionally
   B. cannot avoid physiologic abuse throughout life
   C. is deprived of emotional needs
   D. gets rid of physiological needs

89. From the list of eating habits, we learn that _____.
   A. everyone follows his or her eating pattern to death
   B. one's eating pattern varies with his or her personality
   C. there are no such things as psychosocial environments

D. everybody is born into a conditioned eating environment

90. A Jew or an older Roman Catholic _____.

A. takes an eating habit as a religious belief

B. is conditioned to feel guilty of eating pork in his or her family

C. cannot have a nutritional eating habit conditioned by religious beliefs

D. observes an eating pattern conditioned by his or her psychosocial environment

答案及解析

Passage One

61. 【答案】C

【解析】题目为：作者在第 1 段向人们暗示了什么？ A. 没有科学我们无法生存下去；B. 把科学带来的便利视为理所当然；C. 通过科学我们可以提高生活水平；D. 因为科学进步人们不再被疾病困扰。结合第 1 段最后一句话可知：没有科学，我们的生活将改变得非常缓慢，故 A 项不成立；最后一句话前半部分提到，我们在生活中无视科学带来的便利，故 B 项非暗示；结合第 1 段第 2 句话：没有……所带来的巨大进步，我们的生活水平会下降……人们将会遭受无法治愈的病痛。由此可知，D 项非暗示，而且意思过于绝对，故 C 项为正确答案。

62. 【答案】B

【解析】题目为：作者使用医疗和疫苗为了阐述什么？ A. 科学是如何发展起来的；B. 科学对于社会意味着什么；C. 科学的本质是什么；D. 疾病如何影响社会。此题解题时要联系全文主旨，通篇文章讲述科学对我们生活方方面面的影响和作用。因而第 2 段中的这两个例子也是为了例证文章的中心思想，所以 B 为正确选项。

63. 【答案】C

【解析】题目为：根据作者观点，在哪个方面没有任何东西可以与计算机的发明相媲美？此题解题要点在第 3 段最后一句话，这句话的关键词为 convenience "便利"，所以近义选项为 C。

64. 【答案】B

【解析】题目为：作者对什么感到不满？ A. 人们对文化的无知；B. 人们忽视科学的便利设施；C. 人们对社会毫无贡献；D. 人们对科学进步的误解。此题出处在第 4 段第 1 句。

65. 【答案】C

【解析】此题问作者的语气。A 项 critical "批判的"；B 项 cognizant "认知的"；C 项 appreciative "感激的"；D 项 paradoxical "荒谬的"。全文提到没有科学的进步和发展，人类生活的方方面面就会受到影响，因而作者对于科学以及科学发展持感激的态度。

Passage Two

66. 【答案】D

【解析】此题问生物技术的作用和影响，解题出处在第 1 段。

67. 【答案】B

【解析】此题问污水如何处理。第 1 段第 4 行 "Genetically altered microorganisms can break down a wide range of pollutants by being used, for example, in bio-filters and wastewater-treatment facilities, and in the clean-up of polluted sites." 提到了污水的治理，而这句话体现了生物科技的作用和影响，因而正确选项为 B，意为"通过生物科技手段"。

68. 【答案】D

【解析】题目的原句是在第 2 段的第 5 行。这句话的前一句话阐述了政治家和科学家同样面临识别生态、经济和社会因素之间相互关系和相互作用的挑战，并且当他们寻求解决办法的时候，他们同样面临考虑这些因素的挑战。题目出处进一步阐述为了迎接这一挑战，决策者们需要跨学科的且冲破政治界限的方法和技巧。答案为 D。

69. 【答案】A

【解析】答案出处为第 2 段最后一句话。

70. 【答案】B

【解析】此题解题出处为最后一段的第 1 句话，即各方面要合作执行。

Passage Three

71. 【答案】A

【解析】此题出处为第 4 段最后一句话。

72. 【答案】A

【解析】此题原文出处为第 5 段第 1 句话。

73. 【答案】D

【解析】首先根据人名确定答案在最后一段，然后根据这个专家的话语可以得出正确选项。

74. 【答案】C

【解析】Canadian scientists 的出处在第 2 段，他们的这个试验就是要证明第 1 段的说法，并且第 1 段最后一句话也说明他们的试验就是要证明上述观点。

75. 【答案】B

【解析】根据不同科学家和专家的论证，这一观点得到了科学试验的证实。

Passage Four

76. 【答案】D

【解析】题目为：在信息经济中，什么是挑战？原文第 1 段第 2 行提到 B 选项，但这是一个事实，而不是要面临的挑战。此题解题的原文信息在第 1 段的最后一句话。measure 与 D 项中 quantify 为近义词，因此 D 项为近义改写。

77. 【答案】**D**
　　【解析】此题是关于 Sveiby 对微软公司的阐述。与解题有关的原文信息是此段落中 Sveiby 的话：什么使得微软公司市值达到其记录在案的资产价值的十倍？由市场认定但不是公司记录的额外价值的性质是什么？根据这句话可知，只有 D 项符合原文信息。

78. 【答案】**D**
　　【解析】此题为细节题，解题的原文信息在第 5 段，从第 2 句话开始。

79. 【答案】**D**
　　【解析】原文信息在最后一段的最后一句话，大意是：信息直到成为整合型的知识，才有价值，因而才是有用的。

80. 【答案】**A**
　　【解析】此题为主旨题。全文第一段提到如何衡量无形资产，接下来以微软公司为例，最后进一步讨论知识作为无形资产……，故全文都是在讲知识和资产。

Passage Five

81. 【答案】**A**
　　【解析】此题解题信息在第 1 段最后一句话：...the old "Type A" behavior of a few... into...of the many.

82. 【答案】**C**
　　【解析】题目为：除了＿＿＿＿＿＿，高速生活给我们带来了下列结果。第 2 段最后一句话讲述因为生活节奏加快，我们会有什么样的结果。对比原文信息，只有 C 选项原文没提到，故 C 项为正确选项。

83. 【答案】**A**
　　【解析】题目考查第 3 段的大意。此段落的第 1 句话为段落的主旨句，科技使得我们更希望即时的结果。对比原文信息，A 为正确选项。

84. 【答案】**B**
　　【解析】原文信息在第 4 段。这个段落提到了想得到快速服务的期望使得我们等电梯的短短的时间都显得很漫长。上网时页面打开得慢，也会使得上网人心情烦躁，坐立不安。这些事例都在说明，生活节奏加快，人们的耐心随之减少。B 为正确选项。

85. 【答案】**A**
　　【解析】根据题干关键词，相关原文信息在最后一段的最后一句：我们可以立刻十分灵活地做几件事情，但我们失去了在一件事情上面的深入关注。A 项 scratch the surface of a thing 的含义为"只触及某事的表面"，是原文信息的近义改写。

Passage Six

86. 【答案】**B**
　　【解析】题干的重要关键词"母乳喂养的婴儿"在第 1 段第 3 行开始提到。对比相关信息：the child is more likely to thrive both physically and emotionally，选项 B 为近义改写。

87. 【答案】B

    【解析】原文信息在第 1 段 3 句话，其大意是：如果婴儿可以喝多久就喝多久，而且婴儿和妈妈都在享受这个过程，分享他们彼此的快乐，那么孩子就很可能在身心上都得到很好的发展。这说明喂奶的过程是和妈妈交流的过程，故选项 B 正确。

88. 【答案】A

    【解析】原文信息在第 1 段 "...will begin to show signs of emotional disturbance at an early age."。

89. 【答案】D

    【解析】原文信息在最后一段，第 1 句为主题句。

90. 【答案】D

    【解析】原文信息在最后一段的最后两句话。这道题属于例证处命题，本题出现在例子中，故应该直接找到例子要证明的观点。文章最后一段第 1 句就是主旨句，故选项 D 正确。

三、阅读理解所需语法知识及专项训练

（一）语法基础知识

在阅读理解测试部分，有些考生无法理解作者原意，而且文章中的长难句经常成为考生理解文章的最大障碍。对此，考生的单词量是一个重要因素。另外很重要的一点就是语法知识的欠缺，它使得考生在每个单词都基本认识的情况下，还是无法弄懂句子、段落甚至文章的含义。概括来说，影响阅读理解的语法知识可归纳为：非谓语动词、复合句以及特殊句式。下面将这三个方面的相关语法知识总结如下：

1. 非谓语动词

在英语语法中，按照动词在句中充当的成分，分为谓语动词和非谓语动词。在阅读理解中，解开长难句复杂关系的难点之一就是如何判断句中的动词是谓语动词还是非谓语动词。考生可通过下面的自测题来检测自己对非谓语动词语法知识的掌握情况。

自测题

1. —The last one _____ pays the meal.
   —Agreed!
   A. arrived   B. arrives   C. to arrive   D. arriving

2. I smell something _____ in the kitchen. Can I call you back in a minute?
   A. burning   B. burnt   C. being burnt   D. to be burnt

3. At the beginning of class, the noise of desks _____ could be heard outside the classroom.

    A. opened and closed   B. to be opened and closed

    C. being opened and closed   D. to open and close

4. After a knock at the door, the child heard his mother's voice _____ him.

    A. calling   B. called   C. being called   D. to call

5. There is nothing more I can try _____ you to stay, so I wish you good luck.

    A. being persuaded   B. persuading

    C. to be persuaded   D. to persuade

6. The Town Hall _____ in the 1800's was the most distinguished building at that time.

    A. to be completed   B. having been completed

    C. completed   D. being completed

7. The country has already sent up three unmanned spacecraft, the most recent _____ at the end of last March.

    A. has been launched   B. having been launched

    C. being launched   D. to be launched

8. John received an invitation to dinner, and with his work _____, he gladly accepted it.

    A. finished   B. finishing   C. having finished   D. was finished

9. "Things _____ never come again!" I couldn't help talking to myself.

    A. lost   B. losing   C. to lose   D. have lost

10. —Can I smoke here?

    —Sorry. We don't allow _____ here.

    A. people smoking   B. people smoke

    C. to smoke   D. smoking

11. He is very popular among his students as he always tries to make them _____ in his lectures.

    A. interested   B. interesting   C. interest   D. to interest

12. _____ that she didn't do a good job, I don't think I am abler than her.

    A. To have said   B. Having said   C. To say   D. Saying

13. She wants her paintings _____ in the gallery, but we don't think they would be very popular.

    A. display   B. to display   C. displaying   D. displayed

14. The flowers his friend gave him will die unless _____ every day.

    A. watered   B. watering   C. water   D. to water

15. The children went home from the grammar school, their lessons _____ for the day.

    A. finishing   B. finished   C. had finished   D. were finished

16. Because air pollution has been greatly reduced, this city is still _____.

    A. a good place to live   B. a good place for living in

    C. a good place to be lived in   D. a good place to live in

17. Did you smell something _____?
    A．having burnt　　　　　　　　　　B．to have burnt
    C．burning　　　　　　　　　　　　D．to be burning
18. I don't mind _____ the decision as long as it is not too late.
    A．you to delay making　　　　　　B．your delaying making
    C．your delaying to make　　　　　D．you delay to make
19. _____ from the outer space, our earth looks like a water-covered ball.
    A．Having seen　　　　　　　　　　B．Seeing
    C．Seen　　　　　　　　　　　　　D．Having been seen
20. _____ in an atmosphere of simple living was what her parents wished for.
    A．The girl was educated　　　　　B．The girl educated
    C．The girl's being educated　　　D．The girl to be educated

答案：1-5　CACAD　　6-10　CBAAA　　11-15　ABDAB　　16-20　DCBCD

非谓语动词语法知识重点简要回顾

I.　非谓语动词的形式

	不定式	动名词	现在分词	过去分词
肯定式	to do	doing	doing	done
否定式	not to do	not doing	not doing	not done
完成式	to have done	having done	having done	done
被动式	to be done	being done	being done	done

例如：

I have many things to do. 不定式做定语修饰 things

Seeing these pictures, he thought of those days in Beijing. 现在分词 seeing 做状语

Cheating should be banned thoroughly in exams. 动名词 cheating 做主语

The teacher came into the room, followed by two students. 过去分词 followed 做伴随状语

He is a man loved by all. 过去分词 loved 做定语，修饰 man

II.　非谓语动词所做的成分

	主语	宾语	表语	定语	状语	补语（宾）
不定式	√	√	√	√	√	√
动名词	√	√	√	√		
现在分词			√	√	√	√
过去分词			√	√	√	√

III. 不定式

（1）做主语

To complete the 24-storied building in 10 months was a great achievement.

在 10 个月内建成一座 24 层的大楼是个伟大的成就。

不定式做主语时常把 it 放在句首做形式主语，而将不定式移到谓语后面：

It was a great achievement to complete the 24-storied building in 10 months.

不定式的逻辑主语（for / of + 代词 / 名词），意义有所差别：

It was brave of him to dive from the cliff. (=He was brave to dive from the cliff.)

It is necessary for you to listen to other people's advice. (=It is necessary that you listen to other people's advice.)

常 与 of 搭配的形容词：careless, clever, considerate, foolish, good, impolite, kind, naughty, nice, silly, stupid。

（2）做动词宾语

I hope to improve my English gradually.

I promised not to tell anyone about it.

They asked how to get to the railway station.

后接不定式做宾语的常用动词（往往表示请求、要求、选择、决定、打算、企图等）：

afford	agree	ask	attempt	beg	bother	care	choose
claim	consent	decide	demand	desire	expect	fail	fear
hesitate	intend	plan	manage	learn	pretend	offer	pledge
prepare	refuse	resolve	determine	threaten	undertake	wish	hope

（3）做宾语补足语

His mother advised him not to go out at night.

I asked him to give me a hand.

（4）做后置定语

I never think that I can get the opportunity to work abroad one day.

（5）做表语

The task is to clear up these dishes.

（6）做表语补足语

The water is unfit to drink.

Ann is easy to get along with.

（7）做目的状语

He stopped twice, and leaned on his cane to rest.

He moved to the front row so as to hear the speaker better.

（8）做结果状语

He returned home after the long journey only to find that his house had been broken into.

IV. 动名词

（1）做主语

Milking for once is not a hard job.

It's no use crying over spilt milk.

（2）做宾语

I don't mind telling you the truth.

Let's stop arguing.

① 只能接动名词做宾语的常用动词如下，可通过下列口诀辅助记忆：

喜欢考虑与避免（enjoy, consider, avoid）

停止放弃太危险（stop, quit, risk）

承认理解很值得（admit, understand, be worth）

幻想想象莫拖延（fancy, imagine, delay, postpone）

要求完成时期望（require, finish, look forward to）

建议继续勤操练（suggest, keep on, practice）

不禁原谅是坚持（can't help, excuse, insist on）

继续成功不弃嫌（go on, succeed in, mind）+ deny

② 下列特殊句型中要用动名词的形式

It is no use（no good, no point, no sense, a waste of time 等名词）+ (in) doing sth.

It is good（nice, interesting, useless 等形容词）+(in) doing sth.

There is no point（use, sense, good 等名词）+ (in) doing sth.

have difficulty (trouble, problem, pleasure, a difficult time) + (in) doing sth.

例如：

It's simply a waste of time and money seeing that movie.

There is no point in my going out to date someone.

I find it no good advising him to go with us.

③ 有些动词后既可以接 doing 也可以接 to do，但有区别，如下所示：

➡ forget to do / forget doing

Don't forget to bring pen and paper for the quiz. 考试时别忘了带笔和纸。

I'll never forget meeting you the first time. 我永远不会忘记第一次见你的场景。

➡ remember to do / doing

Remember to take the medicine after dinner. 记得饭后吃药。

I remember switching off the light before I left. 我记得我走前关灯了。

➡ regret to do / doing

I regret to tell you that you failed the exam. 我很遗憾告诉你你考试不及格。

I regret having said that rude word to him. 我后悔对他说了粗话。

⤵ stop doing / to do

He stopped writing and had a talk with me. 他停下笔，和我聊起天来。

He stopped to have a rest. 他停下来，休息了一下。

⤵ mean doing / to do

His nodding means agreeing. 他点头意味着同意了。

He meant to do that work by himself. 他打算自己做那份工作。

⤵ try doing / to do

We try to finish the task on time. 我们试图按时完成任务。

She tried making a dress by herself, but she failed.

她试着自己做衣服，但没成功。

⤵ like / dislike doing / to do

I like watching TV every night, but I don't like to watch TV this evening because I am busy. 每天晚上我都喜欢看电视，但今晚我不想看了，因为太忙。

Ⅴ. 分词

（1）做宾补

Do you see the dark cloud hovering over the surface of the earth?

The shop girl's good intention left the old man feeling better than before.

（2）做定语

All people involved have been questioned.

The factory making trucks is located at the foot of the mountain.

（3）做状语

⤵ 表示时间

Turning around, she saw Tom in tears.

⤵ 表示原因

Being ill, he couldn't go to class.

Seriously injured, Allen was rushed to the hospital.

⤵ 表示让步，由 although / though, even if / though 引入放句首

Even if coming by the subway, you'll need 45 minutes to get here.

Although given the best medical care, he died.

⤵ 表示条件

Unless asked to answer questions, the pupils were not supposed to talk in Mrs Smith's class.

If going there by plane, we'll have to pay twice as much.

❯ 表示伴随

Singing and laughing, the pupils came into the room.

He sat in an armchair, watching TV.

❯ 固定短语

generally (strictly, etc.) speaking	judging from / by
talking of	allowing for
considering	taken as a whole
barring	assuming / supposing
according to	owing to
taking everything into consideration	leaving … on one side
generally / frankly / roughly /strictly / honestly speaking	

（4）分词的独立主格结构

　　①分词可有其独立的逻辑主语

　　②常是名词或代词主格置于分词前

　　③常做句子状语，置于句首或句尾

The river having risen in the night, the crossing was impossible.

Weather permitting, we'll have the match tomorrow.

The work done, we went home.

2. 名词性从句

根据名词性从句所充当的成分，可以分为主语从句、宾语从句、表语从句、同位语从句。

自测题

1. Although there are many predictions about the future, no one knows for sure _____ the world would be like in 50 years.

    A. how   B. that   C. which   D. what

2. I don't think Mr. Watson will come here again today. Please give the ticket to _____ comes here first.

    A. whomever   B. whom   C. who   D. whoever

3. Undoubtedly, _____ wins the election is going to have a tough job getting the economy back on its feet.

    A. anyone   B. who   C. whoever   D. everyone

4. It is a great pity for _____ to be any quarrel in the school board meeting.

    A. where   B. here   C. there   D. why

5. They want to know _____ do to help us.

    A. what can they   B. what they can

    C. how they can   D. how can they

6. These photographs will show you _____.
    A. what does our village look like
    B. what our village looks like
    C. how does our village look like
    D. how our village looks like

7. Can you make sure _____ the gold ring?
    A. where Alice had put
    B. where did Alice put
    C. where Alice has put
    D. where has Alice put

8. Go and get your coat. It's _____ you left it.
    A. there
    B. where
    C. there where
    D. where there

9. _____ the 2012 Olympic Games will be held in London is not known yet.
    A. Whether
    B. If
    C. Whenever
    D. That

10. It worried her a bit _____ her hair was turning grey.
    A. while
    B. that
    C. if
    D. for

11. _____ he said at the meeting astonished everyone present.
    A. When
    B. What
    C. How
    D. That

12. _____ we cannot get seems better than _____ we have.
    A. What; what
    B. What; that
    C. That; that
    D. That; what

13. The fact _____ he has made great progress in this term is quite clear.
    A. why
    B. if
    C. what
    D. that

答案：1-5　D D C C B　　6-10　B C B A B　　11-13　B A D

名词性从句语法知识重点简要回顾

I.　主语从句

分为由 that 引导的主语从句（that 不可省）和由 wh- 引导的主语从句。例如：

What they are after is profit.

That he is a rich man is known to all.

When we shall have our sports meeting is still a question.

Whether we'll go outing depends on the weather.

II.　宾语从句

分为由 that 引导的宾语从句（that 可以省）和由 wh- 引导的宾语从句。例如：

Let's see how we can raise our efficiency.

I don't doubt that they'll be able to overcome the difficulty.

She was never satisfied with what she had achieved.

III.　表语从句

分为 that 引导的表语从句（that 不可省）和 wh- 引导的表语从句。例如：

This is what I want to say.

The fact is that she pretended to be ill yesterday.

IV. 同位语从句

分为 that 引导的同位语从句（that 不可省）和 wh- 引导的同位语从句。

（1）同位语从句在句中做名词的同位语，用以说明名词所表示的具体内容。例如：

An order came that all villagers must leave the village.

（2）同位语从句与定语从句的区别：如果从句所修饰的名词在从句中充当成分，则此从句就是定语从句，反之就是同位语从句。例如：

The order that you gave us is right.（定语从句）

He has the hope that he'll become a college student.（同位语从句）

3. 定语从句

 自测题

1. All of the plants now raised on farms have been developed from plants _____ in the wild.
   A. once they grew
   B. that once grew
   C. they grew once
   D. once grew

2. Scientists can predict regions _____ new species are most likely to be found.
   A. where
   B. when
   C. why
   D. how

3. The only thing _____ really matters to the parents is how soon their children can return home.
   A. what
   B. that
   C. which
   D. this

4. The *Mona Lisa*, _____ in Italy, is now in the Louvre, a museum in Paris.
   A. who painted
   B. who was painted
   C. which painted
   D. which was painted

5. The parents were much kinder to their youngest child than they were to the others, _____, of course, made the others jealous.
   A. which
   B. that
   C. what
   D. who

6. The symbols of mathematics _____ we are most familiar are the signs of addition, subtraction, multiplication, division and equality.
   A. to which
   B. which
   C. with which
   D. in which

7. _____ is often the case with a new idea, much initial activity and optimistic discussion produce no concrete proposal.
   A. It
   B. Which
   C. As
   D. That

答案：1-5 B A B D A   6-7 C C

定语从句语法知识重点简要回顾

I. **定语从句的定义**

修饰名词的从句（修饰名词的句子成分是定语）。例如：

He is a man who is loved by all.

定语从句修饰名词 man。

II. **定语从句的分类**

定语从句分为限制性定语从句和非限制性定语从句（主句和从句之间用逗号隔开）。例如：

She is the nurse who looks after my sick mother.（限制性定语从句）

Football, which is a very interesting game, is played all over the world.（非限制性定语从句）

III. **定语从句的组成部分**

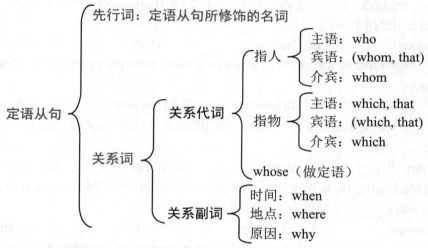

注：关系词所起的作用：

　　① 引导从句

　　② 代替先行词在从句中充当成分

　　关系代词与关系副词的关系：介词 + 关系代词 = 关系副词

请拆分下面的定语从句：

① She is the nurse who looks after my sick mother.
　　　　　　主句　　　　　　　　　　　从句

先行词为 nurse, who 为关系代词并且代替 nurse 在从句中充当主语。

② Do you know the man I spoke to?

③ Do you know the man to whom I spoke?

④ Football, which is a very interesting game, is played all over the world.

⑤ The book you lent me is very interesting.

⑥ The knife with which I used to cut the bread is very sharp.

⑦ She is the student whose mother is a teacher.

⑧ I've lost the dictionary whose cover is blue.

⑨ The day will come when the people all over the world will win liberation.

⑩ I visited the school where my mother taught English ten years ago.

⑪ Do you know the reason why he left here?

4. 状语从句

 自测题

1. You can arrive in Beijing earlier for the meeting _____ you don't mind taking the night train.

   A. if   B. unless   C. though   D. until

2. _____ pollution control measures tend to be money-consuming, many industries hesitate to adopt them.

   A. Although   B. However   C. When   D. Since

3. _____ urgent the situation may be, you will need to make one change at a time, and then move on.

   A. As   B. Whenever   C. However   D. Whatever

4. _____ I admit that the problems are difficult, I don't agree that they cannot be solved.

   A. When   B. Where   C. While   D. Why

5. The ATMs enable bank customers to access their money 24 hours a day and seven days a week _____ ATMs are located.

   A. wherever   B. whenever   C. however   D. whatever

6. It was _____ good weather that we all want to go out for a traveling.

   A. so   B. such   C. because   D. /

7. Although it was raining, _____ still worked in the fields.

   A. but they   B. and they   C. they   D. and yet they

8. I haven't decided _____ I should attend that meeting or not.

   A. if   B. that   C. whether   D. why

9. _____ the weather is fine, I open all the windows.

   A. As   B. For   C. Because of   D. Since that

10. You can also do something great _____ you work very hard at it.

   A. as long as   B. as far as   C. whether   D. so that

11. _____ you have promised him, you should keep your promise.

   A. Now that   B. When   C. After   D. For

12. I was speaking to Ann on the phone about our tour plan _____ suddenly we were cut off.

    A. that   B. while   C. before   D. when

答案：1-5 ADCCA   6-10 BCCAA   11-12 AD

 状语从句语法知识重点简要回顾

I. 状语从句的分类

    分为时间状语从句、地点状语从句、原因状语从句、目的状语从句、结果状语从句、让步状语从句、比较状语从句、方式状语从句、条件状语从句。

II. 时间状语从句

（1）引导时间状语从句的连词：when, while, as, before, after, until, till, as soon as, no sooner… than, since, hardly… when, scarcely… when

    ①when 引导的时间状语从句的动词既可以是延续性动词，又可以是瞬间动词。

        It was 9 o' clock when I got home.

        The doorbell rang when my mother was cooking in the kitchen.

    ②while 所引导的时间状语从句的动词只能是延续性动词。

        While we were watching TV, he came in.

    ③as 所引导的时间状语从句中的动词可以是延续性动词，或是侧重两个动作的同步，译为"一边，一边"。

        As the children walked along the street, they sang happily.

    ④when 的特殊用法：when = at that time something happened suddenly 译为"正在那时突然……"。

        I had just started back for the house to change my clothes when I heard the strange noise.

    ⑤while 的特殊用法：表示对比，译成"而"。

        She likes pop music, while her brother likes light music.

        while 译为"虽然"。

        While I understand your viewpoint, I don't agree with you.

（2）since & before

    ①It is + 一段时间 + since   表示一段时间的起始点，译为"自从"。

        It is + 一段时间 + before   表示一段时间的终止点。

        It is three years since I began to study here.

        It was three years before we met again.

    ②如果 since 引导的时间状语从句中的动词是延续性动词，意为否定。

        It's a long time since Jack lived here. 杰克早不在这儿住了。

        It's a year since I smoked. 我已经有一年不吸烟了。

It's been years since I enjoyed myself so much as last night. 我已经有很多年没有像昨晚那么痛快了。

③before 译为 "就，才"。

It wasn't long before the fire went out. 没过多久，火就熄灭了。

I hadn't gone much farther before I caught up with her. 没走多远，我就赶上了。

（3）hardly… when, no sooner… than, scarcely… when 一……就……

We had hardly got into the village when it began to rain.

我们刚一进村子就下雨了。

= Hardly had we got into the village when it began to rain. 否定词在句首，部分倒装。

He had no sooner arrived home than he was asked to start on another journey.

= No sooner had he arrived home than he was asked to start on another journey.

（4）not… until 直到……才……

She didn't stop crying until her mother came back.

①强调句型

It was not until her mother came back that she stopped crying.

②倒装结构

Not until her mother came back did she stop crying.

（5）其他

Directly I had done it, I knew I had made a mistake.

The moment (that) I saw you, I knew you were angry with me.

Immediately he saw the police, he ran away.

III. 地点状语从句

Make a mark where you have any doubt or question.

区分定语从句和地点状语从句

Put the book where it used to be.（地点状语从句）

I visited the factory where my father worked before.（定语从句，先行词 the factory 在从句中充当地点状语）

IV. 原因状语从句

（1）引导原因状语从句的连词：because, as, since, now that

because：回答 why, 不与 so 连用

since = as = now that 表示众所周知、显而易见的理由，在彼此已知道的事做理由陈述时使用，意为 "既然"。

Since / As / Now that you are here, let's start the meeting.

（2）其他

Considering that they are just beginners, they are doing quite a good job.（考虑到）

Seeing he refused to help us, there is no reason why we should now help him.（鉴于）

（3）for（并列连词），表示原因时，意在解释说明。

I caught a cold, for I had been walking around in the rain.

V. 目的状语从句

（1）引导目的状语从句的连词：so that, in order that, in case, for fear that, etc.

Let's take the front seats so that / in order that we may see more clearly.

You'd better take more clothes in case it is cold.（以免，以防）

He hid his jewelry for fear that it would be stolen.（唯恐）

（2）表示目的的其他说法

to do, in order to do, so as to do（不能放在句首）

So as to catch the bus, he got up early.（×）

He got up early so as to catch the bus.（√）

VI. 结果状语从句

（1）引导结果状语从句的连词：so… that…, such… that…, so … as to do

（2）such… that… & so… that…

①含义：如此……以至于……

②引导结果状语从句

③句型：such + a / an + *a.* + 单数名词 + that … = so + *a.* + a / an + 单数名词 + that…

such + *a.* + 复数名词 + that …

such + *a.* + 不可数名词 + that…

so + *a.* + that…

The teacher set such a difficult examination question that none of us worked it out.

= The teacher set so difficult an examination question that none of us worked it out.

特别关注：注意区分结果状语从句和定语从句。

It is so cold outside that I don't want to go out.

④当名词前有 many, much, few, little 修饰时，用 so 而不用 such。

The house cost <u>so</u> much money that we didn't buy it.

VII. 让步状语从句

（1）引导让步状语从句的连词：though, although, even if, even though, -ever, no matter wh-, as, while

①though = although "虽然"，不与 but 连用，可以与 yet, still 连用。

He still went there, though he didn't feel very well.

②no matter wh- & -ever

No matter where you are, you should work out.

However late he is, his mother will wait for him to have a dinner together.

= No matter how late he is, …

（2）as 引导的让步状语从句

① *a. / ad.*

Clever as he is, he never works hard.

Much as I admire his courage, I don't think he acted wisely.

② *v.*

Try as he does, he never seems able to do the work beautifully.

③ *n.*

Child as he is, he has a lot of knowledge.

VIII. 比较状语从句

同级比较 as... as... 或 so... as...（多用于否定句中）。例如：

Jim is not quite as good a student as his sister.

She is almost as happy here as she was at home.

The horse is getting old and can't run as / so fast as did.

IX. 方式状语从句

as 意为"按照，像"。例如：

Please do it as I tell you to.

As Americans like baseball, the British like soccer.

X. 条件状语从句

（1）引导条件状语从句的连词：if, unless, as long as（只要），注意从句的将来动作用一般现在时表示。

As long as you study hard, you'll get good results.

Unless he comes, I won't come here.

（2）其他

We'll let you use the room on condition that / provided that you keep it clean and tidy.

5. 虚拟语气

 自测题

1. If they had sent a check to the telephone company last week, their telephone _____ out of service at this moment.
   A. will not be
   B. will not have been
   C. would not be
   D. would not have been

2. _____ before we departed last weekend, we would have had a wonderful dinner party.
   A. Had they arrived
   B. Would they arrive
   C. Were they arriving
   D. Were they to arrive

3. Had Paul received six more votes in the last election, he _____ our chairman now.
   A. must be
   B. would have been

C. shall be   D. would be

4. Both approaches require that the actor _____ his or her own personal values as well as the character's.
   A. must understand   B. should understand
   C. has to understand   D. need to understand

5. It is requested that all the students _____ present at the meeting tomorrow.
   A. were   B. will be   C. are   D. be

6. The extensive survey suggested that their assumptions _____ totally wrong.
   A. were   B. be   C. was   D. would be

7. A recent survey suggested that if money were not an issue, most mothers _____ not to work at all.
   A. should prefer   B. prefer   C. would prefer   D. preferred

8. We are sure that _____ to do this face to face, he would find it difficult to express himself without losing his temper.
   A. were he to try   B. would he try
   C. was he trying   D. if he tries

9. Had I been you, I _____ an umbrella with me.
   A. would take   B. had taken
   C. would have taken   D. will take

10. This result suggested that his plan _____ something wrong.
    A. should have   B. have
    C. has   D. has had

11. _____ today, he would get there by Friday.
    A. Would he leave   B. Was he leaving
    C. Were he to leave   D. If he leaves

12. The law requires that everyone _____ his car checked at least once a year.
    A. has   B. had
    C. have   D. have to have

答案：1-5　C A D B D　　6-10　A C A C C　　11-12 A C

虚拟语气语法知识重点简要回顾

I. 虚拟语气在条件句中的应用

条件句的分类 { 真实条件句：假设的情况有可能发生
             虚拟条件句：纯然假设的情况或是发生的可能性不大

251

Ⅱ. 虚拟条件句的应用

	主　句		从　句	
与现在事实相反	would should could might	+ do	动词的过去式	did were
与过去事实相反	would should could might	+ have done	had + 过去分词	
与将来事实相反	would could should might	+ do	动词的过去式	did were were to do should do

（1）一般情况

　　① 与现在事实相反。例如：

　　　　If I had much money, I would buy a house.

　　　　If you were me, how would you deal with the problem?

　　② 与过去事实相反。例如：

　　　　If the hurricane had happened during the daytime, there would have been many more deaths.

　　③ 与将来事实相反。例如：

　　　　If I failed / should fail / were to fail, I would try again.

（2）错综复杂时间条件句：有时条件从句所表示的动作与主句动作发生的时间不一致。例如：

　　If the weather had been more favorable, the crops would be growing still better.

　　注：从句为过去的动作，主句是现在的动作

　　Amy would be alive today if the doctor had come sooner last night.

　　注：从句为过去的动作，主句是现在的动作

（3）if 条件句中 if 的省略（部分倒装）。例如：

　　If we had made enough preparations, we would have succeeded.

　　→ Had we made enough preparations, we would have succeeded.

　　If there would be a flood, what should we do?

　　→ Should there be a flood, what should we do?

（4）表示假设的其他方式。例如：

　　Without music, the world would be a dull place.

　　We could have done better under more favorable conditions.

III.　wish 的名词从句的虚拟语气

（1）用法：退后一个时态

现在→过去

过去→过去的过去

将来→过去的将来

I wish I remembered the address.

We wish we had paid more attention to our pronunciation.

I wish he would try again.

（2）同样用法的其他句型

as if = as though 似乎，好像……

if only 要是……就好了

They talked as if they had been friends for years.

The teacher has loved students as if they were her children.

If only I had listened to your advice.

If only I hadn't lost it.

IV.　(should) + do

（1）suggest, order, demand, propose, command, request, desire, insist（建议、命令、要求、坚持）的名词性从句

I suggest that he（should）give up smoking.

My suggestion is that he (should) give up smoking.

It is suggested that he (should) give up smoking.

My suggestion that he (should) give up smoking was supported by his parents.

特例：suggest 表示"建议"用虚拟语气 (should) do，表示"暗示"不用虚拟语气。

Her surprised impression suggested she didn't know that.

insist 表示"要求"用虚拟语气 (should) do，表示"坚持认为"不用虚拟语气。

I insist that I'm right.

（2）It's a pity, It's a shame, It's incredible, It's strange, It's no wonder, It's natural 等主语从句

It is a great pity that he should be so conceited.

It's incredible that he should have finished the work so soon.

6.　倒装

自测题

1.　Not until recent years _____ a popular means of communication.

   A．e-mail became   B．e-mail has become

   C．did e-mail become   D．will e-mail become

2. _____ shall we forget the day when we received the admission into Harvard University.
   A. No time　　　　　B. Never　　　　C. No sooner　　　D. Nonetheless

3. Scarcely _____ those words when suddenly the monster was transformed into a very handsome youth.
   A. had he uttered　　　　　　　　　B. did he utter
   C. he had uttered　　　　　　　　　D. he did utter

4. Only by understanding the Web deeply _____ hope for people to grasp its full potential.
   A. can there be　　　B. can be there　　C. be there can　　D. there can be

5. _____ will Mr. Forbes be able to regain control of the company.
   A. With hard work　　　　　　　　B. As regards his hard work
   C. Only if he works hard　　　　　　D. Despite his hard work

6. The price here is much higher than in some other stores. Never again _____ here.
   A. I will shop　　　B. will I shop　　　C. shop I　　　　D. I do shop

7. Only _____ solve this problem.
   A. I can　　　　　B. can I　　　　　C. am I　　　　D. I am

8. Not only _____ face it, but also _____ try to conquer it.
   A. we should; we should　　　　　　B. should we; should we
   C. we should; should we　　　　　　D. should we; we should

9. Under his arm _____ a pair of shoes which he had bought from the shop.
   A. is　　B. are　　　C. were　　　　D. was

答案：1-5　C B A A C　　6-9　B A D D

倒装语法知识重点简要回顾

I.　**倒装语序**
　　完全倒装（主语和谓语倒装，主谓→谓主）
　　部分倒装（只是谓语相应的助动词提前）

II.　**完全倒装**
（1）由引导词 there 引起的句子（there be 句型中）。例如：
　　There are many people in the park.
（2）由 there, here 等词引起，谓语为 come, go 的句子。例如：
　　There comes the bus.
　　特例：当句子的主语为代词时，不倒装。例如：
　　Here you are.

There he comes.

（3）由 then 引起，谓语为 come 等词的句子。例如：

Then came a new difficulty.

特例：当句子的主语为代词时，不倒装。

（4）以 out, in, up, down, away 等副词在句首表示强调。例如：

Up went the arrow into the air.

特例：当句子的主语为代词时，不倒装。例如：

Down it flew.

Away they went.

（5）表语置于句首"表语 + 系动词 + 主语"。例如：

表语可以是：

①介词短语

On either side were rows of trees.

②形容词

Very important in students' life is hard-working.

③副词

Below is a restaurant.

④过去分词

Seated on the ground are a group of young men.

⑤现在分词

Watching the performance were mostly foreign guests.

（6）以 so, nor, neither 开头的句子，谓语所表示的情况也适合于另一个人，注意助动词的选择。例如：

He went swimming yesterday. So did I.

He has learned English for 4 years. So have I.

He can't drive a car. Nor / Neither can I.

特例：如果只是强调前面一句话的意思，则不倒装。例如：

It was cold yesterday. So it was.

III.　部分倒装

（1）省略了 if 的虚拟条件句（had, were, should 开头）。例如：

Were she here, she would support the plan.

Had I been informed earlier, I could have done something.

Should anyone call, tell him to wait for me here.

（2）某些表示祝愿的句子。例如：

May you succeed.

（3）as 的让步状语从句。例如：

Angry as he was, he managed to speak calmly.

（4）表示"一……就"的特殊句型

No sooner… than…

Hardly… when…

Scarcely… when…

（5）Not until 的句型。例如：

Not until I began to work did I realize how much time I had wasted.

（6）含有否定意义的词放在句首。例如：

Never shall I forget it.

Little did he know who she was.

（7）做状语的 only 短语位于句首时。例如：

Only in this way can you work out the problem.

特例：当 only 修饰主语时不倒装。例如：

Only a teacher can do it.

（8）So…that 句型中的 so + a. / ad. 位于句首时。例如：

So loudly did he speak that even people in the next room could hear him.

7. 强调句型

（1）强调句型只有 it is / was 两种形式。

（2）区分强调句型和 it 为形式主语的主语从句。例如：

It is important that we should get good command of English.

It is English that we should get good command of.

（二）长难句分析

在正式医学博士英语统考中，很多考生虽然有很好的单词基础，但对于阅读理解，尤其是长难句感到无所适从，进而影响对篇章的理解以及正确解题。这是因为这类考生运用语法背景知识的综合能力欠佳。具备一定的语法知识，考生应付简单句或者单一型的复合句还有信心，但是当语句综合了多种语法现象后，考生就无能为力了。这部分就这一问题给予考生一些启示和帮助。

总的说来，长难句之所以又长又难，是因为在语句中综合运用了如下结构：并列平行结构、非谓语动词、复合句以及特殊句型。下面请考生运用上面所掌握的基本语法知识分析下面的长难句，并且进行翻译。

1. Sveiby's answer is intangible assets, which he defines as employee competence, internal structures (systems, patents, etc.), and external structures (customer and supplier relationships and the organization's image).

_____

_____

_____

_____

【单　　词】intangible asset 无形资产；competence 能力。

【结构分析】由 which 引导非限制性定语从句，在定语从句中，由 and 连接两个并列成分。

【参考译文】Sveiby 的答案是无形资产，他将无形资产界定为员工能力、内部结构（制度、专利品等）以及外部结构（顾客和厂商的关系以及企业形象）。

2. Since knowledge is a key intangible asset, the ability to transfer knowledge from one employee to another, or from outside sources to employees, is a key business capacity, in Sveiby's view.

_____
_____
_____

【单　　词】capacity 能力；transfer...from...to... 将……从……转移到……
【结构分析】since 引导一个原因状语从句，在主句中，由不定式修饰名词 ability。在不定式中有一个由 or 连接的并列成分。
【参考译文】按照 Sveiby 的观点来看，既然知识是个关键的无形资产，将知识从一个员工传递给另一个员工，或者从外部资源传递给员工的能力就是企业的一个重要能力。

3. Like rush-hour drivers fuming when a single accident halts the evening commute, people surfing the Internet squirm if a Web page is slow to load or when access itself is not instantaneous.

_____
_____
_____

【单　　词】fume 发怒；halt 停止；commute 上下班往返；squirm 蠕动；instantaneous 瞬间的。
【结构分析】fuming 现在分词做定语，修饰 driver；when 引导时间状语从句；surfing 现在分词做定语，修饰 people；if 引导的条件状语从句与 when 引导的时间状语从句并列。
【参考译文】就像因事故而被堵在晚高峰路上发怒的司机一样，如果网页打开很慢或者当不能很快进入网页时，上网的人就会坐立不安。

4. Sucking, which is the infant's means of gaining both food and emotional security, conditions the association of eating with well-being or with deprivation.

_____
_____
_____

【单　　词】suck 吸吮；condition 是动词，意为"影响，保持健康"；deprivation 剥夺。
【结构分析】which 引导非限制性定语从句，修饰 sucking。
【参考译文】作为婴儿获得食物和情感安全的一个手段，吸吮决定了吃东西与健康之间的联系或者与剥夺之间的联系。

5. If the child is breast-fed and has supportive body contact as well as good milk intake, if the child is allowed to suck for as long as he or she desires, and if both the child and mother enjoy the nursing experience and share their enjoyment, the child, is more likely to thrive both physically and emotionally.

    _____

    _____

    _____

    _____

    【单　　词】thrive 茁壮成长。

    【结构分析】此句是由 and 连接三个并列 if 引导的条件状语从句。

    【参考译文】如果孩子是母乳喂养并且既能喝到优质的奶水，又可以享受有益的身体接触，如果允许孩子想吸吮多久就多久，如果母婴都能享受哺乳过程并且分享快乐，那么孩子就有可能身心都能茁壮健康地成长。

6. On the other hand, if the mother is nervous and resents the child or cuts him or her off from the milk supply before either the child's hunger or sucking need is satisfied, or handles the child hostilely during the feeding, or props the baby with a bottle rather than holding the child, the child may develop physically but will begin to show signs of emotional disturbance at an early age.

    _____

    _____

    _____

    _____

    【单　　词】resent 愤恨；hostilely 敌对地；prop 支撑；disturbance 扰乱。

    【结构分析】在 if 引导的条件状语从句中，or 连接 5 个并列成分。

    【参考译文】另一方面，如果母亲很紧张并且怨恨孩子或者在孩子仍旧很饿或还没吃够的时候不让孩子吃奶了，再或者在喂奶时对待孩子充满敌意，或者用奶瓶支撑孩子而不是抱着孩子，这个孩子身体会发育但是将会在早期开始出现情绪障碍的迹象。

7. This conditioning to food can remain unchanged through a lifetime unless the individual is awakened to the fact of conditioning and to the possible need for altering his or her eating patterns in order to improve nutritional intake.

    _____

    _____

    _____

    _____

    【单　　词】conditioning 训练，熏陶，习惯；alter 改变；nutritional 有营养的。

    【结构分析】在由 unless 引导的条件状语从句中，altering 为现在分词做介词 for 的宾语，并且 in order to do 为不定式短语做目的状语。

【参考译文】这种饮食习惯可能一生都不会有任何改变，除非一个人对这种习惯的事实有所醒悟，为了改进营养的摄入而改变他或她的饮食方式。

8. Without the vast advances made by chemists, physicists, biologists, geologists, and other diligent scientists, our standards of living would decline, our flourishing, wealthy nation might come to an economic depression, and our people would suffer from disease that could not be cured.

_____

_____

_____

【单　　词】diligent 勤奋的；decline 下降；flourishing 繁荣的；economic depression 经济衰退。

【结构分析】此句为一种特殊句型：虚拟语气。Without the vast advances made by chemists, physicists, biologists, geologists, and other diligent scientists...相当于 if 引导的虚拟条件句，即 if there were not the vast advances made by chemists, physicists, biologists, geologists, and other diligent scientists... 在虚拟条件句的主句中，that 引导的定语从句修饰 disease。

【参考译文】如果没有由化学家、物理学家、生物学家、地质学家以及其他勤奋的科学家所取得的巨大进步，我们的生活水平就会下降，我们繁荣而富有的国家就可能出现经济衰退，我们的人民就会患上无法治愈的疾病。

9. Despite the greatness of present-day innovators and scientists and their revelations, it is requisite to examine the amenities of science that our culture so blatantly disregards.

_____

_____

_____

【单　　词】innovator 创新者；revelation 启示；requisite 必不可少的；amenity 便利设施；blatantly 明目张胆地，公开地；disregard 忽视。

【结构分析】that 引导的定语从句修饰 amenity。

【参考译文】尽管当今创新者们、科学家们以及他们的启示很伟大，但还是有必要审视被我们的文化如此公开漠视的科学带给我们的便利。

10. Political leaders and scientists alike face the challenge of recognizing interrelationships and interactions between ecological, economic, and social factors and taking account of these factors when seeking solution strategies.

_____

_____

_____

【单　　词】challenge 挑战；interaction 相互作用；take account of 考虑。

【结构分析】recognizing 与 taking account of 为并列成分，都做介词 of 的宾语。interrelationships 与 interactions 为并列成分，都做动词 recognizing 的宾语。seeking 为现在分词，做时间状语。

【参考译文】政治家们和科学家们同样面临识别生态、经济和社会因素之间相互关系和相互作用的挑战，并且当他们寻求解决办法的时候，他们同样面临考虑这些因素的挑战。

长难句专项练习

1. A person may relay his or her feelings, thoughts, and reactions through body positioning, body contact, body odors, eye contact, responsive actions, habits, attitudes, interests, state of health, dress and grooming, choice of lifestyle, and use of talents—in fact, through everything the individual says or does.

_____

_____

_____

【单　　词】relay 传递；body odors 体味；grooming 打扮，装束。

【结构分析】此句较长的原因在于 through 后面的并列宾语内容较多。句子主干为：A person may relay his or her feelings, thoughts and reactions through everything the individual says or does.

【参考译文】一个人可以通过身体姿势、身体接触、体味、眼神交流、反应动作、习惯、态度、兴趣、身体状况、穿着打扮、生活方式的选择以及才能的运用，实际上通过所有这个人的所做所说来传递他或她的感受、看法以及反应。

2. The degree to which a person is able to communicate depends upon the extent of his or her conscious awareness, priority of need, and control of this process.

_____

_____

_____

【单　　词】conscious awareness 自觉意识。

【结构分析】此句中 which 引导的定语从句使句子主干的主语与谓语分开，主谓应该为：the degree depends on...

【参考译文】一个人能够交流的程度取决于他或她自觉意识的程度、优先需求以及对于这个过程的控制。

3. The person often projects fears and fantasies onto others, so that no matter what

the real content is of the messages that others relay, the messages received are threatening ones.

_____

_____

_____

【单　词】project 投掷，发送；project sth. onto sb. 将……加诸……；fantasy 幻想。

【结构分析】so that 引导结果状语从句。在该结果状语从句中 no matter what 引导状语从句。在这个状语从句中 that others relay 是定语从句，修饰 messages。

【参考译文】一个人经常将恐惧和幻想加诸别人身上，这样无论别人传递的信息的真正内容是什么，这个人接受的信息都是有威胁性的。

4. Unless such a block is removed shortly after happening, it can have profound and complicating effects that will distort emotional and mental growth and arrest the development potential of the individual.

_____

_____

_____

【单　词】block 妨碍；profound 深远的；complicating 复杂的；distort 扭曲，歪曲；arrest 阻止。

【结构分析】unless 引导条件状语从句，在主句中，that will distort...and arrest... 为定语从句，修饰 effects。

【参考译文】除非这样的障碍在其发生后不久就被消除，否则它会产生深远且复杂的影响。这样的影响将会扭曲情感和心理方面的成长，也会阻碍一个人潜能的开发。

5. Without the vaccines created by doctors, disease such as polio, measles, hepatitis, and the flu would post a threat to our citizens, for although some of these diseases may not be deadly, their side effects can be a vast detriment to an individual affected with the disease.

_____

_____

_____

【单　词】vaccine 疫苗；polio 小儿麻痹症；measles 麻疹；hepatitis 肝炎；detriment 损害。

【结构分析】without 引导的介词短语相当于由 if 引导的虚拟条件句。such as 后面为并列列举 diseases。for 引导表示原因的并列句。在这个并列句中 although 引导让步状语从句。an individual affected 中的 affected 为过去分词做定语，修饰 individual。

【参考译文】如果没有医生们发明的疫苗，像小儿麻痹症、麻疹、肝炎以及流感这些疾病将会威胁到我们的公民。因为尽管这些疾病可能不致命，但它们的副作用对患病人却造成莫大的伤害。

6. Without the presence of this machine, our world could exist, but the conveniences brought into life by the computer are unparalleled.

_____

_____

_____

【单　　词】unparalleled 空前的，无比的。

【结构分析】without 引导的介词短语相当于由 if 引导的条件虚拟句，brought into life... 不是谓语动词，而是过去分词做 conveniences 的定语。

【参考译文】如果没有这个机器的出现，我们的世界或许还存在，但计算机带给我们生活的便利是史无前例的。

7. Research now indicates that blind and sighted people display the same skill at locating a sound's origin when using both ears, but some blind people can home in on sounds more accurately than their sighted counterparts when all have one ear blocked. Canadian scientists describe the work in the Sept. 17 *Nature*.

_____

_____

_____

【单　　词】indicate 指出；counterpart 配对物；home in on sth. 把（注意力等）集中于……

【结构分析】在 that blind and sighted people display 引导的宾语从句中，using 为现在分词做状语，when all have one ear blocked 为状语从句。

【参考译文】如今，研究表明：当使用两只耳朵定位声源时，盲人和有视力的人显示出同样的技能，但是当他们的一只耳朵被堵住时，一些盲人要比同样参加测试的有视力的人更能准确地定位声音。加拿大科学家在 9 月 17 日《自然》杂志上对此有所描述。

8. A survey of news stories in 1996 reveals that the antiscience tag has been attached to many other groups as well, from authorities who advocated the elimination of the last remaining stocks of smallpox virus to Republicans who advocated decreased funding for basic research.

_____

_____

_____

【单　　词】antiscience tag 反科学的标签；be attached to 依附于，被贴在……上；elimination 消除；smallpox 天花。

【结构分析】主句主干结构为：A survey… reveals。that 引导 reveals 的宾语从句。宾语从句的主干为：the antiscience tag has been attached to many other groups… from authorities… to Republicans... 在宾语从句中，who advocated the elimination... 是定语从句，修饰 authorities；而 who advocates decreased... 是另一个定语从句，修饰 Republicans。

【参考译文】1996 年的一篇新闻报道调查显示，反科学的标签也可以贴在许多其他团体上，从鼓吹要消灭最后残留的天花病毒的组织机构到主张削减基础研究经费的共和党人。

9. The great interest in exceptional children shown in public education over the past three decades indicates the strong feeling in our society that all citizens, whatever their special conditions, deserve the opportunity to fully develop their capabilities.

_____

_____

_____

【单　　词】exceptional children 特殊儿童；deserve 值得，应受。

【结构分析】句子主语为 great interest，谓语为 indicates。shown 为过去分词修饰 interest。the strong feeling... 为 indicate 的宾语从句。在宾语从句中，that all citizens... 为同位语从句，whatever their special conditions 为插入语。

【参考译文】在过去 30 年间，公共教育对特殊儿童的极大兴趣表明我们社会中人们的一种强烈感受，即无论公民处于多么特殊的境地，所有人都应该有充分发挥自身才能的机会。

10. Even the folk knowledge in social systems on which ordinary life is based in earning, spending, organizing, marrying, taking part in political activities, fighting and so on, is not very dissimilar from the more sophisticated images of the social system derived from the social sciences, even though it is built upon the very imperfect samples of personal experience.

_____

_____

_____

【单　　词】dissimilar 相异的；sophisticated 久经世故的；derive from 从……衍生出，起源于，来自。

【结构分析】主句主语为 folk knowledge, 谓语为系表结构 is not very dissimilar from...，derived from 为过去分词短语做定语，修饰 images。even though 为让步状语从句。

【参考译文】甚至在基于普通生活的社会体系中，在挣钱、花钱、结社、结婚、参加政治活动及战争等方面的大众知识与那些从社会学衍生而来的社会体系中更高深的描绘并没有很大的不同，尽管这一结论是基于个人经历中那些极不完美的例子的。

11. Foods and medicine, also classified according to their reputed intrinsic nature as Yin (cold) and Yang (hot), may be taken therapeutically to correct the imbalance resulting from ill health, or to correct imbalance due to the overindulgence in a food manifestly excessively "hot" or "cold", or due to age or changed physiological status (for example, pregnancy).

_____

_____

_____

【单　　词】reputed 有名气的；intrinsic 内在的；therapeutically 治疗地；overindulgence 过度嗜好；manifestly 明白地。

【结构分析】主语为 food and medicine, 这个主语由过去分词短语 classified... 修饰；谓语为 may be taken therapeutically...，两个不定式 to correct... 为并列结构，做目的状语；两个 due to... 为介词短语，表示原因，且由 or 连接。

【参考译文】根据其普遍认可的内在性质，食物和药品也被分为"阴"（凉性）和"阳"（热性）；在治疗学上，它们可以用来治疗由疾病引起的失调，也可治疗由对过热或过冷食品的过度嗜好引发的身体失衡，或治疗因年龄或生理变化（如怀孕）所带来的身体失调。

12. It is information systems that affect the scope and quality of health care, make social services more equitable, enhance personal comfort, provide a greater measure of safety and mobility, and extend the variety of leisure forms at one's disposal.

_____

_____

_____

【单　　词】scope 范围；equitable 公正的；mobility 活动性；at one's disposal 任某人支配。

【结构分析】此句为强调句型，强调的内容为 information system。affect，make，enhance，provide，extend 为并列谓语。

【参考译文】正是信息系统影响着人们医疗保健的范围和质量，它使社会服务更加公正，提高了个人的舒适度，为安全和自由行动提供了更多措施，并根据个人的意愿增加闲暇活动的多样性。

13. While larger banks can afford to maintain their own data-processing operations, many smaller regional and community banks are finding that the costs associated

with upgrading data-processing equipment and with the development and maintenance of new products and technical staff are prohibitive.

_____

_____

_____

_____

【单　　词】maintenance 维护；prohibitive 禁止的。

【结构分析】while 引导让步状语从句。主句主干为 banks are finding, 后面紧跟一个由 that 引导的宾语从句。在该宾语从句中，主语为 costs, associated with 为过去分词做定语，且为多个并列结构，谓语为 are prohibitive。

【参考译文】尽管大银行有能力花钱来保持它们自己的数据处理正常运行，但是许多小的地区银行和社区银行却发现：与更新数据处理设备、发展和维护新产品以及技术人员费用等有关的成本费用高不可攀；而且技术人员的费用也非常昂贵。

14. The point at which tool using and tool making acquire evolutionary significance is surely when an animal can adapt its ability to manipulate objects to a wide variety of purposes, and when it can use an object spontaneously to solve a brand-new problem that without the use of a tool would prove insoluble.

_____

_____

_____

_____

【单　　词】evolutionary 进化的；manipulate 操纵，使用；spontaneously 自然地，本能地；insoluble 无法解决的。

【结构分析】句子的框架是：The point...is...when...and when... 两个 when 引导的从句为并列的表语从句。at which tool using and tool making acquire evolutionary significance 为定语从句，修饰主语 the point；第二个 when 引导的表语从句中也有 that 引导的定语从句，修饰 a brand-new problem。ability to manipulate objects 译为"操纵物体的能力"；...a brand-new problem that without the use of a tool would prove insoluble 中 without 和 insoluble 为双重否定，可译成肯定句。

【参考译文】当动物能够使自己操纵物体的能力适用于更广泛的目标范围，并且能够自发地使用物体解决只有通过工具才能解决的崭新问题时，工具的使用和制造就一定达到了具有进化意义的阶段。

15. At the same time, the American Law Institute — a group of judges, lawyers, and academics whose recommendations carry substantial weight — issued new guidelines for tort law stating that companies need not warn customers of obvious

dangers or bombard them with a lengthy list of possible ones.

_____

_____

_____

_____

【单　　词】substantial 实质的；tort law 民事侵权法；bombard 炮轰，轰击。

【结构分析】主语为 the American Law Institute，谓语为 issued, a group of... 为插入语。stating 为现在分词，that companies need not... 为 stating 的宾语从句。

【参考译文】与此同时，美国法律研究所——由一群法官、律师和理论专家组成，他们的建议分量极重，发布了新的民事伤害法令指导方针，宣称公司不必提醒顾客注意显而易见的危险，也不必连篇累牍地一再提请他们注意一些可能会出现的危险。

四、阅读理解考查内容及相应的应试技巧

（一）主要测试题型

1. 主旨题

此类考题主要测试考生对全文中心思想的理解和把握，常用提问方式有：

The main idea of this passage is _____.

The best title of this passage is _____.

The passage mainly discusses _____.

The main purpose of the article is _____.

The general idea of the passage is _____.

当考生根据题目特点判断考题为主旨题时，先不要急于解题。在完成其他细节题后，会对文章有比较深入的了解，这样解题会比较省时省力。另外，解题时，应该重点阅读文章的首段和末段，看是否出现文章的主题句。如果没有出现文章的主题句，则阅读每一段的主题句，然后总结出大意，对比选项。

2. 细节题

此类考题在考试中比重较大，主要有以下几种方式：细节排除题、细节辨析题、细节判断题。细节题测试考生对文章某个特性信息的掌握和理解。如果细节题与某一具体细节有关，则根据线索词在原文寻找答案。如果测试作者对这一现象的看法，就要联系本段落的主题句解题，考虑段落所体现的逻辑关系。在文章中往往能够找到解题看法的线索词，如：

表示列举的线索词：first, second, finally, next, then, meanwhile, besides, also, in addition to 等；

表示因果关系的线索词：because, as a result of, due to, for, since, now that, thus, therefore, consequently, hence, accordingly, on account of, lead to, result in, result from 等；

表示比较的线索词：unlike, like, in comparison, likewise, similarly 等；

表示转折的线索词：but, yet, however, on the other hand, though, although, while, nevertheless, on the contrary, in spite of, despite 等；

表示举例的线索词：for instance, such as, for example, that is, namely 等。

3. 解释题或猜词题

这类考题测试考生对某一个词语、短语或语句的正确理解，通常包括单词释义、短语释义、句子释义。常用提问方式有：

By...the author means / refers to _____.

In this paragraph, the word "..." probably means _____.

The first sentence in Paragraph 5 means _____.

According to the passage, ... can be best defined as _____.

The author uses the word "..." to indicate _____.

这类考题的解题关键在于，一定要在原文信息中理解单词或短语的含义。

4. 态度题

这类考题考查考生对作者针对某现象的看法、观点等的理解。常用提问方式有：

The author's attitude towards something is _____.

What's the writer's attitude to _____?

What's the tone of the passage?

5. 推理题

推理就是对文章的引申义或比喻义进行逻辑推理，从字面理解上升到对文章的宏观把握。题干常见词汇：imply, suggest, infer, assume。这类题型较难。

We can infer from the passage that _____.

It can be assumed that _____.

The passage suggests that _____.

The next paragraph would probably discuss _____.

From the passage, we can see the author feels that _____.

（二）应试技巧提示

无论什么题型，只要是阅读理解题，就离不开对语篇分析能力和做题技巧的强化练习。做阅读理解题的核心是：找（定位）；比（比较定位处与选项、比较选项之间）。

1. 定位的方法

定位是指确定题目考查的内容在原文的位置。因为阅读的做题方法通常是"读题干→

读原文→回原文定位"这样一个顺序，所以定位是在读完题干以后，根据题干的特点，结合原文阅读的重点和所做的标记来确定题目考查内容的位置。

- 原文中出现题干中的关键词

如果原文中出现了题干的关键词，则定位就显得比较容易。我们要提醒考生的是，并不是一个关键词出现，就证明定位成功，而是题干中的关键词、限定词等同时出现的地方，才是题目的定位所在。大家已经充分体会了定位错误是最终选错答案的主要原因，所以我们发现题干关键词后，要与题干再进行比对，然后进行精确定位。

- 原文中没有出现题干中的关键词

为了加大题目的难度，出题人为考生首先设置的障碍就是不让大家在原文中轻易地找到题目的出处。在原文中没有出现题干的关键词的情况下，我们应针对不同题型采取不同的应对措施。具体应对措施见下表。

序号	项目	要点	阅读或解题技巧
1	主题类题	阅读题干，分辨出主题类题即可	定位到全文的中心句
2	态度类题	当原文是转折结构时	定位到转折后的内容，这才是作者真正的态度
3		当原文是说明文时	定位到隐含的优点句和缺点句
4	推断类题	当考查作者的写作目的时	定位到最后一段的内容
5		题干中有 true 或 not true	直接阅读选项，通过选项定位
6	细节类题	细节类题中，若原文无题干原词，则是出题人在写题干时，用近义词对原文进行了改写	利用位置法。一般原文的进展顺序和题目考查顺序是一致的。如果下一道题的原词已经在原文出现，就证明我们错过了上一道题目的原文出处。考生这时不要回读原文，要先看选项，再读上文，看是否出现选项的原词，以此定位
7			利用选项定位。选项中同时出现的词为定位重点；如果选项中没有重复的词，则要找到每一个选项的出处，再比较原文和题干是否一致
8			利用题干近义词定位。原文中出现题干近义词，而不是原词时，停顿一下进行定位。这种方法适用于语言基础较好的学生，在实际考试中，能运用此方法的人并不多

如果是细节类题但定位较困难的话，这样的题目是难题，考生应该给予足够的重视。而在平时解题时，也要有意识地锻炼自己的定位能力。

较难定位的题目有下面几种：

（1）问事物之间的关系（如题干中同时出现了两个事物，则多半是考查这两个事物之间的关系），读者可以先定位到同时标记这两个事物的地方。

例如：The author suggests that the work of Fisher and Hamilton was similar in that both scientists…

（2）问作者的态度，读者可以先定位到有态度词标记的地方。

例如：The author's attitude toward the "activity" and its consequences can best be described as one of…

（3）问事物的缺陷，则可以直接定位到标记缺陷处。

（4）问文章大意类的主旨题可以定位到主题句。

例如：The primary purpose of the passage is to…

其他定位方法：

● 题干核心词定位

如果读完题干，没有发现考点和特征词，或者题干中的专有名词全文皆是，无法分辨所述到底在何处的时候，就要用核心词来定位了。核心词是题干中最能反映其考查点的部分，并且以实义词居多。下面我们罗列出一些题目和其核心词，大家不妨试着找找它们的共同特征：

（1）about/concerning 作为介词时，后面的宾语通常是题干核心词。

1）The passage suggests which of the following **about surges in the Earth's outer core**?

2）Which of the following best states the author's main point **about logical argument**?

3）Which of the following statements **about the use of comedy in Hardy's novels is best supported by the passage**?

4）Which of the following statements **concerning nuclear scientists is most directly suggested in the passage**?

（2）题干中的实义词、短语通常为句子核心部分。

1）According to the passage, **successful game strategy** depends on_____.

2）It can be inferred from the passage that **the mathematical theory of games** has been_____.

3）According to the passage, **widely spaced doses of insulin** can cause_____.

● 替换词定位

例如：It can be inferred from the passage that scientists are currently making efforts to observe which of the following events?

原文：A nucleus that large cannot be stable, but it might be possible to assemble one next to a vacuum for long enough to observe the decay of the vacuum. Experiments attempting to achieve this are now under way.

题干中 currently 在原文中的替换词是 now。

● 选项标志词与题干核心词双重定位

例如：According to the author, glycogen is crucial to the process of anaerobic glycolysis because glycogen _____.

A. increases the organism's need for ATP

B. reduces the amount of ATP in the tissues

C. is an inhibitor of the oxidative metabolic production of ATP

D. ensures that the synthesis of ATP will occur speedily

【解析】这道题的题干中反复出现 glycogen，其自然成为定位的核心词。但是，如果读者稍微扫一下选项就会发现，每个选项都有个很明显的特征词 ATP，用这个专有名词来定位自然更加容易。所以，我们不妨用题干核心词 glycolysis 和选项特征词 ATP 双重定位。

● 段落定位

无论是题干核心词、选项核心词，还是核心词替换词，我们把它们从题目里挑出来，终究还是要到原文中去找，那么长的文章，我们到哪里找这些词呢？用到上面这些定位方法的题目一般为细节类题或者难度稍大的题，这就要求读者对文章结构、内容有更高级的把握，即对段落作用、大意有个大致印象，才好运用段落定位，缩小目标范围。

下面我们列举一篇文章和一些相应的题目为例，初步讲解一下把握段落大意的方法和段落定位的应用。

The term corporate culture refers to an organization's value system. Managerial philosophies, workplace practices, and organizational network are included in the concept of corporate culture. Tyson Food's corporate culture is reflected in the fact that everyone—even CEO Don Tyson wears tan clothes on the job.

The leaders who developed the company and the corporate culture typically shape the corporate culture. One generation of employees passes on a corporate culture to newer employees. Sometimes this is part of formal training; new managers who attend McDonald's Hamburger University may learn skills in management, but they also pick up the basics of the organization's corporate culture. Employees can absorb corporate culture through informal contacts as well, by talking with other workers and through their experiences on the job.

Corporate culture has a major impact on the success of an organization. In organizations with strong cultures, everyone knows and supports the organizations' objectives. In those with weak cultures, no clear sense of purpose exists. In fact, the authors of the classic book *In Search of Excellence* concluded the presence of a strong corporate culture was the single common thread among many diverse but highly successful companies such as General Electric and McDonald's.

As you can imagine, changing a company's corporate culture can be very difficult. But some managers try to do just that when they feel the current culture is weak, or when the organization's objectives change and the old culture no longer fits. Sometimes the competitive situation of a company changes; electric utilities, which once had their profits guaranteed by public regulation, now face capitalist-style competition. Firms that were comfortably competing against other American companies now find themselves fighting competitors from overseas, too.

Management expert Peter Drucker feels that, rather than trying to change culture, managers should focus on changing employees, habits, as follows:

* Define what results are needed. Specify in measurable terms what the organization (or department, or office) needs to achieve.

* Determine where these results are already being achieved within the current organization. Analyze the departments that are already effective and find out what they are doing differently from the rest.

* Determine what top management can do to encourage these good results. Drucker suggests that executives openly ask what they can do to help, and then do it.

* Change the reward system—or develop a new one—to recognize these effective habits. When employees realize that the organization really does reward the new approach, they will adopt it much more quickly.

Whether one wants to change an organization's culture or not, it is important to choose managers and employees whose personal styles fit the organization's goals.

1）According to the author, which of the following is true?

A. The corporate culture of a corporation can be hard to change.

B. The corporate culture of a corporation should never be changed.

C. Strong corporate cultures should not be changed.

D. Strong corporate culture is harder to be changed than weak ones.

2）According to Peter Drucker, when changing employees, a manager should _____.

A. first determine which parts of the organization best meet the corporate culture

B. first determine what is to be achieved by the corporation

C. reward all the employees that best know the organization's corporate culture

D. restructure the organization

【解析】第一题的正确答案是 A。采用的是段落大意定位法。我们从四个选项可以知道，本题考查的是"企业文化改变"的细节。第一段的中心句为第一句，讲述的是"企业文化的定义"，与选项无关；第二段的中心句也是第一句，介绍的是"企业文化的塑造"，与本题无关；第三段还是一个总分关系的段落，说明的是"企业文化的作用"；从第四段的中心句，我们可以得知本段主要论述"企业文化的改变"。中心句的意思是：企业文化是很难改变的，文章中使用了 difficult，选项中的 hard 实际上是对原文的同义替换。

第二题的正确答案是 B。我们首先从文章中找到 Peter Drucker，然后发现对应的词汇回选项定位正确答案。

综合来说，对试题在原文中的位置进行准确定位的前提是抓住试题中的标志词和关键词。关键词是指表达试题内容的中心词，一般是试题中的名词和名词词组。

标志词主要包括：

● 专有名词，是指表示人名、地名和组织机构等的名词，这样的名词在文章中一般首字母都要大写。

● 表示时间或年代的词。

● 专业词汇，这样的词汇一般比较难懂，并且一般是我们不熟悉的词汇。

2. 如何"比"？

在定位处找到原文出处后，我们就要开始在原文和选项之间进行比较了。第一种方法就是正推法，即从原文到选项。这种方法尽管省时，但是使用这种方法需要有以下几个条件：

- 确定正确定位到题目的出处。
- 理解回现点处原文的内容，并能够分析句式。

第二种方法为倒推法，即从选项到原文。与第一种方法相比，这种方法比较费时，因为要去掉错误的选项，留下正确的，而错误的选项有3个，正确的只有1个。但是，这种方法可以帮助我们减少对原文的理解和对定位的要求，我们只需要掌握错误选项的特征即可。所以，这种方法也是大家无计可施时的"蒙题大法"。

3. 正确选项的特征及识别方法

一般来讲，正确选项都是对原文的精确改写或者原文重现。原文重现的对应方式越来越少，甚至有些原文重现，还会是混淆项，用来迷惑考生。因此更多的方式是精确改写。精确改写包含两个层面的含义，一个层面是词汇的改写，指的是同义词、同义词组、同义表达法的替换；另一个层面是指句型和逻辑的一些变化，是在不违背正确逻辑推理的前提下对原文进行的改写，也就是它至少要满足逻辑上的合理性。下面我们就把这些方法总结如下。

（1）最常见的原文改写的方法是词性变换、同义词或同义词组的替换

这些变化往往体现了选项与原文之间文字与文字的精确对应。下面我们通过分类举例，来具体解释原文改写的含义。

例1：Useful as half-sleeping might be, it's only been found in birds and such water mammals as dolphins, whales and seals. Perhaps keeping one side of the brain awake allows a sleeping animal to surface occasionally to avoid drowning.

While sleeping, some water mammals tend to keep half awake in order to _____.

A. alert themselves to the approaching enemy

B. emerge from water now and then to breathe

C. be sensitive to the ever-changing environment

D. avoid being swept away by rapid currents

【解析】原文和答案词汇比较如下：

➢ allows a sleeping animal to surface（浮出水面）= emerge from water（漂浮于水面）

➢ occasionally（偶尔）= now and then（偶尔）

➢ to avoid drowning（防止淹死）= to breathe（呼吸）

答案中的词汇实际上是文中词汇的释义。因此答案是 B。

例2：There is, as Robert Rubin, the treasury secretary, says, a "disjunction" between the mass of business anecdote that points to a leap in productivity and the picture reflected by the statistics.

The official statistics on productivity growth _____.

A. exclude the usual rebound in a business cycle

B. fall short of businessmen's anticipation

C. meet the expectation of business people

D. fail to reflect the truth of economy

【解析】原文和答案词汇与结构比较如下：

➢ a "disjunction" between A and B（A 和 B 分离）= fall short of（不符合）

➢ business anecdote that points to（预测……的商业轶事）= businessmen's anticipation（商人的预料）

答案词汇比文中词汇简单，主要考查考生是否真正理解了原文词汇。答案是 B。

（2）正确选项是原文的总体或局部。

总体和局部（或称一般和特殊）的关系主要表现为：一般是特殊的总和，特殊为一般的属性。这种题型考查考生类比推理的能力。

例如：There are two basic ways to see growth: one as a product, the other as a process. People have generally viewed personal growth as an external result or product that can easily be identified and measured. The worker who gets a promotion, the student whose grades improve, the foreigner who learns a new language—all these are examples of people who have measurable results to show for their efforts.

A person is generally believed to achieve personal growth when _____.

A. he has given up his smoking habit

B. he has made great efforts in his work

C. he is keen on learning anything new

D. he has tried to determine where he is on his journey

【解析】题干中 generally 是关键词，与原文第二句中的 generally 一致。第二句的意思是：人们通常认为个人的成长是外在的成果或产物，是容易辨别和衡量的。所以，正确答案必须符合"外在""易辨别和衡量"这两个一般特征。A 项"当一个人戒了烟"，戒了烟是一种易辨别的、外在的"成果"，与"升职"等相似，属于特殊的情况。故 A 项正确。

（3）正确选项常常是原文长难句的简单化解释。

正如上一章所谈到的，难句是所有考试必考的内容。难句之所以难有三方面的原因：一是句子结构复杂；二是表达抽象；三是单词难。很多题目都围绕长难句做文章，而正确答案却通常使用简单的结构或词汇对难句进行浅显、具体的解释。

例如：But my own worry today is less that of the overwhelming problem of elemental literacy than it is of the slightly more luxurious problem of the decline in the skill even of the middle-class reader, of his unwillingness to afford those spaces of silence, those luxuries of domesticity and time and concentration, that surround the image of the classic act of reading. It has been suggested that almost 80 percent of America's literate, educated teenagers can no longer read without an accompanying noise (music) in the background or a television screen flickering at the corner of their field of perception. We know very little about the brain and how it deals with simultaneous conflicting input, but every commonsense intuition suggests we should be profoundly alarmed. This violation of concentration, silence, solitude goes to the very heart of our notion of literacy; this new form of part-reading, of part-perception against background distraction, renders impossible certain essential acts of apprehension and concentration, let alone that most important tribute any human being can pay to poem or a piece of prose he or she really loves, which is to learn it by heart. Not by brain, by heart; the expression is vital.

1) The author's biggest concern is _____.

A. elementary school children's disinterest in reading classics

B. the surprisingly low rate of literacy in the U.S.

C. the musical setting American readers require for reading

D. the reading ability and reading behavior of the middle class

2) A major problem with most adolescents who can read is _____.

A. their fondness of music and TV programs

B. their ignorance of various forms of art and literature

C. their lack of attentiveness and basic understanding

D. their inability to focus on conflicting input

【解析】第一题考查对第一句话的理解。该句长达 62 个词。全句主干结构为 my worry...is less that of...than... "与其说……不如说……"。句意为：我虽然担心基础读写能力存在问题，但我更担心中产阶级读者的阅读技能也有所下降。接着作者描述了问题所在，从 of his unwillingness 开始，作者说 "他们不愿意在安静的环境里读书，不能集中注意力"。所以 D "中产阶级的阅读能力和阅读行为" 是对整句话的概括。

第二题考查对倒数第二句话的理解，该句长达 66 个词，有两个分句，并用分号隔开。第一个分句大意为：这种阅读时不专心、不安静、不独处的情况是读写最大的问题。go to the heart of 是固定短语，意为 "（问题）最重要的方面"。第二个分句更复杂，难点为作者把 render sth. +adj.（使什么怎么样）句型倒装，形容词提前，名词推后，因为名词部分较长。难词有 apprehension "理解"，pay tribute to "崇敬"。大意为：这种在娱乐背景下边读边理解的阅读新方式，是不可能做到真正理解和专心致志的，更不用说任何一个人对真正喜爱的一首诗或一篇散文所能表现的最重要的赞赏了。所以 C 项 "他们不专心，缺乏基本的理解" 是两个分句的综合，是正确答案。

（4）正确选项是对原文引语的解释。

文章的引语通常较难。作者之所以引述他人的话，是因为自己的话无论怎么说都没有他人说得准确、说得好。引语的目的不是夸耀他人，而是用来论证说明自己的观点。引语是经常考查的内容，题干形式有两种：The author quotes...because... / The author quotes...to illustrate...

例如："Creative thinking may mean simply the realization that there's no particular virtue in doing things the way they have always been done," wrote Rudolph Flesch, a language authority, this accounts for our reaction to seemingly simple innovations like plastic garbage bags and suitcases on wheels that make life more convenient: "How come nobody thought of that before?"

The creative approach begins with the proposition that nothing is as it appears. Innovators will not accept that there is only one way to do anything. Faced with getting from A to B, the average person will automatically set out on the best-known and apparently simplest route. The innovator will search for alternate courses, which may prove easier in the long run and are bound to be more interesting and challenging even if they lead to dead ends.

The author quotes Rudolph Flesch in Paragraph 1 because _____.

A. Rudolph Flesch is the best-known expert in the study of human creativity

B. the quotation strengthens the assertion that creative individuals look for new ways of doing things

C. the reader is familiar with Rudolph Flesch's point of view

D. the quotation adds a new idea to the information previously presented

【解析】这句引语的含义是："创造性思维也许仅仅意味着认识到按常规做事并不一定有什么道理"，下一段的前两句说："创造性思维起始于这样一个命题：一切东西都不是它表现出来的那样。革新家们认为做任何事都不是只有一种方法。"将这两点综合考虑可知，作者引用 Rudolph 的话只不过是为了进一步证明自己的观点，即创新者总是寻找做事的新方法，这与 B 项完全一致。

（5）正确选项是文中例证或事实的归纳总结。

在推断类题中，如下几个特点是正确选项的标志，即：高度概括性、归纳性、总结性、抽象性和推理性。

例如：One hundred and thirteen million Americans have at least one bank-issued credit card. They give their owners automatic credit in stores, restaurants, and hotels, at home, across the country, and even abroad, and they make many banking services available as well. More and more of these credit cards can be read automatically, making it possible to withdraw or deposit money in scattered locations, whether or not the local branch bank is open. For many of us the "cashless society" is not on the horizon—it's already here.

According to the passage, the credit card enables its owner to _____.

A. withdraw as much money from the bank as he wishes

B. obtain more convenient services than other people do

C. enjoy greater trust from the storekeeper

D. cash money wherever he wishes to

【解析】根据对第二句和第三句的概括，信用卡使持卡者比其他人享有更多的便利服务，可知 B 项正确。A、D 两项均过于绝对，且与文意不符；C 项"持卡者得到店主更大的信任"文中未提及，也应排除。

（6）正确选项是对段落中心或者篇章中心的归纳总结。

例如：Few people doubt the fundamental importance of mothers in child rearing, but what do fathers do? Much of what they contribute is simply the result of being a second adult in the home. Bringing up children is demanding, stressful and exhausting. Two adults can support and make up for each other's strengths.

The paragraph points out that one of the advantages of a family with both parents is _____.

A. husband and wife can share housework

B. two adults are always better than one

C. the fundamental importance of mothers can be fully recognized

D. husband and wife can compensate for each other's shortcoming

【解析】本段的主题是抚养子女的过程中母亲或父亲的作用，如果双方互相支持，可以弥补对方的缺陷。由此可见 D 项"夫妇可互相弥补彼此的不足"是对段落中心的概括，符合题意。A 项"夫妇可共同做家务"和 B 项"两个总比一个好"都是根据生活常识编造的选项（合理项，参见前面"错误选项的特征"部分）；C 项"母亲的重要性可以得到充分认可"表达片面。

4. 识别干扰项的方法

读选项的方法因题目类型的不同而不同，一般来说，主题类题目要先看各个选项的主动词，而细节类题目则要逐一看全句。但无论是主题类题还是细节类题，看全句之前都要先着眼于句子主干、主态度，因为快速地扫过主干、判断句子主态度之后，很多选项都可以马上排除；这样花在句子修饰成分上面的时间就可以节省出来。对于那些看了主干之后无法马上排除的选项，不妨再逐词细看。

看选项之后的第一步就是排除，比较典型的排除干扰选项的方法有：

（1）用最高级、唯一性、比较级来排除

使用这种方法来排除干扰选项的前提是原文中凡是最高级、唯一性和比较级的地方都做上标记。用极端性词汇排除选项是一种"少投入、多回报"的方法。此外，原文中关于比较级的记录也是必不可少的，因为比较可以直接反映事物之间的关系，通常为考点，应受到考生的关注（尤其是表示"相同的""不同的"同级比较和带 than 的比较）。如果作者在文中不曾对两者进行过比较，选项说得再像模像样也是错的。

（2）用同性元素来排除

同性元素是指在原文中作用完全一样的事物，当它们同时出现在选项中时，要么都对，要么都错，如果题目是单选题，作用相同的两者同时出现必然同时被排除。

五、阅读理解专项练习及最新真题解析

Passage One

By almost every measure, Paul Pfingst is an unsentimental prosecutor. Last week the San Diego County district attorney said he fully intends to try to suspect Charles Andrew Williams, 15, as an adult for the Santana High School shootings. Even before the tragedy, Pfingst had stood behind the controversial California law that mandates treating murder suspects as young as 14 as adults.

So nobody would have wagered that Pfingst would also be the first D.A. in the U.S. to launch his very own Innocence Project. Yet last June, Pfingst told his attorneys to go back over old murder and rape convictions and see if any unravel with newly developed DNA-testing tools. In other words, he wanted to revisit past victories — this time playing for the other team. "I think people misunderstand being conservative for being biased," says Pfingst. "I consider myself a pragmatic guy, and I have no interest in putting innocent people in jail."

Around the U.S., <u>flabbergasted</u> defense attorneys and their jailed clients cheered his move. Among prosecutors, however, there was an awkward pause. After all, each DNA test costs as much as $5,000. Then there's the unspoken risk: if dozens of innocents turn up, the D.A. will have indicted his shop.

But nine months later, no budgets have been busted or prosecutors ousted. Only the rare case merits review. Pfingst's team considers convictions before 1993, when the city started routine DNA testing. They discard cases if the defendant has been released. Of the 560 remaining files, they have re-examined 200, looking for cases with biological evidence and defendants who still claim innocence.

They have identified three so far. The most compelling involves a man serving 12 years for molesting a girl who was playing in his apartment. But others were there at the time. Police found a small drop of saliva on the victim's shirt — too small a sample to test in 1991. Today that spot could free a man. Test results are due any day. Inspired by San Diego, 10 other counties in the U.S. are starting DNA audits.

1. How did Pfingst carry out his own Innocence Project?
   A. By getting rid of his bias against the suspects.
   B. By revisiting the past victories.
   C. By using the newly developed DNA-testing tools.
   D. By his cooperation with his attorneys.

2. Which of the following can be an advantage of Innocence Project?
   A. To help correct the wrong judgments.
   B. To oust the unqualified prosecutors.
   C. To make the prosecutors in an awkward situation.
   D. To cheer up the defense attorneys and their jailed clients.

3. The expression "flabbergasted" (Paragraph 3) most probably means _____.
   A. excited   B. competent
   C. embarrassed   D. astounded

4. Why was Pfingst an unsentimental prosecutor?
   A. He intended to try a fifteen-year old suspect.

B. He had no interest in putting the innocent in jail.

C. He supported the controversial California law.

D. He wanted to try suspects as young as fourteen.

5. Which of the following is NOT true according to the text?

A. Pfingst's move didn't have a great coverage.

B. Pfingst's move had both positive and negative effect.

C. Pfingst's move didn't work well.

D. Pfingst's move greatly encouraged the jailed prisoners.

本文话题

第一段指出芬斯特作为一位铁面无私的检察官的一些做法；第二段指出芬斯特实施"清白计划"的打算及做法；第三段指出实施"清白计划"造成的反应以及可能存在的问题；第四段和第五段是实施"清白计划"的结果和影响。

难词译注

prosecutor ['prɔsikju:tə(r)] n.	检察官，公诉人，原告律师
controversial [ˌkɔntrə'və:ʃ(ə)l] a.	争论的，争议的
mandate ['mændeit] v.	批准制定一个训令（如通过法律）；发布命令或要求
wager ['weidʒə(r)] v.	下赌注，保证
conviction [kən'vikʃən] n.	定罪，宣告有罪
unravel [ʌn'ræv(ə)l] v.	阐明，解决
flabbergast ['flæbəgɑ:st] v.	<口> 使大吃一惊，哑然失色，使目瞪口呆
indict [in'dait] v.	起诉，控告，指控，告发
bust [bʌst] v.	破产或缺钱
oust [aust] v.	剥夺，取代，驱逐
discard [di'skɑ:d] v.	抛开，遗弃，废弃
molest [mə'lest] v.	骚乱，困扰，调戏
saliva [sə'laivə] n.	口水，唾液

难句译注

1. Even before the tragedy, Pfingst had stood behind the controversial California law that mandates treating murder suspects as young as 14 as adults.

【分析】主体句式：...Pfingst had stood behind ...

结构分析：even before the tragedy 是本句的时间状语；主句是 Pfingst had stood

behind...；that 引导的宾语从句修饰 law；在从句中，as...as 是词组，意思是"和……一样"；出现的第三个 as 是介词，意思是"作为"。

【译文】甚至在这场悲剧发生之前芬斯特就支持加利福尼亚州的一项颇有争议的法律。这项法律规定，以成人身份受审的谋杀嫌疑犯的最低年龄可以降到 14 岁。

答案及解析

1. 【问题】芬斯特是如何开展他的"清白计划"的？
   - A．通过消除他对嫌疑人的偏见。
   - B．通过重提过去的成功。
   - C．通过使用新的 DNA 检测工具。
   - D．通过和律师合作。

   【答案】C

   【解析】事实细节题。文中对应信息"Pfingst told his attorneys to go back over old murder and rape convictions and see if any unravel with newly developed DNA-testing tools."是对第二段第一句的补充说明。

2. 【问题】下列哪一个是"清白计划"的优势？
   - A．纠正过去错判的案件。
   - B．驱逐不合格的检察官。
   - C．使得检察官处于尴尬的境地。
   - D．鼓励辩护律师和入狱的犯人。

   【答案】A

   【解析】推理判断题。从上下文我们可以得知，实施"清白计划"就是使用先进的 DNA 技术来重新审理过去的案件当中可能存在的冤案和错案。

3. 【问题】第三段中 flabbergasted 的意思是_____。
   - A．兴奋的
   - B．胜任的
   - C．尴尬的
   - D．惊讶的

   【答案】D

   【解析】猜词题。从第二段第一句话得知，芬斯特可能是美国第一个实施非常独特的"清白计划"的人，因此他的做法很可能是令人感到吃惊的，从而可猜出该词的含义。

4. 【问题】为什么芬斯特是个铁血检察官？
   - A．他曾经审判过一个 15 岁的嫌疑人。
   - B．他无意将清白的人错判入监。
   - C．他支持有争议的加州法律。
   - D．他想审判小至 14 岁的嫌疑人。

   【答案】B

   【解析】推理判断题。从第一段和第二段给出的事例可以看出，芬斯特不愿放过任何一个犯罪的人，即便他的年龄还不算大；他也不愿使无辜者蒙冤，即便案件已经审理。

5. 【问题】根据文章，下列哪一项不正确？
   - A．芬斯特的行动覆盖面不大。
   - B．芬斯特的行为有正面和负面的效果。
   - C．芬斯特的行为见效不大。

D. 芬斯特的行为很大程度上鼓舞了入狱的犯人。

【答案】C

【解析】推理判断题。正因为"Pfingst's move works well"，美国才又有"ten other counties are starting DNA audits"，而且"no budgets have been busted or prosecutors ousted"。

Passage Two

As you read this, nearly 80,000 Americans are waiting for a new heart, kidney or some other organs that could save their life. Tragically, about 6,000 of them will die this year — nearly twice as many people as perished in the Sept. 11 attacks — because they won't get their transplant in time. The vast majority of Americans (86%, according to one poll) say they support organ donation. But only 20% actually sign up to do it. Why the shortfall?

Part of the problem is the way we handle organ donations. Americans who want to make this sort of gift have to opt in — that is, indicate on a driver's license that when they die, they want their organs to be made available. Many European and Asian countries take the opposite approach; in Singapore, for example, all residents receive a letter when they come of age informing them that their organs may be harvested unless they explicitly object. In Belgium, which adopted a similar <u>presumed-consent</u> system 12 years ago, less than 2% of the population has decided to opt out.

Further complicating the situation in the U.S. is the fact that whatever decision you make can be overruled by your family. The final say is left to your surviving relatives, who must make up their minds in the critical hours after brain death has been declared. There are as many as 50 body parts, from your skin to your corneas, that can save or transform the life of a potential recipient, but for many families lost in grief, the idea of dismembering a loved one is more than they can bear.

The U.S., like all medically advanced societies, has struggled to find a way to balance an individual's rightful sovereignty over his or her body with the society's need to save its members from avoidable deaths. Given America's tradition of rugged individualism and native distrust of Big Brotherly interference, it's not surprising that voters resisted attempts to switch to a presumed-consent system when it was proposed in California, Oregon, Minnesota, Pennsylvania and Maryland. Health Secretary Tommy Thompson last spring announced plans for a new initiative to encourage donations — including clearer consent forms — but its impact is expected to be modest. Given the crying need for organs, perhaps it's time we considered shifting to something closer to the presumed-consent model.

Meanwhile, if you want to ensure that your organs are donated when you die, you should say so in a living will or fill out a Uniform Donor Card (available from the American

Medical Association). Make sure your closest relatives know about it. And if you don't want to donate an organ, you should make your wishes equally explicit.

1. According to the author, one of the reasons for a shortage of organs in America is that _____.
   A. most Americans are reluctant to donate their organs after death
   B. the information about organ donation is not popular in America
   C. the ways to handle organ donation is far from perfect
   D. people waiting for transplant are rapidly increasing in America
2. What is most Americans' attitude towards the organ donation?
   A. Indifferent.　　　B. Indignant.　　　C. Detached.　　　D. Supportive.
3. It can be inferred from Paragraph 4 that _____.
   A. Americans have a long tradition of weak individualism
   B. all the states in America resist the presumed-consent system
   C. it's not easy to find a way to serve the society's need and at the same time to protect the individual's right in the matter of organ donation
   D. the government is not active in solving the problem
4. The term "presumed-consent" probably means _____.
   A. one's organs should be donated whether they agree or not
   B. one is supposed to agree that their organ will be donated after death unless they explicitly object
   C. dismembering a dead body is inhuman
   D. one is assumed to be happy after they decide to donate their organs
5. From the text, we can see the author's attitude towards organ donation is _____.
   A. supportive　　B. indignant　　　C. indifferent　　　D. negative

本文话题

　　本篇文章提出了一个解决美国国内捐献器官严重紧缺问题的办法。第一段以人们的良好愿望和严峻现实的强烈对比开始。第二段找出了产生这一问题的一个原因——运作方式有待提高。第三段找出了产生这一问题的另一个原因——人们的心理承受能力。第四段说明美国必须解决这个问题。最后一段指明目前捐献器官的方式及注意事项。

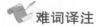

难词译注

perish ['periʃ] v.	死，暴卒；毁灭
donation [dəu'neiʃən] n.	捐赠
shortfall ['ʃɔːtfɔːl] n.	不足之量，短缺的数额
opt [ɔpt] v.	（常与 for 连用）决定做；选择，选取
consent [kən'sent] n & v.	同意

overrule [ˌəuvəˈruːl] v.	驳回，否决
cornea [ˈkɔːniə] n.	角膜
dismember [disˈmembə] v.	肢解
sovereignty [ˈsɔvrinti] n.	完全独立和自我统治，主权
rugged [ˈrʌgid] a.	粗犷的

难句译注

1. There are as many as 50 body parts, from your skin to your corneas, that can save or transform the life of a potential recipient, but for many families lost in grief, the idea of dismembering a loved one is more than they can bear.

   【分析】主体句式：There are…, but the idea…is…

   结构分析：这句是由 but 做连接词连接的两个分句。第一个分句中包含一个由 that 引导的定语从句，修饰 body parts；第二个分句的主语是 the idea。

   【译文】人身上有 50 种可捐献的器官，皮肤和角膜都包括在内。每种都可能救活一个人或改变他们的命运。但对正沉浸在丧失亲人之痛的人来说，把逝去的亲人大卸八块是他们承受不了的。

2. The U.S., like all medically advanced societies, has struggled to find a way to balance an individual's rightful sovereignty over his or her body with the society's need to save its members from avoidable deaths.

   【分析】主体句式：The U.S. … has struggled to find a way to balance …with…

   结构分析：其中短语"balance…with…"的含义是"使……和……相平衡"。

   【译文】像其他医学发达的国家一样，美国也在努力寻求个人和国家之间的最佳平衡点。即让个人对自己的身体有合法的拥有权，又能满足社会救死扶伤的需要。

答案及解析

1. 【问题】根据本文作者的看法，美国器官短缺的原因之一是 _____ 。

   A. 大多数美国人不愿意在死后捐献器官

   B. 关于器官捐献的信息在美国不流行

   C. 处理器官捐献的方式远远不够完善

   D. 等待移植的人在美国迅速增加

   【答案】C

   【解析】事实细节题。从第一、二段可以读出，绝大多数美国人愿意捐出自己的器官，只是运作方式还有待提高。

2. 【问题】大多数美国人对器官捐献的态度是什么？

   A. 冷漠的   B. 愤怒的

   C. 不关注的   D. 支持的

   【答案】D

【解析】推理判断题。从第一段 "The vast majority of Americans say they support organ donation" 可以看出答案。

3. 【问题】从第四段可以推理得知 _____。

    A. 美国人的脆弱的个人主义历史悠久

    B. 美国所有的州都抵制假定捐献人同意的制度

    C. 在器官捐献方面找到满足社会需求，同时保护个人权益的方法是不容易的

    D. 政府在解决问题方面不积极

【答案】C

【解析】属于事实细节题。政府也想改变目前这种状况，只不过措施不那么有效。

4. 【问题】术语 "presumed-consent" 的意思是 _____。

    A. 无论他们是否同意，他们的器官都应该捐献

    B. 人们被认为同意在死后捐出自己器官，除非他们明确地反对

    C. 解剖尸体是不人道的

    D. 人们在决定捐献器官后应该感到高兴

【答案】B

【解析】属于猜测词义题。从第二段对新加坡和比利时的描述中可以得出结论。

5. 【问题】从文中可以看出，作者对器官捐献的态度是 _____。

    A. 支持的   B. 愤怒的

    C. 冷淡的   D. 否定的

【答案】A

【解析】推理判断题。作者认为解决器官短缺这个难题，应该向新加坡和比利时学习，采取新的强有力的措施。最后一段作者给出了想捐献器官的做法以及应注意的问题，这也可以看出作者的态度是支持的。

Passage Three

Many theories concerning the causes of juvenile crime focus either on the individual or on society as the major contributing influence. Theories centering on the individual suggest that children engage in criminal behavior because they were not sufficiently penalized for previous delinquent acts or that they have learned criminal behavior through interaction with others. A person who becomes socially alienated may be more inclined to commit a criminal act. Theories focusing on the role of society in juvenile delinquency suggest that children commit crimes in response to their failure to rise above their socioeconomic status, or as a repudiation of middle-class values.

Most theories of juvenile delinquency have focused on children from disadvantaged families, ignoring the fact that children from affluent homes also commit crimes. The latter may commit crimes because of the lack of adequate parental control, delays in achieving adult status, and hedonistic tendencies. All theories, however, are tentative and are subject to criticism.

Changes in the American social structure may indirectly affect juvenile crime rates. For example, changes in the economy that lead to fewer job opportunities for youth and rising unemployment in general make gainful employment increasingly difficult for young people to obtain. The resulting discontent may in turn lead more youths into criminal behavior.

Families have also experienced changes within the last several decades. More families are one-parent households or have two working parents; consequently, children are likely to have less supervision at home than was common in the traditional family structure. This lack of parental supervision is thought to be an influence on juvenile crime rates.

Other identifiable causes of delinquent acts include frustration or failure in school, the increased availability of drugs, alcohol, and guns, and the growing incidence of child abuse and child neglect. All these conditions tend to increase the probability of a child committing a criminal act, although a direct causal relationship has not yet been established.

No specific treatment has been proven the most effective form. Effectiveness is typically measured by recidivism rates — that is, by the percentage of children treated who subsequently commit additional criminal acts. The recidivism rates for all forms of treatment, however, are about the same. A large percentage of delinquent acts are never discovered, which further complicates this measurement. Thus, an absence of subsequent reported delinquent acts by a treated child may mean nothing more than that the child was not caught.

1. Which of the following is NOT the factor of juvenile crimes according to the theories focusing on individuals?
   A. Insufficient punishment.
   B. Less parental supervision.
   C. Isolation from others.
   D. Lack of self-control.

2. According to the theories centering on society, which of the following is true?
   A. Juveniles could not find his status in the society.
   B. Unemployment leads to juvenile crimes.
   C. Child abuse leads children to engaging in crimes.
   D. Children's discontent with the changes in social structure causes juvenile crimes.

3. The sentence "All theories, however, are tentative and are subject to criticism." implies that _____.
   A. all theories didn't disclose the true reasons for juvenile crimes
   B. contributing factors these theories indicate are not comprehensive and convincing
   C. these theories misled people's attention to the juvenile delinquency
   D. these theories didn't supply the answers for the juvenile crimes

4. What can we know about recidivism rates?
   A．They are used to measure the effectiveness of treatments of juvenile delinquency.
   B．They indicate children's criminal percentage.
   C．They simplified the measurement of treatments.
   D．They are modified in accordance with the specific treatment.

5. What is the tone of the passage?
   A．Critical.　　　　B．Supportive.　　C．Objective.　　　D．Indifferent.

 本文话题

青少年犯罪。

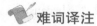 **难词译注**

juvenile [ˈdʒuːvənail] n.		青少年
delinquent [diˈliŋkwənt] a.		违法的
repudiation [riˌpjuːdiˈeiʃən] n.		批判
alienate [ˈeiliəneit] v.		疏远
affluent [ˈæfluənt] a.		富裕的
recidivism [riˈsidivizəm] n.		惯犯

难句译注

1. Theories centering on the individual suggest that children engage in criminal behavior because they were not sufficiently penalized for previous delinquent acts or that they have learned criminal behavior through interaction with others.

   【分析】centering 现在分词做定语，修饰 theories；that 引导宾语从句；because 引导原因状语从句；or 连接两个并列的宾语从句。

   【译文】关注个人的理论认为，儿童因为上一次的犯错没有受到足够的惩罚而参与犯罪，另外，认为儿童通过和他人的交往而学坏。

2. Theories focusing on the role of society in juvenile delinquency suggest that children commit crimes in response to their failure to rise above their socioeconomic status, or as a repudiation of middle-class values.

   【分析】focusing 现在分词做定语，修饰 theories；or 连接两个并列成分，即 in response to… 和 as a repudiation…

   【译文】侧重于社会在青少年犯罪中所处角色的理论认为，儿童犯罪是由于他们在社会经济中无法摆脱命运而引起的，或者是作为对中产阶级价值观的批判而产生。

3. …changes in the economy that lead to fewer job opportunities for youth and rising unemployment in general make gainful employment increasingly difficult for young

people to obtain.

【分析】that 引导定语从句，修饰 changes。

【译文】经济上的变革导致年轻人工作机会减少、失业增加，这使年轻人找到工作变得越来越困难。

答案及解析

1. 【问题】根据个人理论，下面哪一个不是青少年犯罪的原因？

    A．惩罚不够。   B．缺乏父母管教。

    C．孤僻。   D．缺少自控能力。

【答案】D

【解析】细节题。A 项原文信息在第 1 段 "…because they were not sufficiently penalized for previous delinquent acts…"；B 项原文信息在第 2 段 "…because of the lack of adequate parental control…" 以及第 4 段 "…children are likely to have less supervision…"；C 项原文信息在第 1 段 "A person who becomes socially alienated may be more inclined to commit a criminal act." 。由此可知只有 D 项未提及。

2. 【问题】根据社会理论，下面哪一个是正确的？

    A．青少年在社会上无法找到他们的地位。

    B．失业导致青少年犯罪。

    C．儿童受虐促使孩子们参与犯罪。

    D．孩子对社会结构变化不满导致青少年犯罪。

【答案】D

【解析】细节题。D 项原文信息在第 3 段，最后一句话提到，孩子们对因经济变化导致的就业机会少或失业不满，这导致他们的犯罪行为。

3. 【问题】"所有这些理论都是尝试性的，容易遭受批评"这句话暗示我们_____。

    A．所有理论都没有揭示青少年犯罪的真正原因

    B．这些理论提出的原因不够全面，也缺乏说服力

    C．这些理论误导了人们对青少年犯罪的关注

    D．这些理论没能为青少年犯罪提供答案

【答案】B

【解析】推断题。根据全文，这些理论有一定道理，但不能涵盖所有的原因，各自都有不足。故 B 含义与之最为接近。

4. 【问题】关于累犯率我们知道什么？

    A．被用于衡量针对青少年犯罪解决办法的有效程度。

    B．表明儿童犯罪的百分比。

    C．简化解决办法。

    D．被根据特定的解决办法进行修改。

【答案】A

【解析】关于累犯率的信息在原文最后一段。

5. 【问题】这篇文章的语气是什么？

          A．批评的。   B．支持的。   C．客观的。   D．漠不关心的。

【答案】C

【解析】态度题。综观全文，作者只是在客观地罗列各种理论，没有体现任何个人的偏爱和喜好，因而 C 为正确答案。

Passage Four

There's a species of smoker among us that is common yet poorly understood. Their habitat consists of parties, barbecues, and the sidewalks outside bars and restaurants. They prefer to scrounge for their cigarettes, and if they do buy a pack, they're apt to nurse it for a week or more. You may hear them say, "I'm not a smoker," or "Only on weekends." These are "social smokers" — and there are more of them than you might think.

Smoking is often characterized as an all-or-nothing activity — on doctor's office questionnaires it's usually a yes-or-no question, for instance — but by some estimates, anywhere from one-fifth to one-third of adults who smoke don't light up every day. While some of these so-called nondaily smokers smoke regularly but sparingly, up to 30% likely fall into the social-smoker category.

Hard numbers are difficult to come by, in part because the definition of a social smoker is so vague. A 2007 study of social smoking among college students — one of very few that have been published on the subject — found the term was used "loosely and inconsistently", even among researchers. But most people know a social smoker when they see one. They smoke occasionally, almost always in groups, and more often than not while drinking alcohol. By definition, they do not consider themselves addicted to nicotine. Many started smoking casually in high school or college but never graduated to a daily habit.

While the overall number of smokers in the United States is dropping, the proportion of occasional smokers appears to be on the rise. News reports and studies have also provided anecdotal（传闻的）evidence that social smoking is increasing, especially among young people.

The reasons for this apparent trend haven't been fully explained. Some suggest that the growing awareness of health risks, the stigma surrounding smoking (which may explain why the smokers interviewed for this article didn't want their full names used), and the smoking bans in public places are causing heavy smokers to cut back. Vickie, for instance, wouldn't be caught dead smoking around her two young children, and the restrictions against smoking at work or inside bars and restaurants are often enough to extinguish her urges, she says — especially in the wintertime.

Another popular theory is that social smokers, unlike social drinkers, don't really exist. Social smokers, the thinking goes, are low-level addicts either in denial or on the brink of addiction. It's a bit like the old saying about there being two types of motorcyclists: those who have had accidents and those who are going to. And research indicates that there may be something to this: In the recent study of college students, 60% of the students surveyed who denied that they were smokers did identify themselves as social smokers; roughly 10% of these alleged nonsmokers in fact smoked at least every other day.

1. What can be known about social smokers?
   A. They tend to light up on weekends.
   B. They are not real smokers.
   C. They tend to nurse a pack for several days or more.
   D. They only appear in parties or restaurants.

2. Which of the following words is closest in meaning with the underlined word "sparingly" in Paragraph 2?
   A. Economically.   B. Prudently.   C. Extravagantly.   D. Indulgently.

3. What can be inferred from the phrase "loosely and inconsistently" in Paragraph 3?
   A. Researchers are not convinced of the reasons for social smokers.
   B. There is no consensus about the definition of social smokers.
   C. Social smokers are hard to be characterized by people.
   D. There is no definite standard for distinguishing social smokers from others.

4. According to the passage, what may be the explanation for the trend that occasional smokers are on the rise while the overall number of smokers is decreasing?
   A. The growing awareness of health.
   B. Bans on smoking at home.
   C. Advice from medical professionals.
   D. The increasing self-discipline.

5. What can be implied from the old saying about there being two types of motorcyclists?
   A. Social smokers are in danger of addiction to nicotine.
   B. Social smokers don't addict to smoking at all.
   C. Social smokers don't consider themselves as smokers.
   D. Social smokers either deny their addiction or are at the risk of addiction.

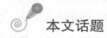 本文话题

社交型吸烟者。

🖊 **难词译注**

habitat [ˈhæbitæt] *n.*	聚集处
scrounge [skraundʒ] *v.*	白要，白拿
vague [veig] *a.*	含糊的
nicotine [ˈnikəti:n] *n.*	尼古丁

🖊 **难句译注**

In the recent study of college students, 60% of the students surveyed who denied that they were smokers did identify themselves as social smokers; roughly 10% of these alleged nonsmokers in fact smoked at least every other day.

【分析】surveyed 是过去分词做定语，修饰 students；that 引导宾语从句。

【译文】在最近针对大学生的研究中，60% 被调查的学生否认自己是烟民，同时视自己为社交型吸烟者；事实上，那些声称自己为非烟民的人中，约 10% 的人每隔一天会吸一次烟。

✝ **答案及解析**

1. 【问题】有关社交型吸烟者我们可以知道什么？
   　　A．他们总是在周末吸烟。
   　　B．他们不是真正的吸烟者。
   　　C．他们总是几天或更长的时间吸一包（烟）。
   　　D．他们只出现在聚会和餐馆。

   【答案】C

   【解析】细节题，选项 C 相关原文信息在第一段 "…they're apt to nurse it for a week or more…"。

2. 【问题】下面哪一个词的意思和画线词 "sparingly" 最接近？
   　　A．节约地。　　　B．谨慎地。　　　C．挥霍无度地。　　　D．放任地。

   【答案】A

   【解析】猜词题。画线词的含义为 "节俭地"。根据上下文信息也可以得出答案。

3. 【问题】从 "loosely and inconsistently" 这个词组可以推断出什么？
   　　A．研究者们不相信社交型吸烟者的理由。
   　　B．关于社交型吸烟者的定义没有一致看法。
   　　C．人们很难定义社交型吸烟者。
   　　D．没有区分社交型吸烟者和其他吸烟者确定的标准。

   【答案】B

   【解析】推断题。根据本段第 1 句话 "Hard numbers are difficult to come by, in part because the definition of a social smoker is so vague…" 就可以解题，这句话是这一段的

主题句。vague 的含义为"含糊的，不清楚的"。

4. 【问题】根据文章所述，针对偶尔吸烟者人数在上升而整体吸烟者人数在下降这一趋势的解释是什么？

    A. 健康意识的增强。   B. 家中禁烟。

    C. 医学专业人士的建议。   D. 自律增强。

【答案】A

【解析】细节题。在文章第 4 段提到题目所说的这一现象，虽然第 5 段第一句话中没有完整的解释，但是人们健康意识的增强可以作为一个解释，因而答案为 A。

5. 【问题】从那个有关两种骑摩托车者的古老谚语中可以得到什么暗示？

    A. 社交型吸烟者处于尼古丁上瘾的危险中。

    B. 社交型吸烟者对吸烟根本不会上瘾。

    C. 社交型吸烟者自认为不是吸烟者。

    D. 社交型吸烟者要么否认他们上瘾，要么否认他们处于上瘾的危险中。

【答案】D

【解析】推断题。这个比喻出现在最后一段，根据对这一比喻的解释和最后一段有关 social smokers 的相关信息可以解题。

Passage Five

Is there any beverage that's more versatile than beer? The malted barley brew can provide a way to bond with buddies, celebrate victories, mourn defeats, and is almost a prerequisite for watching sports. However, if your waistline has started to expand into the stereotypical beer belly zone, you may be looking with disdain at that pint in your hand.

It's commonly assumed that there is a direct correlation between the amount of beer men consume and the size of their beer bellies, but how accurate is this perception? We've investigated the connection between beer and beer bellies, so read on to learn the truth.

Despite the common "beer belly" moniker, excess belly flab is not always caused by swigging too many pints of liquid bread. Beer, at around 140 calories per 12-ounce bottle, is high in calories and frequent imbibing can result in the extra calories that lead to a distended waistline. So, in this case, there is a link. However, like fat that appears in other areas of the body, it has more to do with how many overall calories you consume versus how many you're burning through regular exercise. Your body can't tell the difference between beer-related calories and extra calories from any other food. So, the answer is also, no.

Calories certainly hold part of the answer, but so does age: metabolism slows down after the age of 35, so you may find that the further the calendar advances, the more trouble you have keeping a trim figure. Another part of the reason has to do with your gender. While most women tend to keep their extra flab on their hips, thighs and buttocks, men commonly store fat around the waist. So combine your age and gender with an excess of calories, and the result can be a charming pot belly.

Not only is it an unattractive accessory, belly fat — or visceral fat — is now getting extra attention as one of the riskiest kinds of extra flab a person can sport. People with excess belly fat have a tendency to develop nasty conditions such as insulin resistance, diabetes, high blood pressure, heart disease, and high cholesterol over and above the already increased risk a person receives from other forms of obesity.

So, how do you know if your spare tire is overinflated? Use a measuring tape. Keeping in mind that everybody is different, a general guideline some doctors use for men is a maximum waist measurement of 40 inches. Anything over that and your chances of developing nasty health problems will escalate. To see how you compare, wrap a tape measure around the area above your hipbone. Make sure the tape is level all the way around your midsection, hold it snug, breathe out, and see what the damage is.

1. According to the passage, which of the following statements is true?
    A. Beer belly is in proportion to the amount of beer consumed.
    B. The excess belly flab is not caused by beer.
    C. A complex factor along with age and gender may lead to distended waistline.
    D. Compared with women, men store more fat around the waist.

2. Which of the following statements is true about reasons for fat deposited in the belly?
    A. Age correlates with fat stored in the belly.
    B. Males tend to store fat around the waist.
    C. Extra calories lead to a distended waistline.
    D. All of the above.

3. According to the passage, as a risk of health, beer belly may develop some diseases EXCEPT _____.
    A. diabetes   B. hepatitis
    C. hypertension   D. cardiovascular disease

4. According to the passage, the way to know how much belly is too much is _____.
    A. measuring the waistline
    B. blood routine
    C. urine routine
    D. consulting medical professionals

5. The next paragraph would probably discuss _____.
    A. how to give up drinking beer
    B. how to get rid of beer belly
    C. how to know whether you are addicted to beer
    D. how to deal with the diseases in relation to beer belly

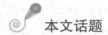 本文话题

啤酒肚。

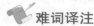 难词译注

versatile [ˈvəːsətail] a.		通用的，万能的
malted barley		麦芽
prerequisite [ˌpriːˈrekwizit] n.		先决条件
stereotypical [ˌsteriəˈtipikəl] a.		模式化观念的
pint [paint] n.		品脱
moniker [ˈmɔnikə(r)] n.		绰号
flab [flæb] n.		松弛的肌肉，赘肉
swig [swig] v.		痛饮
imbibe [imˈbaib] v.		吸收
distend [diˈstend] v.		使扩大
metabolism [meˈtæbəlizəm] n.		新陈代谢
visceral fat		内脏脂肪
insulin [ˈinsjulin] n.		胰岛素
cholesterol [kəˈlestərɔl] n.		胆固醇
obesity [əuˈbiːsəti] n.		肥胖

难句译注

1. Beer, at around 140 calories per 12-ounce bottle, is high in calories and frequent imbibing can result in the extra calories that lead to a distended waistline.

   【分析】that 引导定语从句，修饰 calories。

   【译文】啤酒含有很高的热量，每 12 盎司的瓶装啤酒大约含有 140 卡路里的热量，经常喝啤酒会使腰围增大。

2. However, like fat that appears in other areas of the body, it has more to do with how many overall calories you consume versus how many you're burning through regular exercise.

   【分析】that 引导定语从句，修饰 fat。versus 是介词，此处意为"相对，相比"。

   【译文】然而，与身体其他部位的脂肪一样，腹部脂肪的多少更取决于你摄入的热量与通过锻炼而燃烧掉的热量的差值。

答案及解析

1. 【问题】根据文章，下面哪一个表述是正确的？

   A．啤酒肚和喝的啤酒量成正比。

B．大啤酒肚不是由啤酒造成的。

C．包括年龄和性别在内的复杂因素可能导致腰围增大。

D．与女性相比，男性在腰上囤积更多的脂肪。

【答案】C

【解析】细节题。原文第 3 段和第 4 段提到造成啤酒肚的原因：卡路里摄入、年龄以及性别等。

2．【问题】下面哪一个关于腹部脂肪堆积的原因是正确的？

  A．年龄与腹部脂肪堆积相关。 B．男性总是在腰上囤积脂肪。

  C．热量过多可能导致腰围增大。 D．以上都是。

【答案】D

【解析】细节题。解题信息依然在原文第 3 段和第 4 段。

3．【问题】根据文章，作为一个健康的危险因素，啤酒肚可能导致疾病，除了_____。

  A．糖尿病 B．肝炎

  C．高血压 D．心血管疾病

【答案】B

【解析】细节题。原文信息在第 5 段最后一句话：...develop nasty conditions such as insulin resistance, diabetes, high blood pressure, heart disease, and high cholesterol over and above the already increased risk a person receives from other forms of obesity.

4．【问题】根据文章，知道多大的肚子算超标的方法是_____。

  A．量腰围 B．血常规

  C．尿常规 D．咨询医学专业人士

【答案】A

【解析】细节题。原文相关信息在最后一段。

5．【问题】下一个段落可能讨论_____。

  A．如何戒啤酒 B．如何消除啤酒肚

  C．如何知道你是否对啤酒上瘾 D．如何应对和啤酒肚相关的疾病

【答案】B

【解析】推理题。综观全文，提到啤酒肚的成因、危害以及如何判断腹部腰围，按照逻辑推理，下一个段落应该讲述如何消除啤酒肚。

Passage Six

Can the Internet help patients jump the line at the doctor's office? The Silicon Valley Employers Forum, a sophisticated group of technology companies, is launching a pilot program to test online "virtual visits" between doctors at three big local medical groups and about 6,000 employees and their families. The six employers taking part in the Silicon Valley initiative, including heavy hitters such as Oracle and Cisco Systems, hope that online visits will mean employees won't have to skip work to tend to minor ailments or to follow up on chronic conditions. "With our long commutes and traffic, driving 40 miles to your doctor in your hometown can be a big chunk of time," says Cindy Conway, benefits director at Cadence Design Systems, one of the participating companies.

Doctors aren't clamoring to chat with patients online for free; they spend enough unpaid time on the phone. Only 1 in 5 has ever e-mailed a patient, and just 9 percent are interested in doing so, according to the research firm Cyber Dialogue. "We are not stupid," says Stirling Somers, executive of the Silicon Valley employers group. "Doctors getting paid is a critical piece in getting this to work." In the pilot program, physicians will get $20 per online consultation, about what they get for a simple office visit.

Doctors also fear they'll be swamped by rambling e-mails that tell everything but what's needed to make a diagnosis. So the new program will use technology supplied by Healinx, an Alameda, Calif.-based start-up. Healinx's "Smart Symptom Wizard" questions patients and turns answers into a succinct message. The company has online dialogues for 60 common conditions. The doctor can then diagnose the problem and outline a treatment plan, which could include e-mailing a prescription or a face-to-face visit.

Can e-mail replace the doctor's office? Many conditions, such as persistent cough, require a stethoscope to discover what's wrong — and to avoid a malpractice suit. Even Larry Bonham, head of one of the doctor's groups in the pilot, believes the virtual doctor's visits offer a "very narrow" sliver of service between phone calls to an advice nurse and a visit to the clinic.

The pilot program, set to end in nine months, also hopes to determine whether online visits will boost worker productivity enough to offset the cost of the service. So far, the Internet's record in the health field has been underwhelming. The experiment is "a huge roll of the dice for Healinx," notes Michael Barrett, an analyst at Internet consulting firm Forester Research. If the "Web visits" succeed, expect some HMOs (Health Maintenance Organizations) to pay for online visits. If doctors, employers, and patients aren't satisfied, figure on one more e-health start-up to stand down.

1. The Silicon Valley employers promote the e-health program for the purpose of _____ .
   A. rewarding their employees
   B. gratifying the local hospitals
   C. boosting worker productivity
   D. testing a sophisticated technology
2. What can be learned about the on-line doctors' visits?
   A. They are a quite promising business.
   B. They are funded by the local government.

C. They are welcomed by all the patients.

D. They are very much under experimentation.

3. According to Paragraph 2, doctors are _____.

A. reluctant to serve online for nothing

B. not interested in Web consultation

C. too tired to talk to the patients online

D. content with $20 paid per Web visit

4. "Smart Symptom Wizard" is capable of _____.

A. making diagnoses

B. producing prescriptions

C. profiling patients' illness

D. offering a treatment plan

5. It can be inferred from the passage that the future of online visits will mostly depend on whether _____.

A. the employers would remain confident in them

B. they could effectively replace office visits

C. HMOs would cover the cost of the service

D. new technologies would be available to improve the e-health project

本文话题

虚拟网上问诊。

难词译注

sophisticated [sə'fistikeitid] a.		老练的；复杂巧妙的
ailment ['eilmənt] n.		疾病
chunk [tʃʌŋk] n.		大块
clamor ['klæmə] v.		大声要求
swamp [swɔmp] v.		淹没
rambling ['ræmbliŋ] a.		凌乱的；不切题的；蔓生的
succinct [sək'siŋkt] a.		简洁的
stethoscope ['steθəskəup] n.		听诊器
dice [dais] n.		骰子
malpractice [ˌmæl'præktis] n.		玩忽职守
offset [ˌɔf'set] v.		抵消

答案及解析

1. 【问题】硅谷的老板们推广电子医疗项目有什么目的？

        A. 奖励员工。   B. 使当地医院满意。

        C. 提高工人生产力。   D. 测试一个复杂的技术。

【答案】C

【解析】 细节题。原文信息首先出现在第 1 段：…hope that online visits will mean employees won't have to skip work to tend to minor ailments of to follow up on chronic conditions. 这句话告诉我们，这些参与其中的老板们希望网上问诊，这意味着他们的员工不必翘班去看病。在最后一段第 1 句话也提到：The pilot program, set to end in nine months, also hopes to determine whether online visits will boost worker productivity enough to offset the cost of the service. 此句意为：这一试验项目九个月后就将结束，同样希望能确定网上问诊是否能提高工人生产力，以抵消这项服务的费用。故选 C。

2. **【问题】** 有关网上问诊我们可以知道什么？

    A．这是很有前景的生意。   B．由当地政府资助。

    C．深受所有患者的欢迎。   D．还处于试验阶段。

【答案】D

【解析】 细节题。此题用排除法较容易解题。文章第 4 段和第 5 段阐述这一项目的不足和担心，很多参与者还持观望态度，无法判断这个项目是否有发展前途，故 A 错误。B 为错误选项，文章没有提到该项目由政府资助；C 为错误选项，理由与 B 相同。最后一段提到该项目是 pilot program，意思就是"试验性的，试点的"。故 D 正确。

3. **【问题】** 在第 2 段，医生们对网上会诊的态度是_____。

    A．不愿意免费进行网上会诊

    B．对网上会诊不感兴趣

    C．太疲劳了，以至于不愿意在网上和患者交流

    D．对每次网上会诊 20 元的费用感到满意

【答案】A

【解析】 段落大意。根据第 2 段的内容，可以首先排除 C 和 D，因为没有相关信息。第 2 段第 1 句话 "Doctors aren't clamoring to chat with patients online for free." 意思是，医生们不情愿在网上和患者免费交流。因而选项 A 为正确答案。

【问题】 SSW 能够做什么？

    A．进行诊断。   B．开处方。

    C．扼要介绍病人病情。   D．提供治疗方案。

4. **【答案】C**

【解析】 细节题。有关 SSW 的原文信息在第 3 段。第 3 段提到，这个项目使用称为 SSW 的新技术。该技术可以询问病人，并将病情简要记录下来，然后由医生诊断病情，确定治疗方案。这个方案可以是将处方发邮件给病人或者面对面的问诊。

5. 【问题】从文章中可以推断网上问诊的前景主要依靠什么？

        A．老板们是否对它有信心。

        B．是否能有效取代面对面的问诊。

        C．HMOs 是否负担费用。

        D．新的技术是否能改进该项目。

【答案】B

【解析】推断题。根据全文内容以及上面几道细节题可知：硅谷老板们推广电子医疗为了提高工人的生产力，但医生们对于网上问诊的态度很不情愿，因而可以推断，网上问诊在今后的前景取决于是否能有效地取代面对面的问诊，故选项 B 正确。

Passage Seven

There must be few questions on which responsible opinion is so utterly divided as on that of how much sleep we ought to have. There are some who think we can leave the body to regulate these matters for itself. "The answer is easy," says Dr. A. Burton. "With the right amount of sleep you should wake up fresh and alert five minutes before the alarm rings." If he is right many people must be undersleeping, including myself. But we must remember that some people have a greater inertia than others. This is not meant rudely. They switch on slowly, and they are reluctant to switch off. They are alert at bedtime and sleepy when it is time to get up, and this may have nothing to do with how fatigued their bodies are, or how much sleep they must take to lose their fatigue.

Other people feel sure that the present trend is towards too little sleep. To quote one medical opinion, thousands of people drift through life suffering from the effects of too little sleep; the reason is not that they can't sleep. Like advancing colonists, we do seem to be grasping ever more of the land of sleep for our waking needs, pushing the boundary back and reaching, apparently, for a point in our evolution where we will sleep no more. This in itself, of course, need not be a bad thing. What could be disastrous, however, is that we should press too quickly towards this goal, sacrificing sleep only to gain more time in which to jeopardize our civilization by actions and decisions made weak by fatigue.

Then, to complete the picture, there are those who believe that most people are persuaded to sleep too much. Dr. H. Roberts, writing in *Every Man in Health*, asserts: "It may safely be stated that, just as the majority eat too much, so the majority sleep too much." One can see the point of this also. It would be a pity to retard our development by holding back those people who are gifted enough to work and play well with less than the average amount of sleep, if indeed it does them no harm. If one of the trends of evolution is that more of the life span is to be spent in gainful waking activity, then surely these people are in the van of this advance.

1. The author seems to indicate that _____.
   A. there are many controversial issues like the right amount of sleep
   B. among many issues the right amount of sleep is the least controversial
   C. people are now moving towards solving many controversial issues
   D. the right amount of sleep is a topic of much controversy among doctors

2. The author disagrees with Dr. Burton because _____.
   A. few people can wake up feeling fresh and alert
   B. some people still feel tired with enough sleep
   C. some people still feel sleepy with enough sleep
   D. some people go to bed very late at night

3. The underlined word "jeopardize" is closest in meaning to _____.
   A. endeavor   B. endanger   C. endorse   D. endow

4. In the last paragraph the author points out that _____.
   A. sleeping less is good for human development
   B. people ought to be persuaded to sleep less than before
   C. it is incorrect to say that people sleep too little
   D. those who can sleep less should be encouraged

5. We learn from the passage that the author _____.
   A. comments on three different opinions
   B. favours one of the three opinions
   C. explains an opinion of his own
   D. revises someone else's opinion

本文话题

人们的睡眠长短。

难词译注

jeopardize ['dʒepədaiz] v.   危害

答案及解析

1. 【问题】作者似乎要指出_____。
   A. 有很多有争议的话题，例如睡眠量
   B. 在众多话题中适当的睡眠量是最不具争议的话题
   C. 现在人们转向解决许多有争议的问题
   D. 多少睡眠量是适当的在医生中很有争议

   【答案】D

【解析】此题为主旨题。文章首句揭示主题：There must be few questions on which responsible opinion is so utterly divided as on that of how much sleep we ought to have. 此句意为：很少有问题像我们应该睡多长时间那样引起如此大的分歧。

2. 【问题】作者不同意 Burton 博士的观点，因为_____。

 A．很少有人醒来感到精力充沛并思维敏捷

 B．一些睡眠足的人仍旧感到劳累

 C．一些睡眠足的人仍旧感到困

 D．一些人很晚才上床睡觉

【答案】A

【解析】细节题。原文中能够体现作者对 Dr. Burton 的观点的态度信息在第 1 段：If he is right many people must be undersleeping, including myself. 此句意为：如果他（Dr. Burton）是对的话，许多人都一定是睡眠不足，包括我在内。这句话体现作者与 Dr. Burton 的观点不一致。

3. 【问题】与画线词 "jeopardize" 含义最接近的是_____。

 A．努力 　　　B．危及 　　　C．签署 　　　D．捐赠

【答案】B

【解析】猜词题。由上下文可知，画线词的含义为 "危害"。

4. 【问题】在最后一段，作者指出_____。

 A．睡眠不足对人体发育有好处 　　　B．应该劝说人们要比以前睡得少一些

 C．人们睡得太少的说法不正确 　　　D．应该鼓励那些可以少睡觉的人

【答案】D

【解析】细节题。原文信息为最后一段：It would be a pity to retard our development by holding back those people who are gifted enough to work and play well with less than the average amount of sleep, if indeed it does them no harm. 有些人天生就可以少睡觉，并且不耽误工作和玩乐，如果确实对他们无害，那么因阻止他们这样做而延误我们整个社会发展的话，就太遗憾了。

5. 【问题】从文章中我们可以知道作者_____。

 A．对于三种不同观点进行评论 　　　B．赞成三个不同观点中的一个

 C．解释他自己的一个观点 　　　D．修正其他人的观点

【答案】A

【解析】主旨题。综观全文，作者就对睡眠的三种观点进行阐述，并且针对这三种观点进行了评论，最终提出自己的看法。因而选项 A 为正确答案。

Passage Eight

In the world of entertainment, TV talk shows have undoubtedly flooded every inch of space on daytime television. And anyone who watches them regularly knows that each one varies in style and format. But no two shows are more profoundly opposite in content, while at the same time standing out above the rest, than the Jerry Springer and the Oprah

Winfrey shows.

Jerry Springer could easily be considered the king of "trash talk". The topics on his show are as shocking as shocking can be. For example, the show takes the ever-common talk show themes of love, sex, cheating, guilt, hate, conflict and morality to a different level. Clearly, the Jerry Springer show is a display and exploitation of society's moral catastrophes（灾难）, yet people are willing to eat up the intriguing（有迷惑力的）predicaments（困境）of other people's lives.

Like Jerry Springer, Oprah Winfrey takes TV talk show to its extreme, but Oprah goes in the opposite direction. The show focuses on the improvement of society and an individual's quality of life. Topics range from teaching your children responsibility, managing your work week, to getting to know your neighbors.

Compared to Oprah, the Jerry Springer show looks like poisonous waste being dumped on society. Jerry ends every show with a "final word". He makes a small speech that sums up the entire moral of the show. Hopefully, this is the part where most people will learn something very valuable.

Clean as it is, the Oprah show is not for everyone. The show's main target audiences are middle-class Americans. Most of these people have the time, money, and stability to deal with life's tougher problems. Jerry Springer, on the other hand, has more of an association with the young adults of society. These are 18-to 21-year-old ones whose main troubles in life involve love, relationship, sex, money and peers. They are the 18-to 21-year-old ones who see some value and lessons to be learned underneath the show's exploitation.

While the two shows are as different as night and day. Both have ruled the talk show circuit for many years now. Each one caters to a different audience while both have a strong following from large groups of fans. Ironically, both could also be considered pioneers in the talk show world.

1. Compared with other TV talk shows, both the Jerry Springer and the Oprah Winfrey are _____.
   A. more family-oriented   B. unusually popular
   C. more profound   D. relatively formal

2. Though the social problems Jerry Springer talks about appear distasteful, the audiences _____.
   A. remain fascinated by them   B. are ready to face up to them
   C. remain indifferent to them   D. are willing to get involved in them

3. Which of the following is likely to be a topic of the Oprah Winfrey show?
   A. A new type of robot.   B. Racist hatred.
   C. Family budget planning.   D. Street violence.

4. Despite their different approaches, the two talk shows are both _____.

　　A．ironical　　　　　B．sensitive　　　　C．instructive　　　D．cynical

5. We can learn from the passage that the two talk shows _____.

　　A．have monopolized the talk show circuit

　　B．exploit the weaknesses in human nature

　　C．appear at different times of the day

　　D．are targeted at different audiences

本文话题

脱口秀。

难词译注

ironically [ai'rɔnikli] ad.　　　　　　　　　　　　　　　　讽刺地

答案及解析

1. 【问题】和其他电视脱口秀相比，杰瑞和奥普拉的节目_____。

　　A．更加面向家庭　　　　　　　　B．非常受人欢迎

　　C．更深刻　　　　　　　　　　　D．相对正式

【答案】B

【解析】推断题。第 1 段最后一句话提到 standing out above the rest，说明他们两个的节目与其他节目相比十分出类拔萃。文章最后一段提到：Each one caters to a different audience while both have a strong following from large groups of fans. 此句意为：两个节目都有大量不同的但很固定的支持者。

2. 【问题】尽管杰瑞谈到的社会问题看上去令人不愉快，但是观众_____。

　　A．仍旧被它们所吸引　　　　　　B．自愿面对它们

　　C．仍旧漠不关心　　　　　　　　D．自愿牵涉其中

【答案】A

【解析】细节题。原文出处在第 2 段最后一句话。原文大意是：无疑，他的节目是展示和挖掘社会的道德灾难，但人们对其他人在生活中令人好奇的困境却很感兴趣。

3. 【问题】下面哪一个可能成为奥普拉节目的题目？

　　A．新型机器人。　　　　　　　　B．种族仇恨。

　　C．家庭预算计划。　　　　　　　D．街头暴力。

【答案】C

【解析】推理题。在第 3 段阐述了她节目的风格，与 Jerry Springer 的截然不同，她的节目致力于改进社会和提高个人生活质量。话题从教育孩子有责任感、安排一周的工作到逐渐了解邻居。从这段可以看出她的节目更关注家庭。因而选 C。

4. 【问题】尽管这两个脱口秀方法不同，但它们都是_____。

    A．讽刺的   B．敏感的   C．有益的   D．愤世嫉俗的

【答案】C

【解析】推理题。第4段和第5段的最后一句话分别认为两个节目都会让人有所回味和领悟。

5. 【问题】从文章我们可以知道这两个脱口秀_____。

    A．独霸脱口秀节目   B．揭露人性弱点

    C．出现在白天的不同时段   D．定位不同的观众

【答案】D

【解析】细节题。此题用排除法比较简单。由最后一段提到两个节目名列前茅但不是独霸，所以排除A；根据两个节目的风格就可以知道B项错误；原文中没有C项相关的信息。因而答案为D。

Passage Nine

It is said that in England death is pressing, in Canada inevitable and in California optional. Small wonder. Americans' life expectancy has nearly doubled over the past century. Failing hips can be replaced, clinical depression controlled, cataracts（白内障） removed in a 30-minute surgical procedure. Such advances offer the aging population a quality of life that was unimaginable when I entered medicine 50 years ago. But not even a great health-care system can cure death and our failure to confront that reality now threatens this greatness of ours.

Death is normal; we are genetically programmed to disintegrate and perish, even under ideal conditions. We all understand that at some level, yet as medical consumers we treat death as a problem to be solved. Shielded by third-party payers from the cost of our care, we demand everything that can possibly be done for us, even if it's useless. The most obvious example is late-stage cancer care. Physicians frustrated by their inability to cure the disease and fearing loss of hope in the patient too often offer aggressive treatment far beyond what is scientifically justified.

In 1950, the U.S. spent $ 12.7 billion on health care. In 2002, the cost will be $ 1,540 billion. Anyone can see this trend is unsustainable. Yet few seem willing to try to reverse it. Some scholars conclude that a government with finite resources should simply stop paying for medical care that sustains life beyond a certain age — say 83 or so. Former Colorado governor Richard Lamm has been quoted as saying that the old and infirm "have a duty to die and get out of the way", so that younger, healthier people can realize their potential.

I would not go that far. Energetic people now routinely work through their 60s and beyond, and remain dazzlingly productive. At 78, Viacom chairman Sumner Redstone jokingly claims to be 53. Supreme Court Justice Sandra Day O'Connor is in her 70s, and former surgeon general C. Everett Koop chairs an Internet start-up in his 80s. These leaders are living proof that prevention works and that we can manage the health problems that come naturally with age. As a mere 68-year-old, I wish to age as productively as they have.

Yet there are limits to what a society can spend in this pursuit. Ask a physician, I know the most costly and dramatic measures may be ineffective and painful. I also know that people in Japan and Sweden, countries that spend far less on medical care, have achieved longer, healthier lives than we have. As a nation, we may be overfunding the quest for unlikely cures while underfunding research on humbler therapies that could improve people's lives.

1. What is implied in the first sentence?
    A. Americans are better prepared for death than other people.
    B. Americans enjoy a higher life quality than ever before.
    C. Americans are over confident of their medical technology.
    D. Americans take a vain pride in their long life expectancy.

2. The author uses the example of cancer patients to show that _____.
    A. medical resources are often wasted
    B. doctors are helpless against fatal diseases
    C. some treatments are too aggressive
    D. medical costs are becoming unaffordable

3. The author's attitude toward Richard Lamm's remark is one of _____.
    A. strong disapproval   B. reserved consent
    C. slight contempt   D. enthusiastic support

4. In contrast to the U.S., Japan and Sweden are funding their medical care _____.
    A. more flexibly   B. more extravagantly
    C. more cautiously   D. more reasonably

5. The text intends to express the idea that _____.
    A. medicine will further prolong people's lives
    B. life beyond a certain limit is not worth living
    C. death should be accepted as a fact of life
    D. excessive demands increase the cost of health care

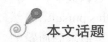 **本文话题**

针对死亡的不同看法。

难词译注

disintegrate [dis'intigreit] *v.*　　　　　　　　　　使分裂，使解体
perish ['periʃ] *v.*　　　　　　　　　　　　　　　　凋谢，消亡
extravagantly [ik'strævəgəntli] *ad.*　　　　　　　奢侈地，挥霍无度地

答案及解析

1. 【问题】第一句暗示了什么？
    A. 美国人比其他国家的人为死亡做了更好的准备。
    B. 美国人享受了比以前更好的生活质量。
    C. 美国人对他们的医疗技术过于自信。
    D. 美国人对他们的长寿很自负。
   【答案】C
   【解析】推断题。原文中第 1 句话：It is said that in England death is pressing, in Canada inevitable and in California optional. 此句意为：据说，死亡在英国迫在眉睫，在加拿大不可避免，在加利福尼亚可以选择。从第 1 段后面的阐述中可以得知，美国的医疗技术有了显著的进步，这使美国年纪大的人可以享受更好的生活，这也符合原文信息中的关键词 optional，人们因为医疗水平的进步可以控制死亡，延缓生命。故选项 C 更接近原文信息。

2. 【问题】作者用癌症患者的例子是要说明＿＿＿＿＿＿。
    A. 医疗资源总是被浪费　　　　　　　B. 医生对于致命疾病束手无策
    C. 一些治疗方法太激进　　　　　　　D. 医疗成本日益让人支付不起
   【答案】A
   【解析】细节题中的例证题。癌症的例子出现在第 2 段。这个例子是为证明作者在本段的观点。在第 2 段，作者一开始便提出观点：死亡是很正常的，但人们视死亡为要解决的问题。因而人们要求使用任何方法来解决这一难题，尽管这样做是毫无意义的。根据这些有关观点的原文阐述，对比选项就可以得出答案。

3. 【问题】作者对于理查德的评论持何种态度？
    A. 强烈反对。　　B. 有所保留地赞成。　　C. 有点轻蔑。　　D. 大力支持。
   【答案】B
   【解析】态度题。首先 Richard Lamm's remark 出现在第 3 段最后一句：…the old and infirm "have a duty to die and get out of the way". 含义是年老体衰的人有义务死亡，并且（为年轻健康的人）腾地方。作者对此的态度出现在第 4 段以及第 5 段：第 4 段第 1 句话 "I would not go that far.（还以为我不会这么极端。）"第 5 段第 1 句话 "Yet there are limits to what a society can spend in this pursuit…（然而，社会在这一追求中的花费是有限制的。）"这一追求指的是追求高质量的老年生活。根据这两个主题句可以推断，作者对 Richard 的观点是不完全赞同的，但与其观点有些近似。故选 B。

4. 【问题】与美国对比，日本和瑞典投资医疗服务_____。

    A．更灵活   B．更奢侈

    C．更谨慎   D．更合情合理

【答案】D

【解析】细节题。信息在原文第 5 段：I also know that people in Japan and Sweden, countries that spend far less on medical care, have achieved longer, healthier lives than we have. 此句意为：我也知道在日本和瑞典，人们在医疗方面的开销很少，但比我们活得更长更健康。这说明这两个国家的人在医疗方面的开销更为有效，更为合理，不会造成过度浪费。符合此意的是选项 D。

5. 【问题】文章试图表达的想法是_____。

    A．医药将会进一步延长人们的寿命

    B．超过一定限制的生活不值得过

    C．死亡应该作为生活的事实被人们接受

    D．过度的需求增加医疗成本

【答案】C

【解析】主旨题。综观全文，作者的观点是：死亡很正常，我们不应该在解决死亡的问题上过度投入，这样的投入是毫无意义的，换句话说，我们应该坦然地接受死亡。

Passage Ten

If you intend to use humor in your talk to make people smile, you must know how to identify shared experiences and problems. Your humor must be relevant to the audience and should help to show them that you are one of them or that you understand their situation and are in sympathy with their point of view. Depending on whom you are addressing, the problems will be different. If you are talking to a group of managers, you may refer to the disorganized methods of their secretaries; alternatively if you are addressing secretaries, you may want to comment on their disorganized bosses.

Here is an example, which I heard at a nurses' convention, of a story which works well because the audience all shared the same view of doctors. A man arrives in heaven and is being shown around by St. Peter. He sees wonderful accommodations, beautiful gardens, sunny weather, and so on. Everyone is very peaceful, polite and friendly until, waiting in a line for lunch, the new arrival is suddenly pushed aside by a man in a white coat, who rushes to the head of the line, grabs his food and stomps over to a table by himself. "Who is that?" the new arrival asked St. Peter. "Oh, that's God," came the reply, "but sometimes he thinks he's a doctor."

If you are part of the group which you are addressing, you will be in a position to know the experiences and problems which are common to all of you and it'll be appropriate for you to make a passing remark about the inedible canteen food or the chairman's notorious bad taste in ties. With other audiences you mustn't attempt to cut in with humor as they will resent an outsider making disparaging remarks about their canteen or their chairman. You will be on safer ground if you stick to scapegoats like the Post Office or the telephone system.

If you feel awkward being humorous, you must practice so that it becomes more natural. Include a few casual and apparently off-the-cuff remarks which you can deliver in a relaxed and unforced manner. Often it's the delivery which causes the audience to smile, so speak slowly and remember that a raised eyebrow or an unbelieving look may help to show that you are making a light-hearted remark. Look for the humor. It often comes from the unexpected. A twist on a familiar quote "If at first you don't succeed, give up" or a play on words or on a situation. Search for exaggeration and understatements. Look at your talk and pick out a few words or sentences which you can turn about and inject with humor.

1. To make your humor work, you should _____.
   A. take advantage of different kinds of audience
   B. make fun of the disorganized people
   C. address different problems to different people
   D. show sympathy for your listeners

2. The joke about doctors implies that, in the eyes of nurses, they are _____.
   A. impolite to new arrivals
   B. very conscious of their godlike role
   C. entitled to some privileges
   D. very busy even during lunch hours

3. It can be inferred from the text that public services _____.
   A. have benefited many people
   B. are the focus of public attention
   C. are an inappropriate subject for humor
   D. have often been the laughing stock

4. To achieve the desired result, humorous stories should be delivered _____.
   A. in well-worded language   B. as awkwardly as possible
   C. in exaggerated statements   D. as casually as possible

5. The best title for the text may be _____.
   A. Use Humor Effectively   B. Various Kinds of Humor
   C. Add Humor to Speech   D. Different Humor Strategies

本文话题

如何在发言中使用幽默。

难词译注

stomp [stɔmp] *n.*		迈着重重的步子走
inedible [in'edəbl] *a.*		不可食用的
notorious [nəu'tɔ:riəs] *a.*		声名狼藉的
off-the-cuff [ˌɔfðə'kʌf] *a.*		即席的
disparaging [di'spæridʒiŋ] *a.*		轻视的
scapegoat ['skeipgəut] *n.*		替罪羊

难句译注

1. Your humor must be relevant to the audience and should help to show them that you are one of them or that you understand their situation and are in sympathy with their point of view.

   【分析】must be relevant to 与 should help 为并列谓语，两个 that 为平行并列的宾语从句。

   【译文】你的幽默要和听众相关，要借助幽默表明你是他们中的一员，或者让他们知道，你理解他们的处境并且同意他们的观点。

2. If you are part of the group which you are addressing, you will be in a position to know the experiences and problems which are common to all of you and it'll be appropriate for you to make a passing remark about the inedible canteen food or the chairman's notorious bad taste in ties.

   【分析】if 引导了一个条件状语从句，which 引导定语从句修饰 group；在主句中 and 连接两个并列句，其中 which are common… 作为定语从句修饰 experiences and problems。

   【译文】如果你是正在听你发言的听众中的一员，你就可以站在他们的角度了解你们共有的经历和存在的问题，也会使你很恰当地对饭厅难以下咽的食物和主席着装的低品位进行评论。

3. Often it's the delivery which causes the audience to smile, so speak slowly and remember that a raised eyebrow or an unbelieving look may help to show that you are making a light-hearted remark.

   【分析】which causes the audience to smile 是定语从句，修饰 delivery。or 连接两个并列主语。

   【译文】通常这是引起观众发笑的话，因而语速要慢，记得挑起眉毛或者一副不相信的面部表情都有助于表明你正在进行一个轻松愉快的发言。

答案及解析

1. 【问题】为了使幽默产生效果，你应该_____。

   A．利用各种听众　　　　　　　　B．取笑无条理的人

   C．有区别地对待不同的听众　　　D．对听众表现出同情

【答案】C

【解析】细节题。原文信息在第 1 段。在第 1 段里，作者提到：如果你想在发言中使用幽默，让人发笑，你就必须让你的听众感觉到你是他们中的一分子，针对不同的听众，问题也不同。根据对这些细节的理解，选项中只有 C 项正确。

2.　【问题】有关医生的笑话暗示，在护士眼中，医生们_____。

A．对新来的人很不礼貌

B．很在意他们像上帝一样的角色

C．享有特权

D．很忙，甚至午饭时间也是

【答案】B

【解析】推断题。有关医生的笑话出现在原文第 2 段。既然题目是这个有关医生的笑话给我们什么暗示，因而表示笑话表面含义的选项都不选。故 B 项为正确选项。

3.　【问题】文章暗示公共服务_____。

A．造福了很多人　　　　　　　　B．是公众的焦点

C．不适合成为幽默的话题　　　　D．经常被当作笑料

【答案】D

【解析】推断题。原文中和公共服务有关的信息在第 3 段最后一句话：With other audiences you mustn't attempt to cut in with humor. You will be on safer ground if you stick to scapegoats like the Post Office or the telephone system. 在这句话中 post office 以及 the telephone system 指的就是公共服务。最后一句话的含义是：如果你执意拿邮局或电话局这样的替罪羊开玩笑，那么你是安全的。换句话说拿公共服务开玩笑没关系，故选 D。

4.　【问题】要想达到想要的结果，幽默的故事应该_____讲述。

A．用精辟的语言　　　　　　　　B．尽可能笨拙地

C．用夸张的手法　　　　　　　　D．尽可能轻松地

【答案】D

【解析】细节题。信息在原文第 4 段第 1 句话：If you feel awkward being humorous, you must practice so that is becomes more natural. 这里的 natural 为关键词，D 项与它相对应。

5.　【问题】本文最好的题目是_____。

A．有效地使用幽默　　　　　　　B．多种多样的幽默

C．在发言中增加幽默　　　　　　D．不同的幽默技巧

【答案】A

【解析】主旨题。根据各段的主题句就可以总结概括出文章的主题思想。文章从如何有针对性地使用幽默，到要想达到理想效果，该如何做。这些信息都是围绕如何使用幽默而展开的，故选 A。

2018 年医学博士统考阅读理解部分真题

Passage One

When Tony Wagner, the Harvard education specialist, describes his job today, he says he's "a translator between two hostile tribes"—the education world and the business world, the people who teach our kids and the people who give them jobs. Wagner's argument in his book "Creating *Innovators: The Making of Young People Who Will Change the World*" is that our K-12 and college tracks are not consistently "adding the value and teaching the skills that matter most in the marketplace".

This is dangerous at a time when there is increasingly no such things as a high-wage, middle-skilled job—the thing that sustained the middle class in the last generation. Now, there is only a high-wage, high-skilled job. Every middle-class job today is being pulled up, out or down faster than ever. That is, it either requires more skill or can be done by more people around the world or is being buried—made obsolete—faster than ever. Which is why the goal of education today, argues Wagner, should not be to make every child "college ready" but "innovation ready"—ready to add value to whatever they do.

That is a tall task. I tracked Wagner down and asked him to elaborate ."Today," he said via e-mail, "because knowledge is available on every Internet-connected device, what you know matters far less than what you can do with what you know. The capacity to innovate—the ability to solve problems creatively or bring new possibilities to life—and skills like critical thinking, communication and collaboration are far more important than academic knowledge. As one executive told me, 'We can teach new hires the content. And we will have to because it continues to change, but we can't teach them how to think—to ask the right questions—and to take initiative.'"

My generation had it easy. We got to "find" a job. But, more than ever, our kids will have to "invent" a job. Sure, the lucky ones will find their first job, but, given the pace of change today, even they will have to reinvent, re-engineer and reimagine that job much often than their parents if they want to advance in it.

"Finland is one of the most innovative economies in the world," Wagner said,"and it is the only country where students leave high school 'innovation-ready'. They learn concepts and creativity more than facts, and have a choice of many electives—all with a shorter school day, little homework, and almost no testing. There are a growing number of 'reinvented' colleges like the Olin College of Engineering, the M.I.T. Media Lab and the 'D-school' Stanford where students learn to innovate."

61. In his book, Wagner argues that _____.

    A. the education world is hostile to our kids

B. the business world is hostile to those seeking jobs

C. the business world is too demanding on the education world

D. the education world should teach what the marketplace demands

62. What does the "tall task" refer to in the third paragraph?

    A. Sustaining the middle class.

    B. Saving high-wage, middle-skilled jobs.

    C. Shifting from "college ready" to "innovation ready".

    D. Preventing middle-class jobs from becoming obsolete fast.

63. What is mainly expressed in Wagner's e-mail?

    A. New hires should be taught the content rather than the ways of thinking.

    B. Knowledge is more readily available on Internet-connected devices.

    C. Academic knowledge is still the most important to teach.

    D. Creativity and skills matter more than knowledge.

64. What is implied in the fourth paragraph?

    A. Jobs favor the lucky ones in every generation.

    B. Jobs changed slowly in the author's generation.

    C. The author's generation led an easier life than their kids.

    D. It was easy for the author's generation to find their first job.

65. What is the purpose of the last paragraph?

    A. To orient future education.

    B. To exemplify the necessary shift in education.

    C. To draw a conclusion about the shift in education.

    D. To criticize some colleges for their practices in education.

 本文话题

如今的就业市场是需要创造工作的地方。作者认为，教育领域，尤其是高等教育领域应该随其革新，不能再固步自封，与世界变化隔绝。

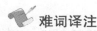 **难词译注**

| consistently [kən'sistəntli] *ad.* | 一贯地，坚持地 |
| obsolete ['ɔbsəli:t] *a.* | 废弃的；老式的，已过时的 |

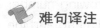 **难句译注**

1. This is dangerous at a time when there is increasingly no such things as a high-wage, middle-skilled job — the thing that sustained the middle class in the last generation.

   【分析】at a time when... 是常见的 "先行词 + 定语从句" 的结构，when 引导的定语从句中主干结构为 there be 句型。破折号后为"名词 + 定语从句结构",作为 job 的同位语来进行解释说明。

【译文】这是很危险的,因为现在高工资、中等技能之类的工作越来越见不着了,而这些工作曾维持上一代的中产阶级。

2. Which is why the goal of education today, argues Wagner, should not be to make every child "college ready" but "innovation ready"—ready to add value to whatever they do.

【分析】该句的主谓结构为 Wagner argues,倒装后插入表语从句中的主谓之间。表语从句中有 not...but... 的并列结构。

【译文】瓦格纳认为,这就是为什么今天的教育目标不应该让每个孩子都"准备好上大学",而是"准备好创新",准备为他们所做的任何事情增加价值。

答案及解析

61.【问题】瓦格纳在他的书中认为_____。

A. 教育领域对孩子们充满了敌意

B. 商业世界对求职者充满敌意

C. 商业世界对教育领域过于苛刻

D. 教育领域应该教授市场所需要的技能

【答案】D

【解析】细节题。由题干中的 book 定位到第一段:Wagner's argument in his book …is that our K-12 and college tracks are not consistently "adding the value and teaching the skills that matter most in the marketplace". 即他认为教育应该教给孩子市场最需要的技术。因此本题正确答案为 D。

62.【问题】第三段中的 tall task 指的什么?

A. 维持中产阶级。

B. 保留高工资、中等技能的工作。

C. 从"准备好上大学"转向"准备好创新"。

D. 防止中产阶级的工作太快被废弃。

【答案】C

【解析】指代题。定位到第三段首句:That is a tall task. 这里的 that 指代的是上一段的末尾,不难判断 C 为本题的正确答案。

63.【问题】瓦格纳的邮件主要表达了什么?

A. 新的求职者应该被教授内容,而不是思维方式。

B. 知识在连接互联网的设备上更容易获得。

C. 学术知识仍然是最重要的教学内容。

D. 创造性和技巧比知识更重要。

【答案】D

【解析】细节题。通过 email 可定位到文中第三段:… what you know matters far less than what you can do with what you know … and collaboration are far more important than academic knowledge. 即学术知识远没有创造性解决问题的能力和在生活中创造新可能性重要，因此本题正确答案为 D。

64. 【问题】第四段隐含了什么意义？
    A．工作垂青于每一代人中的幸运者。
    B．工作在作者这一代改变很慢。
    C．作者这一代比其子女生活更为容易。
    D．作者这一代人更容易找到自己的第一份工作。

【答案】D

【解析】推理题。从第四段中得知，作者说他们这一代很容易。他们必须"找到"一份工作。但是，他们的孩子比以往任何时候都需要"发明"一份工作。当然，幸运儿们会找到他们的第一份工作，但是，考虑到今天的变化速度，若他们想要进步，他们也不得不重新设计和重新构思这项工作。从这里不难看出，作者这一代的压力比下一代要小多了。因此本题正确答案为 D。

65. 【问题】最后一段的目的是什么？
    A．引导教育的方向。
    B．举例说明教育转型的必要性。
    C．对教育转型的总结。
    D．谴责某些大学的教育实践。

【答案】B

【解析】写作目的题。最后一段作者讲到了芬兰、奥林工程学院，M.I.T. 媒体实验室和"D 学校"斯坦福大学的教学模式，也是举例说明现有的教学模式改革。因此 B 选项是作者的写作目的。

2017 年医学博士统考阅读理解部分真题

This issue of *Science* contains announcements for more than 100 different Gordon Research Conferences, on topics that range from atomic physics to developmental biology. The brainchild（某人的主意）of Neil Gordon of Johns Hopkins University, these week-long meetings are designed to promote intimate, informal discussions of frontier science. Often confined to fewer than 125 attendees, they have traditionally been held in remote places with minimal distractions. Beginning in the early 1960s, I attended the summer Nucleic Acids Gordon Conference in rural New Hampshire, sharing austere（简朴的）dorm facilities in a private boy's school with randomly assigned roommates. As a beginning scientist, I found the question period after each talk especially fascinating, providing valuable insights into the personalities and ways of thinking of many senior scientists whom I had not encountered previously. Back then, there were no cellphones and no Internet, and all of the speakers seemed to stay for the entire week. During the long, session-free afternoons, graduate students mingled freely with professors. Many lifelong friendships were begun, and—as Gordon intended—new scientific collaborations began. Leap forward to today, and every scientist can gain immediate access to a vast store of scientific thought and to millions of other scientists via the Internet. Why, nevertheless, do in-person scientific meetings remain so valuable for a life in science?

Part of the answer is that science works best when there is a deep mutual trust and understanding between the collaborators, which is hard to develop from a distance. But most important is the critical role that face-to-face scientific meetings play in stimulating a random collision of ideas and approaches. The best science occurs when someone combines the Knowledge gained by other scientists in non-obvious ways to create a new understanding of how the world works. A successful scientist needs to deeply believe, whatever the problem being tackled, that there is always a better way to approach that problem than the path currently being taken. The scientist is then constantly on the alert for new paths to take in his or her work, which is essential for making breakthroughs. Thus, as much as possible, scientific meetings should be designed to expose the attendees to ways of thinking and techniques that are different from the ones that they already know.

66. Assembled at Gordon Research Conference are those who _____.
    A. are physicists and biologists
    B. just start doing their sciences
    C. stay in the forefront of science
    D. are accomplished senior scientists
67. Speaking of the summer Nucleic Acids Gordon Conference, the author thinks highly of _____.
    A. the personalities of senior scientists
    B. the question period after each talk
    C. the austere facilities around
    D. the week-long duration
68. It can be inferred from the author that the value of the in-person scientific conference _____.
    A. does not change with time
    B. can be explored online exclusively
    C. lies in exchanging the advances in life science
    D. is questioned in establishing a vast store of ideas
69. The author believes that the face-to-face scientific conferences can help the attendees better _____.
    A. understand what making a breakthrough means to them
    B. expose themselves to novel ideas and new approaches
    C. foster the passion for doing science

D. tackle the same problem in science

70. What would the author most probably talk about in the following paragraphs?

A. How to explore scientific collaborations.

B. How to make scientific breakthroughs.

C. How to design scientific meetings.

D. How to think like a genius.

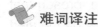

本文话题

现场科学会议的重要意义。

难词译注

frontier science	前沿科学
randomly ['rændəmli] ad.	随便地，未加计划地
mingle [miŋgl] v.	混合，混淆

答案及解析

66. 【问题】聚集在戈登研究会议的是那些_____.

　　A. 物理学家和生物学家　　　　B. 刚在科学研究上起步的人

　　C. 科学前沿的人　　　　　　　D. 功成名就的资深科学家

【答案】C

【解析】推理题。从首段中 designed to promote intimate, informal discussions of frontier science 可知，与会者都是前沿科学的参与者。C 为正确答案。

67. 【问题】说到夏季核酸戈登会议，作者高度赞扬了_____。

　　A. 资深科学家们的性格

　　B. 每个发言后的提问时间

　　C. 周围简朴的设备

　　D. 长达一周的时间

【答案】B

【解析】细节题。首段中讲到 I found the question period after each talk especially fascinating，他发现提问环节非常棒，因为他可以充分了解未曾谋面的科学家们的思想和个性。因此 B 为正确答案。

68. 【问题】可推理得知，作者认为现场科学会议的价值_____。

　　A. 不会随着时间的改变而改变

　　B. 只能在线开发

　　C. 存在于生命科学进步成果的交流中

　　D. 在树立一系列观点时被质疑

【答案】A

【解析】推理题。从第一段中的最后一句"Why, nevertheless, do in-person scientific meetings remain so valuable for a life in science"可知，无论在过去还是在互联网时代，现场会议的价值是保持不变的。因此正确答案为A。

69.【问题】作者认为面对面的科学会议能帮助参会者更好地_____。

A．理解突破性进展的含义

B．接触新颖的观点和方法

C．培养科研热情

D．处理科学中相通的问题

【答案】B

【解析】细节题。从第二段中"But most important is the critical role that face-to-face scientific meetings play in stimulating a random collision of ideas and approaches"可知，面对面的科学会议在刺激思想和方法的随机碰撞方面发挥关键作用，B选项符合文意。

70.【问题】下一段作者最可能谈到什么？

A．如何开展科研协作。

B．如何进行科技创新。

C．如何设计科研会议。

D．如何像天才一样思考。

【答案】C

【解析】推理题。第二段末尾讲到科学会议的设计应该尽最大可能让与会者充分接触不同的思维方式和技巧，由此可推断，作者极有可能在第三段讲述如何安排一场好的现场科学会议。故本题正确答案为C。

2016 年医学博士统考阅读理解部分真题

Passage One

Parents are on a journey of discovery with each child whose temperament, biology, and sleep habits result in a unique sleep-wake pattern. It can be frustrating when children's sleep habits do not conform to the household schedule. Helping the child develop good sleep habits in childhood takes time and parental attention, but it will have beneficial results throughout life. An understanding of the changing patterns of the typical sleep-wake cycle in children will help alleviate any unfounded concerns. Maintaining a sleep diary for each child will provide the parents with baseline information in assessing the nature and severity of childhood sleep problems. Observant patents will come to recognize unusual sleep disruptions or those that persist or intensify.

Developmental changes throughout childhood bring differences in the sleep-wake cycle and in the type and frequency of parasomnias that may interrupt sleep. Medical consultation to rule out illness, infection or injury is prudent if the child's sleep problems prevent adequate sleep and result in an ongoing sleep deficit. As reported by *News-Medical* in Child Health News, children's sleep problems should be taken seriously as they may be a "marker" for predicting later risk of early adolescent substance use. In the same article, University of Michigan psychiatry professor Kirk Brower, who has studied "the interplay of alcohol and sleep in adults", stressed that " The finding does not mean there's a cause-and-effect relationship."

Consultation with a child psychologist may be helpful if frightening dreams intensity and become more frequent as this may indicate a particular problem or life circumstance that needs to be changed or one that the child may need extra help working through.

Most childhood sleep disturbance will diminish over time as the brain matures and a regular sleep-wake cycle is established. Parental guidance is crucial to development of healthy sleep habits in children.

61. To have journey of discovery with each child, according to the passage, is_____.
    A. to discover their unique sleep-wake cycles
    B. to follow their behavioral preferences
    C. to alleviate their sleeping problems
    D. to explore their asset

62. In the first paragraph, the author suggests that parents_____.
    A. seek professional consultation for their child's sleep problem
    B. adjust their household schedule to the child's sleeping habit
    C. take their child's unfounded concerns into consideration
    D. keep a diary on sleep pattern for their child

63. Where there exists a "marker" in the child, according to the passage_____.
    A. it might lead to his or her early substance use
    B. he or she will carry it all his or her life
    C. it might interrupt his or her sleep pattern
    D. he or she is destined to be an alcoholic

64. What is the author trying to tell us in the third paragraph?
    A. It takes time to combat sleeping problem in children.
    B. Sometimes parents need to seek professional assistance.
    C. Parents cannot afford to neglect their child's sleeping problem.
    D. Much importance should be attached to the child's life circumstance.

65. What is the main idea of the passage?
    A. Child sleep disturbance and its future impact.
    B. Child sleep disturbance and its family history.
    C. Parent's role in building their child's healthy sleeping habit.

D. A psychological perspective on sleep disturbance in children.

Passage Two

The United States and England each has a major—and unique—health-care challenge, according to a study comparing the health of senior citizens in the two countries. The study, conducted by researchers from RAND Corporation in the United States and Institute for Fiscal Studies in the United Kingdom, found that disease and health disorder incidence was higher among U.S. senior citizens, but mortality rates were higher among English senior citizens.

Americans aged 65 and older have almost twice the rate of diabetes found among their English counterparts and more than double the rate of cancer. Nevertheless, death rate among Americans 65 and older is lower.

"Americans are a sicker group of people who tend to live longer," says James Smith, a study co-author. He attributes the U.S. health problems to lifestyle factors, including poor eating habits and inadequate exercise. Americans tend to eat much larger servings of food, for example, "There is what I call an American plate. When we go to a restaurant, it's a plate I can't even eat any more. It's a plate with so much food on if it's not even appealing to me."

Smith also says that English adults are generally much more physically active than Americans. Biking and walking are much common in everyday life in England. He observes that "there is a lot of walking in London, and there is a lot of bicycle riding. I don't see people in downtown Los Angeles on their bicycles".

On the other hand, England's problem is that doctors fail to diagnose serious conditions each enough. American doctors tend to screen patients for cancer, diabetes, and other illnesses more frequently. Smith notes, "American medicine is much more aggressive. It leads to high costs, but it has benefits, too. "

66. The study's results indicated _____.
    A. an urgent call for health promotion among English and American senior citizens
    B. health disparities between English and American senior citizens
    C. a close relation between disease incidence and mortality rate
    D. a significant rise in mortality rates among senior citizens
67. Which of the following is a unique health care challenge for English senior citizens when compared with their American counterparts?
    A. A higher death rate.
    B. A higher rate of cancer.
    C. A higher incidence of disease.
    D. A lower tendency to have diabetes.
68. What does James Smith imply by "an American plate"?

A．A sedentary American lifestyles.

B．American junk foods on the table.

C．A large portion of food consumed by Americans.

D．Severe malnutrition among American senior citizens.

69. The Americans' unique health-care challenge according to James Smith, is derived from _____．

A．their unusual forms of physical activities

B．their different geographic locations

C．their genetic likelihood of obesity

D．their unhealthy lifestyle factors

70. Even though it is much more aggressive, the American medicine _____．

A．better improves the quality of life among its senior citizens

B．benefits more seniors who need medical care

C．facilitates its senior citizens to live longer

D．helps its senior citizens live healthier

Passage One

 本文话题

孩子睡眠状况以及父母的作用。

 难词译注

temperament ['temprəmənt] *n.*		性格
parasomnia ['pærəsɒmniə] *n.*		深眠状态
prudent ['pru:dnt] *a.*		小心谨慎的

答案及解析

61.【问题】根据文章，探索发现每一个孩子的过程是_____。

A．发现他们独特的睡眠——觉醒周期　　B．遵循他们的行为喜好

C．缓解他们的睡眠问题　　　　　　　　D．挖掘他们的潜力

【答案】A

【解析】此题为细节理解题。根据题干可以定位到文章第一段第一句。此句提到家长正在探索发现孩子的过程中，孩子的性格和睡眠习惯都会产生独特的睡眠觉醒周期。因而我们可以得知父母探索孩子是为了了解他们的睡眠——觉醒周期。所以答案为A。

62.【问题】在第一段，作者建议父母_____。

A．为孩子的睡眠问题寻求专业咨询

B．根据孩子的睡眠习惯调整家庭作息

  C. 重视孩子未被发现的问题

  D. 记录孩子的睡眠模式

【答案】D

【解析】此题为细节理解题。第一段提到帮助孩子在童年时期建立很好的睡眠习惯虽然费时费力，但终身受益。对孩子睡眠习惯的了解也能缓解他们的睡眠问题。随后作者建议父母记录孩子的睡眠情况就能识别睡眠问题以及严重程度。因而答案为 D。

63. 【问题】根据文章，当孩子出现"标记物"时_____。

  A. 这可能导致孩子过早吸毒   B. 孩子终身携带

  C. 可能影响孩子的睡眠模式   D. 孩子注定要酗酒

【答案】A

【解析】此题为细节理解题。文章第二段第三句出现题干关键词 marker，这句话也提到 marker 的出现，预示着孩子在青少年时期开始吸毒的危险性。因而答案为 A。

64. 【问题】第三段作者想告诉我们什么？

  A. 解决孩子的睡眠问题是需要时间的。

  B. 有时父母需要寻求专业帮助。

  C. 父母绝不能忽视孩子的睡眠问题。

  D. 孩子的生活环境至关重要。

【答案】C

【解析】此题为推断题。本段提到如果父母发现孩子噩梦情况严重或者频繁发生，有必要咨询医生，因为这些变化可能预示着一个病症，或者生活环境需要改变，也或者表示孩子的问题需要更多帮助。这些都说明作为父母一定要密切关注孩子的睡眠状况，出现情况要及时寻求专业人士的帮助，因而答案为 C。

65. 【问题】全文主要内容是什么？

  A. 孩子的睡眠问题及对其今后的影响。

  B. 孩子的睡眠问题及家族史。

  C. 父母在建立孩子正确睡眠习惯中的作用。

  D. 从心理学视角看孩子的睡眠问题。

【答案】C

【解析】此题为主旨题，解题可结合段落含义或者综合前几道细节题的答案。文章最后一段也提到大多数孩子的睡眠问题随着年龄增长而逐渐消失，但在这一过程中父母的指导作用至关重要。因而答案为 C。

Passage Two

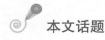

本文话题

英美两国各自老年人健康问题及对比。

66. 【问题】研究结果表明_____。

A．提高英美两国老年人健康水平迫在眉睫

B．英美两国老年人健康水平相差悬殊

C．发病率与死亡率之间紧密相关

D．老年人死亡率显著上升

【答案】A

【解析】第一段第一句提到英美两国各有各的主要医疗问题。随后对两国老年人的健康状况进行研究，结果表明在美国老年人的患病率偏高，而在英国老年人的死亡率偏高。这说明两国老年人的健康状况均不乐观，因而答案为A。尽管对比两国老年人健康状况，但都不乐观，因而选项B错误。选项C和D文章没有提到。

67．【问题】与美国老年人相比，下列哪一项是英国老年人特有的健康问题？

A．较高的死亡率。

B．较高的患癌率。

C．较高的发病率。

D．患糖尿病的可能性较低。

【答案】A

【解析】此题为细节定位题。根据题干，可以定位到第一段第一句。具体到英国老年人的健康问题是在第一段最后一句话提到该国老年人死亡率偏高。因而答案为A。

68．【问题】通过"An American Plate"，James Smith暗示什么？

A．美国人不爱运动的生活方式。

B．美国人餐桌上的垃圾食品。

C．美国人食量大。

D．美国老人严重营养不良。

【答案】C

【解析】根据题干关键词，定位到文章第三段。研究者James Smith将美国人的健康问题归因为不健康的生活方式，例如不良的饮食习惯和不爱运动。作者随后谈到美国人食量很大，用an American plate作为实例。因而答案为C。

69．【问题】根据James Smith的看法，美国人特有的健康问题来源于_____。

A．不寻常的体育锻炼形式　　　　B．不同的地理位置

C．基因肥胖概率　　　　　　　　D．不健康的生活方式

【答案】D

【解析】此题为细节定位题。此题定位在第三段。第二句提到他认为美国人的健康问题来源于生活方式，因而答案为D。

70．【问题】尽管过于激进，但是美国医学_____。

A．能更好地提高美国老年人的生活质量

B．惠及更多有需要的老年人

C．帮助老年人延年益寿

D．帮助老年人活得更健康

【答案】C

【解析】此题根据题干定位到文章最后一段。本段提到英国的问题在于疾病的早期筛查，

而在这方面美国做得好多了。文章最后提到虽然美国医学激进，成本高，但也有好处。这里的益处指的就是疾病的早期筛查。因而答案为 C。

2015 年医学博士统考阅读理解部分真题

Passage One

The American Society of Clinical Oncology wrapped its annual conference this week, going through the usual motions of presenting a lot of drugs that offer some added quality or extension of life to those suffering from a variety of as-yet incurable diseases. But buried deep in an AP story are a couple of promising headlines that seems worthy of more thorough review, including one treatment study where 100 percent of patients saw their cancer diminish by half.

First of all, it seems pharmaceutical companies are moving away from the main cost-effective one-size-fits-all approach to drug development and embracing the long cancer treatments, engineering drugs that only work for a small percentage of patients but work very effectively within that group.

Pfizer announced that one such drug it's pushing into late-stage testing is targeted for 4% of lung cancer patients. But more than 90% of that tiny cohort responded to the drug initial tests, and 9 out of ten is getting pretty close to the ideal ten out of ten. By gearing toward more boutique treatments rather than broad umbrella pharmaceuticals that try to fit for everyone it seems cancer researchers are making some headway. But how can we close the gap on that remaining ten percent?

Ask Takeda Pharmaceutical and Celgene, two drug makers who put aside competitive interests to test a novel combination of their treatments. In a test of 66 patients with the blood disease multiple myeloma, a full 100 percent of the subjects saw their cancer reduced by half. Needless to say, a 100 percent response to a cancer drug (or in this case a drug cocktail) is more or less unheard of. Moreover, this combination never would've been tried if two competing companies hadn't sat down and put their heads together.

Are there more potentially effective drug combos out there separated by competitive interest and proprietary information? Who's to say, but it seems like with the amount of money and research being pumped into cancer drug development, the outcome is pretty good. And if researchers can start pushing more of their response numbers toward 100 percent, we can more easily start talking about oncology's favorite four-letter word: cure.

61. Which of the following can be the best title for the passage?
    A. Competition and Cooperation.
    B. Two Competing Pharmaceutical Companies.

C. The Promising Future of Pharmaceuticals.

D. Encouraging News: A 100% Response to a Cancer Drug.

62. In cancer drug development, according to the passage, the pharmaceuticals now _____.

    A. are adopting the cost-effective one-size-fits-all approach

    B. are moving towards individualized and targeted treatments

    C. are investing the lion's shares of their money

    D. care only about their profits

63. From the encouraging advance by the two companies, we can infer that _____.

    A. the development can be ascribed to their joint efforts and collaboration

    B. it was their competition that resulted in the accomplishment

    C. other pharmaceutical companies will join them in the research

    D. the future cancer treatment can be nothing but cocktail therapy

64. From the last paragraph it can be inferred that the answer to the question _____.

    A. is nowhere to be found   B. can drive one crazy

    C. can be multiple   D. is conditional

65. The tone of the author of this passage seems to be _____.

    A. neutral   B. critical   C. negative   D. optimistic

Passage Two

Liver disease is the 12th-leading cause of death in the U.S., chiefly because once it's determined that a patient needs a new liver it's very difficult to get one. Even in case where a suitable donor match is found, there's no guarantee a transplant will be successful. But researchers at Massachusetts General Hospital have taken a huge step toward building functioning livers in the lab, successfully transplanting culture-grown livers into rats.

The livers aren't grown from scratch, but rather within the infrastructure of a donor liver. The liver cells in the donor organ are washed out with a detergent that gently strips away the liver cells, leaving behind a biological scaffold of proteins and extracellular architecture that is very hard to duplicate synthetically.

With all of that complicated infrastructure already in place, the researchers then seeded the scaffold（支架）with liver cells isolated from healthy livers, as well as some special endothelial cells to line the bold vessels. Once repopulated with healthy cells, these livers lived in culture for 10 days.

The team also transplanted some two-day-old recellularized livers back into rats, where they continued to thrive for eight hours while connected into the rats' vascular systems. However, the current method isn't perfect and cannot seem to repopulate the blood vessels quite densely enough and the transplanted livers can't keep functioning for more than about 24 hours (hence the eight-hour maximum for the rat transplant).

But the initial successes are promising, and the team thinks they can overcome the blood vessel problem and get fully functioning livers into rats within two years. It still might be a decade before the tech hits the clinic, but if nothing goes horribly wrong — and especially if stem-cell research establishes a reliable way to create health liver cells from the very patients who need transplants — lab-generated livers that are perfect matches for their recipients could become a reality.

66. It can be inferred from the passage that the animal model was mainly intended to _____.
    A. investigate the possibility of growing blood vessels in the lab
    B. explore the unknown functions of the human liver
    C. reduce the incidence of liver disease in the U.S.
    D. address the source of liver transplants

67. What does the author mean when he says that the livers aren't grown from scratch?
    A. The making of a biological scaffold of proteins and extracellular architecture.
    B. A huge step toward building functioning livers in the lab.
    C. The building of the infrastructure of a donor liver.
    D. Growing liver cells in the donor organ.

68. The biological scaffold was not put into the culture in the lab until _____.
    A. duplicated synthetically
    B. isolated from the healthy liver
    C. repopulated with the healthy cells
    D. the addition of some man-made blood vessels

69. What seems to be the problem in the planted liver?
    A. The rats as wrong recipients.
    B. The time point of the transplantation.
    C. The short period of the recellularization.
    D. The insufficient repopulation of the blood vessels.

70. The research team holds high hopes of _____.
    A. creating lab-generated livers for patients within two years
    B. the timetable for generating human livers in the lab
    C. stem-cell research as the future of medicine
    D. building a fully functioning liver into rats

Passage One

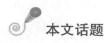

本文话题

制药公司在治疗癌症药物研发方面取得的成就。

难词译注

cost-effective [kɔst iˈfektiv] a.	划算的
one-size-fits-all	一刀切，万全之策
headway [ˈhedwei] n.	进展，前进
proprietary [prəˈpraiətri] a.	专有的，专利的

答案及解析

61.【问题】下列哪一个是文章最好的标题？

A．竞争与合作。

B．两家竞争的制药公司。

C．制药业的光明前景。

D．令人兴奋的消息：某种抗癌药物的 100% 回应。

【答案】C

【解析】主旨题。本文的中心思想是制药公司在治疗癌症的问题上的努力以及取得的成就。因此，C 选项（制药业的光明前景）是正确答案。

62.【问题】在抗癌药物的开发中，制药公司现在 _____。

A．正在采用有成本效益的一刀切方式

B．正朝个性化和针对性的治疗方式发展

C．正在进行巨大的投资

D．只在乎他们的利益

【答案】B

【解析】通过 cancer drug development 回到原文定位到第二段，一些制药公司正由成本效益高的"一刀切"的发展模式向注重药物发展方面转变，并且接受长期癌症治疗，以及研发适用于特定患者群的高效药物。由此可知，制药公司正向治疗个体化和目标特定化前进。individualized and targeted 与原文中的 work for a small percentage of patients 对应。

63.【问题】从两大公司令人鼓舞的进步中，我们可推理得知 _____。

A．所取得的进展是共同努力和合作的结果

B．正是他们的竞争才有后来的成绩

C．其他制药公司会参与研究

D．将来癌症的治疗方案只不过是鸡尾酒疗法

【答案】A

【解析】细节题。用 two companies 回到原文定位到倒数第二段，从最后一句可知，如果两家公司不坐下来商榷，就不会有这项研究。故本题答案为 A（归因于两家公司的共同努力和协作）。

64.【问题】从最后一段可推理得知，对该问题的答案 _____。

A．无处可寻   B．能使人疯狂

　　　　C．可以多元化　　　　　　　　D．是有条件的

【答案】A

【解析】细节题。最后一段中讲到，（对这个问题）谁都说不准，因为两家竞争公司之间存在竞争效益和信息专有的问题。由此可知，没人能告知答案。

65.【问题】本文作者的语气是_____。

　　　　A．中立的　　　　B．批判的　　　　C．负面的　　　　D．积极的

【答案】D

【解析】细节题。从末段最后一句可知，如果研究人员开始把药物效率向百分之百推进，那我们也能更加容易地开始探讨肿瘤界最令人神往的一个词：治愈。即作者很乐观，充满了希望。故本题答案为D。

Passage Two

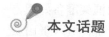 **本文话题**

人工培植肝脏可能成为肝脏疾病的治疗方法。

难词译注

culture ['kʌltʃə] n.	养殖；（微生物等的）培养
detergent [di'tə:dʒənt] n.	洗涤剂
endothelial [ˌendə'θi:liəl] adj.	内皮的
recipient [ri'sipiənt] n.	接受者；容器

答案及解析

66.【问题】从文中可推理得知，动物模型的主要目的是_____。

　　　　A．检验实验室中血管生长的可能性

　　　　B．研究人类肝脏未知的功能

　　　　C．减少美国肝脏疾病的发生概率

　　　　D．解决肝脏移植的肝源问题

【答案】D

【解析】推理题。从文中首段可知，目前美国第十二大致命杀手便是肝脏疾病，主要是因为一旦患上这种疾病，患者需要移植一颗新的肝脏，但是要找到完全匹配的肝脏非常困难。因此动物模型主要是为了解决肝脏来源的问题。故本题答案为D。

67.【问题】作者说肝脏无法"无中生有"的意思是什么？

A．蛋白质的生物支架和细胞外结构的形成。

B．在实验室中培养功能性肝脏的巨大一步。

C．捐赠者肝脏的基本框架。

D．在捐赠者器官里生长的肝脏细胞。

【答案】C

【解析】细节题。通过 grow from scratch 回到原文定位到第二段首句，大意是"这些肝脏不是无中生有，而是在供体肝的框架里培养出来的"。因此首先要搭建这样一个 infrastructure。故本题答案为 C。

68.【问题】生物支架先要 _____，然后才会放进实验室的培养液中。

A．合成复制
B．从健康的干细胞中分离

C．植入健康的肝脏细胞
D．增加一些人造血管

【答案】C

【解析】细节题。用 culture 回到原文定位到第三段，可知这些复杂的基础框架准备好后，研究者将从健康肝脏里分离出来的肝脏细胞和粗血管上的内皮细胞植入蛋白质支架之中。健康的肝脏细胞植入之后，肝脏便能够在培养基中存活 10 天。因此正确答案应该是"植入健康的肝脏细胞"。故本题答案为 C。

69.【问题】移植肝脏的问题是什么？

A．白鼠是不合适的受体。
B．移植的时间点。

C．再细胞化的时间短。
D．血管的密度不够。

【答案】D

【解析】细节题。答案在第四段：目前采用的这种肝脏移植的方法并不尽善尽美，因为血管再生密度不够。另外，移植肝脏发挥正常功能的时间不超过 24 小时。因此本题正确答案为 D。

70.【问题】研究团队对 _____ 报以很大希望。

A．两年内为病人创造实验室培育的肝脏

B．实验室培育人类肝脏的时间表

C．医学未来的干细胞研究

D．将正常功能的肝脏移植到白鼠体内

【答案】D

【解析】细节题。文章最后一段首句讲到，研究团队认为他们能在两年之内解决肝脏移植过程中遇到的血管问题，从而培养出功能完全正常的肝脏，并移植入老鼠体内。因此正确答案为 D。

2014 年医学博士统考阅读理解部分真题

Passage One

I have just returned from Mexico, where I visited a factory making medical masks. Faced with fierce competition, the owner has cut his costs by outsourcing some of his production. Scores of people work for him in their homes, threading elastic into masks by hand. They are paid below the minimum wage, with no job security and no healthcare provision.

Users of medical masks and other laboratory gear probably give little thought to where their equipment comes from. That needs to change. A significant proportion of these products are made in the developing world by low-paid people with inadequate labor rights. This leads to human misery on a tremendous scale.

Take lab coats. Many are made in India, where most cotton farmers are paid an unfair price for their crops and factory employees work illegal hours for poor pay.

One-fifth of the world's surgical instruments are made in northern Pakistan. When I visited a couple of a years ago I found most workers toiling 12 hours a day, seven days a week, for less than a dollar a day, exposed to noise, metal dust and toxic chemicals. Thousands of children, some as young as 7, work in the industry.

To win international contracts, factory owners must offer rock-bottom prices, and consequently drive down wages and labor conditions as far as they can. We laboratory scientists in the developed world may unwittingly be encouraging this: we ask how much our equipment will cost, but which of us asks who made it and how much they were paid?

This is no small matter. Science is supposed to benefit humanity, but because of the conditions under which their tools are made, many scientists may actually be causing harm.

What can be done? A knee-jerk boycott of unethical goods is not the answer; it would just make things worse for workers in those manufacturing zones. What we need is to start asking suppliers to be transparent about where and how their products are manufactured and urge them to improve their manufacturing practices.

It can be done. Many universities are committed to fair trade in the form of ethically sourced tea, coffee or bananas. That model should be extended to laboratory goods.

There are signs that things are moving. Over the past few years I have worked with health services in the UK and in Sweden. Both have recently instituted ethical procurement practices. If science is truly going to help humanity, it needs to follow suit.

1. From the medical masks to the lab coats, the author is trying to tell us _____.
   A. the practice of occupational protection in the developing world
   B. the developing countries plagued by poverty and disease
   C. the cheapest labor in the developing countries
   D. the human misery behind them
2. The concerning phenomenon the author had observed, according to the passage _____.
   A. is nothing but the repetition of the miserable history
   B. could have been even exaggerated
   C. is unfamiliar to the wealthy west
   D. is prevailing across the world

3. The author argues that when researchers in the wealthy west buy tools, they should _____.
    A. have the same concern with the developing countries
    B. be blind to their sources for the sake of humanity
    C. pursue good bargains in the international market
    D. spare a thought for how they were made

4. A proper course of action suggested by the author is _____.
    A. to refuse to import the unethical goods from the developing world
    B. to ask scientists to tell the truth as the prime value of their work
    C. to urge the manufacturers to address the immoral issues
    D. to improve the transparency of international contracts

5. By saying at the end of the passage that if science is truly going to help humanity, it needs to follow suit, the author means that _____.
    A. the scientific community should stand up for all humanity
    B. the prime value of scientists' work is to tell the truth
    C. laboratory goods also need to be ethically sourced
    D. because of science, there is hope for humanity

Passage Two

A little information is a dangerous thing. A lot of information, if it's inaccurate or confusing, even more so. This is a problem for anyone trying to spend or invest in an environmentally sustainable way. Investors are barraged with indexes purporting to describe companies eco-credentials, some of dubious quality Green labels on consumer products are ubiquitous, but their claims are hard to verify. **The confusion** is evident from the *New Scientists*' analysis of whether public perception of companies' green credentials reflect reality. It shows that many companies considered "green" have done little to earn that reputation, while others do not get sufficient credit for their efforts to reduce their environmental impact. Obtaining better information is crucial, because decisions by consumers and big investors will help propel us towards a green economy.

At present, it is too easy to make unverified claims. Take disclosure of greenhouse gas emission, for example. There are voluntary schemes such as a Carbon Disclosure Project, but little scrutiny of the figures companies submit, which means investors may be misled.

Measurements can be difficult to interpret, too, like those for water use. In this case, context is crucial: a little from rain-soaked Ireland is not the same as a little drawn from the Arizona desert.

Similar problems bedevil "green" labels attached to individual products. Here, the computer equipment rating system developed by the Green Electronics Council show the way forward. Its criteria come from the IEEE, the world's leading, professional association for technology.

Other schemes, such as the "sustainability index" planned by US retail giant Walmart, are broader. Devising rigorous standards for a large number of different types of product will be tough, placing a huge burden on the academic-led consortium that is doing the underlying scientific work.

Our investigation also reveals that many companies choose not to disclose data. Some will want to keep it that way. This is why we need legal requirements for full disclosure of environmental information, with the clear message that the polluter will eventually be required to pay. They market forces will drive companies to lean up their acts.

Let's hope we can rise to this challenge. Before we can have a green economy we need a green information economy — and it's the quality of information, as well as its quality, that will count.

6. "The confusion" in the first paragraph refers to _____.
   A. where to spend or invest in a sustainable way
   B. an array of consumer products to choose
   C. a fog of unreliable green information
   D. little information on eco-credibility
7. From the *New Scientists* analysis it can be inferred that in many cases _____.
   A. eco-credibility is abused
   B. a green economy is crucial
   C. an environment impact is lessened
   D. green credentials promote green economy
8. From unverified claims to difficult measurements and then to individual products, the author suggests that _____.
   A. eco-credibility is a game between scientists and manufactures
   B. neither scientists nor manufactures are honest
   C. it is vital to build a green economy
   D. better information is critical
9. To address the issue, the author is crying for _____.
   A. transparent corporate management   B. establishing sustainability indexes
   C. tough academic-led management   D. strict legal weapon
10. Which of the following can be the best inference from the last paragraph?
   A. The toughest challenge is the best opportunity.
   B. It is time for another green revolution.
   C. Information should be free at all.
   D. No quantity, no quality.

Passage One

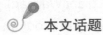 **本文话题**

医用物品的生产环境堪忧。

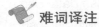 **难词译注**

outsource ['autsɔ:s] v.		将……外包
gear [giə] n.		装备
toil [tɔil] v.		辛苦工作
unwittingly [ʌn'witiŋli] ad.		不知不觉地，不经意地
knee-jerk		膝反射

答案及解析

1. 【问题】从医用口罩到实验服，作者想要告诉我们 _____。

    A．发展中国家对职业保护的做法

    B．发展中国家饱受贫穷和疾病的困扰

    C．发展中国家最廉价的劳动力

    D．背后的人类疾苦

【答案】D

【解析】此题为信息理解题。本文第一段作者在工厂观察到医用器具生产的恶劣环境，由此作者产生忧虑，因而答案是 D。

2. 【问题】根据文章，作者过去所观察到的令人关注的现象 _____。

    A．只是悲惨历史的重现

    B．可能被夸大了

    C．在富有的西方不常见

    D．在全世界都普遍存在

【答案】C

【解析】此题为细节信息题。根据第一至第四段我们得知，西方国家的医疗用品都是来源于发展中国家，因而答案为 C。

3. 【问题】作者认为当西方富国的研究者购买工具时，他们应该 _____。

    A．与发展中国家有同样的担心

    B．出于人道考虑，对他们的材料源头视而不见

    C．在国际市场追求赚钱的买卖

    D．想想这些器具是如何制成的

【答案】D

【解析】此题为细节信息题。原文出处是在第五段最后一句话，这一问句说明我们关心的是产品价格，但很少关心产品的出产地和生产状况，这一问题应该引起我们的关注。因而答案为 D。

4. 【问题】作者建议的恰当做法是 _____。

    A．禁止进口来自发展中国家的不道德的产品

    B．作为他们工作的首要价值，科学家要告知真相

    C．敦促生产商解决不道德的问题

    D．提高国际合同的透明度

【答案】C

【解析】此题为细节信息题。原文信息在文章第七段最后一句话：我们需要做的是让货品提供商在产品产地和制作方法上更加透明，敦促他们改善生产做法。因而答案为 C。

5. 【问题】在文章结尾，作者提到：如果科学是真的要造福人类，它就应该照着做。作者的意思是 _____。

    A．科学界应该支持所有人类

    B．科学家工作的首要价值就是告知真相

    C．实验室用品也需要有公德

    D．科学给人类带来了希望

【答案】C

【解析】此题为信息理解题。文章最后一段提到在英国和瑞典，他们已经开始了更为符合道德的采购做法，作为造福人类的科学也应如此，即关注实验室用品的来源，因而答案为 C。

Passage Two

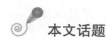

本文话题

为了环保绿色经济，信息的数量和准确性事关重要。

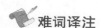

难词译注

barrage [ˈbærɑːʒ] *n.*		密集轰炸
dubious [ˈdjuːbiəs] *a.*		可疑的
ubiquitous [juːˈbikwitəs] *a.*		普遍存在的
propel [prəˈpel] *v.*		激励，促使
thorny [ˈθɔːni] *a.*		苦恼的；多刺的
bedevil [biˈdevl] *v.*		使痛苦，使苦恼
consortium [kənˈsɔːtiəm] *n.*		财团，合伙

答案及解析

6. 【问题】第一段中的"The confusion"指的是 _____。

   A. 在哪里以可持续的方式进行投资消费

   B. 大量的产品供选择

   C. 不可靠的环保信息

   D. 环保资质信息很少

   【答案】C

   【解析】此题为指代题。confusion 指代的应该是前句中提到的 dubious quality green labels, 再根据文章首句告诉我们信息量虽然很大，但不准确或者迷惑人可能更加危险。因而答案为 C。

7. 【问题】从《新科学人》的分析可以推断出在很多情况下 _____。

   A. 环保信誉被滥用

   B. 绿色环保经济很重要

   C. 环境影响弱化了

   D. 环保资质促进绿色环保经济

   【答案】A

   【解析】此题为细节信息题。根据题干定位到文章第一段第五句。第六句话告诉我们该分析表明大多数企业被认为是环保型的，但名不副实，因而答案为 A。

8. 【问题】从未经证实的说法到测量的困难，再到个人产品，作者想说 _____。

   A. 环保信誉是科学家和生产商之间的较量

   B. 科学家和生产商都不诚实

   C. 建立绿色环保经济很重要

   D. 更完善的信息很重要

   【答案】D

   【解析】根据题干提到的三个方面，可以定位到文章的第二、三、四段。这三个方面都是举例说明，为的是证明文章第一段最后一句话：获取更完善的信息很重要。因而答案为 D。

9. 【问题】为了解决问题，作者呼吁 _____。

   A. 透明的企业管理　　　　　　　B. 确立可持续性指标

   C. 严格的以学术为先导的管理　　D. 严格的法律武器

   【答案】D

   【解析】文章第五段提到为各种产品制定严格的标准很难，而且也会给学术机构造成很大负担，所以可以排除选项 B 和 C。答案的原文出处在最后一段，作者提到对企业环保信息公开提出法律要求很必要，因而答案为 D。

10. 【问题】下面哪一项是对最后一段最好的推测？

    A. 难度最大的挑战是最好的机会。

    B. 是开始另一场绿色革命的时候了。

    C. 信息应该完全免费。

D. 没数量，就没质量。

【答案】B

【解析】本题的解题要结合文章的主题，文章开头就提到不准确且迷惑人的信息尽管数量很大，但造成的结果更危险。因而为了实现绿色环保经济，首当其冲要确保信息的正确性，因而答案为B。

2013 年医学博士统考阅读理解部分真题

Passage One

There is plenty we don't know about criminal behavior. Most crime goes unreported so it is hard to pick out trends from the data, and even reliable sets of statistics can be difficult to compare. But here is one thing we do know: those with a biological predisposition to violent behavior who are brought up in abusive homes are very likely to become lifelong criminals.

Antisocial and criminal behavior tends to run in families, but no one was sure whether this was due mostly to social-environmental factors or biological ones. It turns out both are important, but the effect is most dramatic when they act together. This has been illustrated in several studies over the past six years which found that male victims of child abuse are several times as likely to become criminals and abusers themselves if they were born with a less-active version of a gene for the enzyme monoamine oxidase A (MAO-A), which breaks down neurotransmitters crucial to the regulation of aggression.

Researchers recently made another key observation: kids with this "double whammy" of predisposition and an unfortunate upbringing are likely to show signs of what's to come at a very early age. The risk factors for long-term criminality — attention deficit hyperactivity disorder, low IQ, language difficulties — can be spotted in kindergarten. So given what we now know, shouldn't we be doing everything to protect the children most at risk?

No one is suggesting testing all boys to see which variant of the MAO-A gene they have, but what the science is telling us is that we should redouble efforts to tackle abusive upbringings, and even simple neglect. This will help any child, but especially those whose biology makes them vulnerable. Thankfully there is already considerable enthusiasm in both the US and the UK for converting the latest in behavioral science into parenting and social skills: both governments have schemes in place to improve parenting in families where children are at risk of receiving poor care.

Some people are uncomfortable with the idea of early intervention because it implies our behavior becomes "set" as we grow up, compromising the idea of free will. That view is understandable, but it would be negligent to ignore what the studies are telling us. Indeed, the cost to society of failing to intervene — in terms of criminal damage, dealing with offenders and helping victims of crime — is bound to be greater than the cost of improving parenting. The value to the children is immeasurable.

1. Researchers have come to a consensus: to explain violent behavior _____.
   A. in terms of physical environment
   B. from a biological perspective
   C. based on the empirical data
   D. in a statistical way

2. When we say that antisocial and criminal behavior tends to run in families, as indicated by the recent findings, we can probably mean that _____.
   A. a particular gene is passed on in families
   B. child abuse will lead to domestic violence
   C. the male victims of child abuse will pass on the tendency
   D. the violent predisposition is exclusively born of child abuse

3. The recent observation implicated that to check the development of antisocial and criminal behavior _____.
   A. boys are to be screened for the biological predisposition
   B. high-risk kids should be brought up in kindergarten
   C. it is important to spot the genes for the risk factors
   D. active measures ought to be taken at an early age

4. To defend the argument against the unfavorable idea, the author makes it a point to consider _____.
   A. the immeasurable value of the genetic research on behavior
   B. the consequences of compromising democracy
   C. the huge cost of improving parenting skills
   D. the greater cost of failing to intervene

5. Which of the following can be the best title for the passage?
   A. Parenting Strategies for Kids.
   B. The Making of a Criminal.
   C. Parental Education.
   D. Abusive Parenting.

Passage Two

After 25 years battling the mother of all viruses, have we finally got the measure of HIV? Three developments featured in this issue collectively give grounds for optimism that would have been scarcely believable a year ago in the wake of another failed vaccine and continuing problems supplying drugs to all who need them.

Perhaps the most compelling hope lies in the apparent "cure" of a man with HIV who had also developed leukemia. Doctors treated his leukemia with a bone marrow transplant that also vanquished the virus. Now US Company Sangamo Biosciences is hoping to emulate the effect using gene therapy. If it works, and that is still a big if, it would open up the possibility of patients being cured with a single shot of gene therapy, instead of taking antiretroviral drugs for life.

Antiretroviral therapy (ART) is itself another reason for optimism. Researchers at the World Health Organization have calculated that HIV could be effectively eradicated in Africa and other hard-hit places using existing drugs. The trick is to test everyone often, and give those who test positive ART as soon as possible. Because the drugs rapidly reduce circulating levels of the virus to almost zero, it would stop people passing it on through sex. By blocking the cycle of infection in this way, the virus could be virtually eradicated by 2050.

Bankrolling such a long-term program would cost serious money — initially around $3.5 billion a year in South Africa alone, rising to $85 billion in total. Huge as it sounds, however, it is peanuts compared with the estimated $1.9 trillion cost of the Iraq war, or the $700 billion spent in one go propping up the US banking sector. It also looks small beer compared with the costs of carrying on as usual, which the WHO says can only lead to spiraling cases and costs.

The final bit of good news is that the cost of ART could keep on falling. Last Friday, GlaxoSmithKline chairman Andrew Witty said that his company would offer all its medicines to the poorest countries for at least 25 percent less than the typical price in rich countries. GSK has already been doing this for ART, but the hope is that the company may now offer it cheaper still and that other firms will follow their lead.

No one doubts the devastation caused by AIDS. In 2007，2 million people died and 2.7 million more contracted the virus. Those dismal numbers are not going to turn around soon — and they won't turn around at all without huge effort and investment. But at least there is renewed belief that, given the time and money, we can finally start riddling the world of this most fearsome of viruses.

6. Which of the following can be most probably perceived beyond the first paragraph?
   A. The end of the world.　　　　　　B. A candle of hope.
   C. A Nobel prize.　　　　　　　　　D. A quick fix.

7. According to the passage, the apparent "cure" of the HIV patient who had also developed leukemia would _____.
   A. make a promising transition from antiretroviral medication to gene therapy
   B. facilitate the development of effective vaccines for the infection
   C. compel people to draw an analogy between AIDS and leukemia
   D. change the way we look at those with AIDS

8. As another bit of good news, _____.
   A. HIV will be virtually wiped out first in Africa
   B. the cycle of HIV infection can be broken with ART
   C. the circulating levels of HIV have been limited to almost zero
   D. the existing HIV drugs will be enhanced to be more effective in 25 years

9. The last reason for optimism is that _____.
   A. governments will invest more in improving ART
   B. the cost of antiretroviral therapy is on the decline
   C. everybody can afford antiretroviral therapy in the world
   D. the financial support of ART is coming to be no problem
10. The whole passage carries a tone of _____.
   A. idealism B. activism C. criticism D. optimism

Passage Three

Archaeology can tell us plenty about how humans looked and the way they lived tens of thousands of years ago. But what about the deeper questions? Could early humans speak? Were they capable of self-conscious reflection? Did they believe in anything?

Such questions might seem to be beyond the scope of science. Not so. Answering them is the focus of a burgeoning field that brings together archaeology and neuroscience. It aims to chart the development of human cognitive powers. This is not easy to do. A skull gives no indication of whether its owner was capable of speech, for example. The task then is to find proxies（替代物）for key traits and behaviors that have stayed intact over millennia.

Perhaps the most intriguing aspect of this endeavor is teasing out the role of culture as a force in the evolution of our mental skills. For decades, development of the brain has been seen as exclusively biological. But increasingly, that is being challenged.

Take what the Cambridge archaeologist Colin Renfrew calls "the sapient（智人的）paradox（矛盾）". Evidence suggests that the human genome, and hence the brain, has changed little in the past 60,000 years. Yet it wasn't until about 10,000 years ago that profound changes took place in human behavior: people settled in villages and built shrines. Renfrew's paradox is why, if the hardware was in place, did it take so long for humans to start changing the world?

His answer is that the software — the culture — took a long time to develop. In particular, the intervening time saw humans vest（赋予）meaning in objects and symbols. Those meanings were developed by social interaction over successive generations, passed on through teaching, and stored in the neuronal connections of children.

Culture also changes biology by modifying natural selection, sometimes in surprising ways. How is it, for example, that a human gene for making essential vitamin C became blocked by junk DNA? One answer is that our ancestors started eating fruit, so the pressure to make vitamin C "relaxed" and the gene became unnecessary. By this reasoning, early humans then became addicted to fruit, and any gene that helped them to find it was selected for.

Evidence suggests that the brain is so plastic that, like genes, it can be changed by relaxing selection pressure. Our understanding of human cognitive development is still fragmented and confused, however. We have lots of proposed causes and effects, and hypotheses to explain them. Yet the potential pay-off makes answers worth searching for. If we know where the human mind came from and what changed it, perhaps we can gauge where it is going. Finding those answers will take all the ingenuity the modern human mind can muster.

11. The questions presented in the first paragraph _____.
    A. seem to have no answers whatever
    B. are intended to dig for ancient human minds
    C. are not scientific enough to be answered here
    D. are raised to explore the evolution of human appearance

12. The scientists find the proxy to be _____.
    A. the role of culture   B. the passage of time
    C. the structure of a skull   D. the biological makeup of the brain

13. According to Renfrew's paradox, the transition from 60,000 to 10,000 years ago suggests that _____.
    A. human civilization came too late
    B. the hardware retained biologically static
    C. it took so long for the software to evolve
    D. there existed an interaction between gene and environment

14. From the example illustrating the relation between culture and biology, we might conclude that _____.
    A. the mental development has not been exclusively biological
    B. the brain and culture have not developed at the same pace
    C. the theory of natural selection applies to human evolution
    D. vitamin C contributes to the development of the brain

15. Speaking of the human mind, the author would say that _____.
    A. its cognitive development is extremely slow
    B. to know its past is to understand its future
    C. its biological evolution is hard to predict
    D. as the brain develops, so as the mind

Passage One

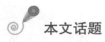 本文话题

犯罪行为的原因。

难词译注

predisposition [ˌpriːdispəˈziʃən] n.   倾向
double whammy [ˈdʌbl] [ˈwæmi]   祸不单行
neurotransmitter [ˌnjuərətrænzˈmitə] n.   神经递质

 难句译注

　　This has been illustrated in several studies over the past six years which found that male victims of child abuse are several times as likely to become criminals and abusers themselves if they were born with a less-active version of a gene for the enzyme monoamine oxidase A (MAO-A), which breaks down neurotransmitters crucial to the regulation of aggression.

【分析】此句为复合句，句中有多个定语从句。主句为：This has been illustrated in several studies over the past six years. 后面 which 引导定语从句（which found…oxidase A）修饰 studies。在定语从句中有一个 if 引导的条件状语从句。最后 which 引导的非限制性定语从句（which breaks down…）修饰 MAO-A。

【译文】过去的六年间多个研究已经阐述了这个观点。研究发现，如果虐待儿童案件中受害的男孩出生时就带有相对不活跃的单胺氧化酶基因，（那么）他们将来成为罪犯和施暴者的可能性多达几倍。而这种酶可以分解为对控制人的进攻行为至关重要的神经传递素。

 答案及解析

1. 【问题】研究者已经达成共识：从 _____ （方面）解释犯罪行为。
　　　　　A．自然环境　　　　　　　　B．生物角度
　　　　　C．经验数据　　　　　　　　D．统计方法
　　【答案】B
　　【解析】此题为细节定位题。根据第一段得知，对于犯罪行为，由于多数未报道，因而采集数据或者用可靠的统计方法都很困难，故排除选项C和D，选项A也没提到。第一段最后一句话是此题的有效信息。

2. 【问题】当说到"正如最近的研究结果指出，反社会和犯罪行为通常发生在家族中"，我们的意思可能是_____。
　　　　　A．由家族中一个特殊的基因遗传下来
　　　　　B．虐待儿童会导致家庭暴力
　　　　　C．虐待儿童案件中受害的男孩将会继续这种倾向
　　　　　D．暴力倾向仅仅出现在虐待儿童的家庭
　　【答案】A
　　【解析】此题为细节理解题。根据题干信息，可以定位到文章的第二段，最后一句话是解题的有效信息，句义理解详见难句译注。

3. 【问题】最近的观察暗示，为了探究反社会和犯罪行为的发展，_____。

  A．要筛查男孩的生理倾向性 B．高危孩子应该在幼儿园养育

  C．发现危险因素基因很重要 D．在早期应采取积极措施

【答案】D

【解析】此题为细节定位题。根据题干信息，可以定位到第三段。解题有效信息为最后一句。根据本段主题句可以得知有暴力倾向的孩子在早期会出现迹象。而最后一句用反问的方式提出，我们是否应该就我们目前了解的知识，采取措施保护那些处于危险中的孩子们。因而答案为 D。

4. 【问题】为了支持反对不利观点的论点，作者认为要考虑_____。

  A．行为基因研究的无限价值。 B．妥协民主的后果。

  C．提高父母教育的技巧。 D．干涉失败成本更大。

【答案】D

【解析】此题为细节理解题。根据题干信息，可以定位到文章最后一段。解题有效信息是第三句，句意为：事实上，社会干预失败所付出的成本必定大于提高父母教育能力的成本。考虑到成本的差异，作者指出，尽管不利观点可以理解，但对于孩子来说家庭教育提升这一早期介入意义重大。因而答案为 D。

5. 【问题】文章最恰当的题目是什么？

  A．父母对子女教育的策略。 B．罪犯的形成。

  C．父母教育。 D．虐待型的父母教育。

【答案】B

【解析】此题为主旨题。根据文章第一段的主题句以及每段的主题句可以得知，文章围绕犯罪行为的形成因素展开讨论，因而选项 B 为答案。

Passage Two

本文话题

HIV 的治疗进展。

难词译注

leukemia [luːˈkiːmiə] *n.*		白血病
vanquish [ˈvæŋkwiʃ] *v.*		征服，抑制
emulate [ˈemjuːleit] *v.*		仿效
antiretroviral drug [ˌæntiˌretrəuˈvairəl] [drʌg]		抗逆转录病毒药
bankroll [ˈbæŋkrəul] *n./v.*		资助
spiral [ˈspaiərəl] *n./v.*		螺旋，盘旋
devastation [ˌdevəˈsteiʃən] *n.*		毁坏

难句译注

Three developments featured in this issue collectively give grounds for optimism that would have been scarcely believable a year ago in the wake of another failed vaccine and continuing problems supplying drugs to all who need them.

【分析】主句为：Three developments give grounds for optimism。featured 做定语修饰 development。"that would have been…" 是定语从句，修饰 optimism。in the wake of 的意思是 "随着……而来"。

【译文】以这个问题为主的三个进展共同为这个问题的乐观态度提供理由，这在一年前随着另一个疫苗的失败和给予人们的药物不断出现问题的情况下是几乎不可想象的。

答案及解析

6. 【问题】下列哪一个是通过第一段可以得知的？

    A．世界的灭亡。   B．希望之光。

    C．诺贝尔奖。   D．快速修复。

【答案】B

【解析】此题为细节定位题。根据第一段最后一句话可以得知，针对 HIV 病毒，研究进展又带给我们希望，因而答案为 B。

7. 【问题】根据文章，对已经患上白血病的 HIV 病毒病人表面上的治愈将 _____。

    A．有望从抗逆转录病毒治疗转向基因疗法

    B．有助于有效的抗感染疫苗的研制

    C．迫使人们将艾滋病与白血病进行类比

    D．改变我们看待艾滋病患者的方式

【答案】A

【解析】此题为细节定位题。根据题干信息可定位到第二段，解题有效信息为最后一句，意思是希望仿效那些仅采用单一基因疗法患者的疗效，取代终身服用抗逆转录病毒的药物。因而答案为 A。

8. 【问题】另一个好消息是 _____。

    A．HIV 病毒将在非洲首先被消灭

    B．HIV 病毒感染的循环可以被 ART 打破

    C．HIV 病毒的流行程度已经几乎降为零

    D．现有的 HIV 病毒药物将在 25 年后效力更强

【答案】B

【解析】此题为细节理解题。根据题干和第三段首句信息可以得知，解题有效信息就在第三段。首先，根据第三段第二句话可以排除选项 A，原文信息中没有提到 HIV 病毒首先将在非洲被消灭；另外，根据第四句可排除选项 C，原文信息是 "因为药物能快速将病毒流行程度降到零，这就防止人们通过性传播病毒"。选项

D 在文章中没有相应信息。

9. 【问题】乐观的最后一个原因是 _____。

      A. 政府将为提高 ART 给予更多投资

      B. ART 的成本在下降

      C. 世界上的每个人都能承受 ART（费用）

      D. 对 ART 的资金支持将不成问题

【答案】B

【解析】此题为细节定位题。根据题干信息，可定位至第五段。本段首句为有效信息，其含义与选项 B 吻合。

10. 【问题】全篇的语气是 _____。

      A. 理想化   B. 行动性   C. 批评   D. 乐观

【答案】D

【解析】此题为态度推断题，根据每段的主题句内容以及上述细节题可以得出，全篇语气态度为乐观积极的，因而答案为 D。

Passage Three

本文话题

人类大脑思维的形成与进化。

难词译注

archaeology [ˌɑːkiˈɔlədʒi] *n.*	考古学
burgeoning [ˈbəːdʒəniŋ] *a.*	增长迅速的，生机勃勃的
intact [inˈtækt] *a.*	完整的，原封不动的
millennia [miˈleniə] *n.*	千年
intriguing [inˈtriːgiŋ] *a.*	有趣的，迷人的
endeavor [enˈdevə] *n./v.*	努力，尽力
gauge [geidʒ] *n./v.*	测量
ingenuity [ˌindʒəˈnjuːəti] *n.*	心灵手巧，独创性
muster [ˈmʌstə] *n./v.*	召集，集合

答案及解析

11. 【问题】第一段提出的问题 _____。

      A. 似乎没有答案   B. 想要挖掘古人类的思维

      C. 不够科学，无法回答   D. 为探究人类相貌进化而提出

【答案】B

【解析】此题为细节定位题，解题有效信息在第一段最后一句话。

12. 【问题】科学家们寻找的替代物是 _____。
      A. 文化的作用   B. 时间推移
      C. 头颅的结构   D. 大脑的生理结构

【答案】A

【解析】此题为细节定位题。根据题干可以定位到第二段最后一句话，而解题有效信息是第三段的第一句话，因而答案为 A。

13. 【问题】根据 Renfrew 的悖论，从 6 万年前到 1 万年前的转变说明 _____。
      A. 人类文明来得太晚了   B. 硬件仍旧在生理上没有变化
      C. 软件的进化经历了太长时间   D. 基因和环境间存在着联系

【答案】C

【解析】此题为推断题，根据题干定位到第四段。段落大意是：证据表明，人类基因组及大脑在过去的 6 万年间几乎没有变化，然而直到 1 万年前人类行为才发生深远的变化……如果硬件保持不变，人类为什么要花费如此长的时间才开始改变世界呢？因而答案为 C。

14. 【问题】从文化和生理关系的实例中我们可以得出的结论是 _____。
      A. 心智发展已不仅仅是生理上的
      B. 大脑和文化不是同步发展的
      C. 自然选择理论适用于人类进化
      D. 维生素 C 有助于大脑发育

【答案】C

【解析】此题为推论题。解题有效信息在第六段，这两段主要论述文化与人类生理变化的关系。本段首句指出：文化也通过修改自然选择而改变生理。因而选项 C 为答案。

15. 【问题】提到人类思维，作者想要说 _____。
      A. 认知发展十分地缓慢   B. 知晓过去就是了解未来
      C. 生理进化很难预测   D. 随着大脑的发育，心智也随之发育

【答案】B

【解析】此题为推断题，解题有效信息在最后一段。解题有效信息是最后三句：可能的回报使得探寻答案是有意义的，如果我们知道人类的思维从何而来并且如何改变，也许我们就可以测算它今后的发展方向……选项 B 与此句含义吻合。

2012 年医学博士统考阅读理解部分真题

Passage One

As the defining epidemic of a modern age notable for overconsumption and excess, obesity is hard to beat. The increased availability of high-fat, high-sugar foods, along with more sedentary lifestyles, has helped push the number of obese people worldwide to beyond 400 million, and the number of overweight to more than 1.6 billion. By 2015, those figures are likely to grow to 700 million and 2.3 billion respectively, according to the World Health Organization. Given the health implications — increased risk of heart disease, stroke, diabetes and some cancers — anything that helps people avoid piling on the pounds must be a good thing, right?

Those who agree will no doubt welcome the growing success of researchers striving to develop "diet pills" that provide a technical fix for those incapable of losing weight any other way. Last week a study published in *The Lancet* showed that tesofensine, which works by inducing a sense of fullness, is twice as effective as any other drug at enabling patients to lose weight.

There is no question that advances such as this are good news for those with a strong genetic predisposition to obesity. But for the rest of us it is dangerous to see treatment as a more effective solution than prevention. There are several reasons for this. For a start, the traditional ways of maintaining a safe weight, such as limiting what you eat, increasing consumption of fruit and vegetables and taking more exercise, are beneficial for our health in many ways.

Second, overindulgence in fatty foods has implications for the entire planet. Consider the deleterious environmental effects of the rising demand for meat. As demonstrated in our special issue on economic growth, technological fixes will not compensate for excessive consumption. Third, interfering with the brain circuits that control the desire for food can have an impact on other aspects of a person's personality and their mental and physical health.

We need two approaches: more research into the genetics of obesity to understand why some people are more susceptible, and greater efforts to help people avoid eating their way to an early death. Cynics will say we've tried education and it hasn't worked. That is defeatist: getting people to change their behavior takes time and effort, held back as we are by our biological tendency to eat more than we need, and by the food industry's ruthless opportunism in exploiting that.

Drugs will be the saving of a few — as a last resort. But the global obesity problem is one of lifestyle, and the solution must be too.

1. In the first paragraph all the figures surrounding obesity reflect _____.
   A. a close link between growing obese and developing disease
   B. the inevitable diseases of modern civilization
   C. the war against the epidemic we have lost
   D. the urgency of the global phenomenon

2. When it comes to the recently reported diet pills, the author would say that _____.
   A. drugs are no replacement of prevention
   B. the technical advance is not necessarily good news
   C. the technical fix does help reverse the obesity epidemic
   D. the mechanism of tesofensine still remains to be verified

3. Which of the following can be referred to as the environmental perspective of the author's argument?

    A. Belittling good health behavior.

    B. Imposing a heavy burden on our planet.

    C. Making trouble for our social environment.

    D. Having implications for mental and physical health.

4. The author argues that we make greater efforts to help people fight against _____.

    A. their biological overeating tendency and aggressively marketed foods

    B. the development of diet pills as a technical fix for obesity

    C. their excuses for their genetic susceptibility to obesity

    D. the defeatism prevailing in the general populations

5. Which of the following can be the best title for the passage?

    A. No Quick Fix.

    B. Disease of Civilization.

    C. Pursuing a Technical Fix.

    D. A War on Global Obesity.

Passage Two

An abandoned airfield near a former Nazi concentration camp may soon feature pagodas and Tai Chi parks. A $700 million project aims to give Germany its own Chinatown 22 miles north of Berlin in the town of Oranienburg, housing 2,000 residents by 2010.

The investor group behind the scheme hopes the new Chinatown will attract tourists and business to rival the famed Chinatowns of San Francisco and New York by delivering an "authentic Chinese experience". "You'll be able to experience China, go out for a Chinese meal, and buy Chinese goods," says Stefan Kunigam, managing director of Bandenburg-China-Project-Management GmbH.

The project has attracted investors in both Germany and China, reports Christoph Lang of Berlin's Trade and Industry Promotion Office. "Chinese investors have already asked if we have a Chinatown here." He says. "The cultural environment is very important for them. You cannot build a synthetic Chinatown."

Germany is home to about 72,000 Chinese migrants (2002 Federal Statistical Office figures), but the country has not had a Chinatown since the early 1930s in Hamburg, when most of the city's 2,000 Chinese residents fled or were arrested by the Nazis.

German's more-recent history with anti-foreigner extremism remains a problem even within the government, reports Deutsche Welle (DW), Germany's international broadcaster. DW notes that National Democratic Party lawmaker Holger Apfel's xenophobic（恐外的）comments about "state-subsidized Oriental mega-families" at first went largely uncriticized.

"Every fourth German harbors anti-foreigner sentiments," DW quotes Miriam Gruss, a Free Democratic Party parliamentarian. "Right-wing extremism is clearly rooted in the middle of society. It's not a minor phenomenon." The German government initiated a special youth for Democracy and Tolerance program in January 2007 as part of its tolerance-building efforts.

While it is not clear how many Chinese migrants will ultimately settle in the new German Chinatown, developers hope the project will increase Germans' understanding for China and Chinese culture.

6. If set up, according to the passage, the new German Chinatown will probably be _____.
   A. a rival to the Chinatowns of San Francisco and New York
   B. mainly made of pagodas and Tai Chi parks
   C. located in the north suburbs of Berlin
   D. the biggest one in Germany

7. When he says that you cannot build a synthetic Chinatown, Lang means _____.
   A. the real imported goods made in China
   B. the authoritative permission for the project
   C. the importance of the location for a Chinatown
   D. the authentic environment to experience Chinese culture

8. By mentioning the population of Chinese migrants in Germany, the author most probably means that _____.
   A. it is too late to build a Chinatown
   B. it is their desire to save a Chinatown
   C. it is important to create jobs for them
   D. it is necessary to have a Chinatown there

9. According to the passage, German anti-foreigner extremism _____.
   A. can seed the new community with hatred
   B. could be an obstacle to the project
   C. will absolutely kill the plan
   D. is growing for the scheme

10. The message from the plan is clear _____.
   A. to build a new community
   B. to fight against right-wing extremism
   C. to promote more cultural understanding
   D. to increase Chinese's understanding of Germany

Passage One

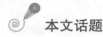

本文话题

减肥药的危害以及如何应对肥胖的方式。

难词译注

predisposition [ˌpriːdispəˈziʃən] *n.*　　　　　　　　　倾向；易染病的体质
deleterious [ˌdeliˈtiəriəs] *a.*　　　　　　　　　　　　有毒的，有害的

答案与解析

1. 【问题】第一段中有关肥胖的所有数据反映出_____。
　　　A. 越来越胖与患病的密切关系　　　　B. 现代文明不可避免的疾病
　　　C. 我们已经输掉了抗争流行病的战役　　D. 这一全球现象的紧迫性
　　【答案】D
　　【解析】此题为总结概括题。第一段的数据清楚地表明肥胖已经成为全球性的趋势，解
　　　　　决该问题刻不容缓，因而答案为 D。

2. 【问题】当谈到最近报道的减肥药时，作者认为_____。
　　　A. 药物无法取代预防
　　　B. 科技进步不一定是好消息
　　　C. 技术手段确实有助于逆转肥胖的流行趋势
　　　D. tesofensine 的原理仍需证实
　　【答案】B
　　【解析】此题为转折处命题。根据减肥药的专有名词定位到第二段，第二段主要讲述该
　　　　　药的作用。第三段第二句话转折后说，对于其他人（没有明显的遗传肥胖基因
　　　　　的人）来说，将治疗看作比预防更有效的手段是很危险的。因而答案为 B。对
　　　　　于有遗传肥胖基因的人来说这种药确实有效，因而 A 过于绝对。

3. 【问题】下列哪一个指的是作者对环境方面的观点？
　　　A. 轻视有利于健康的行为。　　　　　　B. 对我们的星球添加过重的负担。
　　　C. 给我们的社会环境增添麻烦。　　　　D. 对身心健康有意义。
　　【答案】B
　　【解析】此题参看文章第四段。

4. 【问题】作者认为我们要更努力帮助人类抵抗_____。
　　　A. 生理上饮食过度的趋势和被过度营销的食品
　　　B. 减肥药这一技术手段的发展
　　　C. 以遗传导致肥胖为借口

D．大众中流行的挫败心理

【答案】C

【解析】根据题干定位到第五段的第一句话：...greater efforts to help people avoid eating their way to an early death. 这句话说明更多的人将自己的肥胖归因于有肥胖的遗传基因，而忽视了生活方式的影响。因而选项 C 正确。

5. 【问题】下列哪一个是文章最好的标题？

A．没有快速的办法。　　　　　　　B．文明病。

C．寻求技术上的办法。　　　　　　D．针对全球肥胖的斗争。

【答案】D

【解析】此题为主旨题。本文利用众多数据表明肥胖问题刻不容缓，随后阐述了减肥药的作用。但作者对于这一药物的弊端进行了分析，最后指出两种应对措施：一是研究肥胖基因，二是努力避免人们消极对待这一问题而坐以待胖。文章最后作者提到减肥药可以救助一些人，但全球肥胖的问题是生活方式问题，因而其解决方法也应由此入手。选项 D 为答案。

Passage Two

 本文话题

德国准备建造唐人街。

✝答案与解析

6. 【问题】根据文章，如果建立，新的德国唐人街将可能 _____。

A．是旧金山和纽约唐人街的劲敌　　B．主要由古塔和太极公园组成

C．位于柏林的北部郊区　　　　　　D．是德国最大的一个

【答案】A

【解析】此题为细节定位题，原文信息参考第二段的第一句话。文章第一段提到这个唐人街将以古塔和太极公园为特征，但并没有说由古塔和太极公园组成，所以选项 B 错误；同时第一段提到新建的唐人街位于柏林以北 22 英里的 Oranienburg，因而选项 C 错误；选项 D 没提到。

7. 【问题】当 Lang 说你不能建造一个综合性的唐人街时，他的意思是 _____。

A．真正进口中国制造的物品　　　　B．该项目的官方准许

C．唐人街位置的重要性　　　　　　D．感受中国文化的真实环境

【答案】D

【解析】此题参见文章第三段。倒数第二句提到文化环境很关键，因而我们可以推断出 Lang 的意思指的是文化氛围，故选项 D 正确。

8. 【问题】通过提及德国的中国移民者，作者最可能的意思是 _____。

A．建议安全权威部门使用更重的碰撞测试假人

B．迫切呼吁碰撞测试假人的标准化

C．减少碰撞测试假人的重量

D．鼓励肥胖者减肥

【答案】A

【解析】此题为细节信息定位题，根据人名定位到文章第六段。本段最后一句提到，他认为问题答案可能就在于要检验汽车行驶安全时，权威部门应该使用更重的碰撞测试假人。

14．【问题】当探究重伤和致死率的原因时，Mock 最可能的观点是 _____。

A．汽车要更安全，以避免车祸

B．肥胖者最好不要饮酒驾车

C．不仅是总重量的问题，而是肥胖本身很危险

D．问题背后的主要原因是饮酒者的过重体重

【答案】C

【解析】此题为推断题。文章最后一段提到 Mock 推断汽车内部设计不太适合体重较大的人，或者有高血压、糖尿病等疾病的肥胖者很难从事故受伤中康复。因此我们可以推断 Mock 的观点在于肥胖本身可能是该问题的原因。

15．【问题】下面哪一个问题与文章紧密联系？

A．车内确实有必要安装气囊吗？   B．汽车真的能保证安全驾驶了吗？

C．碰撞测试假人重量不够？   D．车祸可以避免吗？

【答案】C

【解析】此题参考文章主旨：文章第一段。并且可以参考第 13 题。

D．大众中流行的挫败心理

【答案】C

【解析】根据题干定位到第五段的第一句话：...greater efforts to help people avoid eating their way to an early death. 这句话说明更多的人将自己的肥胖归因于有肥胖的遗传基因，而忽视了生活方式的影响。因而选项 C 正确。

5. 【问题】下列哪一个是文章最好的标题？

    A．没有快速的办法。   B．文明病。

    C．寻求技术上的办法。   D．针对全球肥胖的斗争。

【答案】D

【解析】此题为主旨题。本文利用众多数据表明肥胖问题刻不容缓，随后阐述了减肥药的作用。但作者对于这一药物的弊端进行了分析，最后指出两种应对措施：一是研究肥胖基因，二是努力避免人们消极对待这一问题而坐以待胖。文章最后作者提到减肥药可以救助一些人，但全球肥胖的问题是生活方式问题，因而其解决方法也应由此入手。选项 D 为答案。

Passage Two

 本文话题

德国准备建造唐人街。

🏹 答案与解析

6. 【问题】根据文章，如果建立，新的德国唐人街将可能＿＿＿＿＿＿。

    A．是旧金山和纽约唐人街的劲敌   B．主要由古塔和太极公园组成

    C．位于柏林的北部郊区   D．是德国最大的一个

【答案】A

【解析】此题为细节定位题，原文信息参考第二段的第一句话。文章第一段提到这个唐人街将以古塔和太极公园为特征，但并没有说由古塔和太极公园组成，所以选项 B 错误；同时第一段提到新建的唐人街位于柏林以北 22 英里的 Oranienburg，因而选项 C 错误；选项 D 没提到。

7. 【问题】当 Lang 说你不能建造一个综合性的唐人街时，他的意思是＿＿＿＿＿＿。

    A．真正进口中国制造的物品   B．该项目的官方准许

    C．唐人街位置的重要性   D．感受中国文化的真实环境

【答案】D

【解析】此题参见文章第三段。倒数第二句提到文化环境很关键，因而我们可以推断出 Lang 的意思指的是文化氛围，故选项 D 正确。

8. 【问题】通过提及德国的中国移民者，作者最可能的意思是＿＿＿＿＿＿。

A. 建造唐人街太晚了　　　　　　B. 拯救唐人街是他们的愿望

C. 为他们创造工作机会很重要　　D. 在那里有个唐人街很有必要

【答案】D

【解析】此题参见文章第四段，德国有很多中国移民者，但没有一个唐人街，因而作者的意思是 D 项。

9.【问题】根据文章，德国排外极端主义＿＿＿＿＿＿。

A. 可能充满仇恨地建造这个新社区　　B. 可能阻碍这个项目

C. 一定会扼杀这个计划　　　　　　　D. 正为这个计划发展壮大

【答案】B

【解析】文章倒数第二段提到德国的右翼极端排外主义扎根于社会中，并且不是一个小问题。因此我们可以推断德国排外极端主义可能会阻碍建唐人街的计划。

10.【问题】这个计划传递出的信息很清楚：＿＿＿＿＿＿。

A. 建立一个新的社区　　　　　　　B. 对抗右翼极端主义

C. 更好地促进文化上的理解　　　　D. 增进中国人对德国的了解

【答案】C

【解析】此题参见文章最后一句：建造者们希望这个建造唐人街的计划能增进两国之间的文化了解，所以选项 C 正确。

2011 年医学博士统考阅读理解部分真题

Passage One

Patients can recall what they hear while under general anesthetic even if they don't wake up, concludes a new study.

Several studies over the past three decades have reported that people can retain conscious or subconscious memories of thinks that happened while they were being operated on. But failure by other researchers to confirm such findings has led skeptics to speculate that the patients who remembered these events might briefly have regained consciousness in the course of operations.

Gitta Lubke，Peter Sebel and colleagues at Emory University in Atlanta measured the depth of anesthesia using bispectral analysis, a technique which measures changes in brainwave pattern in the frontal lobes moment by moment during surgery. Before this study researchers only took an average measurement over the whole operation, says Lubke.

Lubke studied 96 trauma patients undergoing emergency surgery, many of whom were too severely injured to tolerate full anesthesia. During surgery, each patient wore headphones through which a series of 16 words was repeated for 3 minutes each. At the same time bispectral analysis recorded the depth of anesthesia.

After the operation Lubke tested the patients by showing them the first three letters of a word such as "limit", and asking them to complete it. Patients who had had a word starting with these letters played during surgery — "limit", for example — chose that word an average of 11 per cent more often than patients who had been played a different word list. None of the patients had any conscious memory of hearing the word lists.

Unconscious priming was strongest for words played when patients were most lightly anaesthetized. But it was statistically significant even when patients were fully anaesthetized when the word was played.

This finding which will be published in the journal *Anesthesiology* could mean that operating theatre staff should be more discreet. What they say during surgery may distress patient afterwards, says Philip Merikle, a psychologist at the University of Waterloo, Ontario.

1. Scientists have found that deep anesthesia _____.
    A. is likely to affect hearing
    B. cannot block surgeons' words
    C. can cause serious damages to memory
    D. helps retain conscious or subconscious memories

2. By the new study the technique of bispectral analysis helps the scientists _____.
    A. acquire an average measurement of brainwave changes over the whole surgery
    B. decide whether the patient would retain conscious or subconscious memories
    C. relate their measurements and recordings to the verbal sounds during surgery
    D. assure the depth of anesthesia during surgery

3. To test the patients the scientists _____.
    A. prepared two lists of words
    B. used 96 headphones for listening
    C. conducted the whole experiment for three minutes
    D. voiced only the first three letters of 16 words during surgery

4. The results from the new study indicate that it was possible for the patients _____.
    A. to regain consciousness under the knife
    B. to tell one word from another after surgery
    C. to recall what had been heard during surgery
    D. to overreact to deep anesthesia in the course of operations

5. What can we infer from the finding?
    A. How surgery mispractice can be prevented.
    B. Why a surgeon cannot be too careful.
    C. Why surgeons should hold their tongues during surgery.
    D. How the postoperative patients can retain subconscious memories.

Passage Two

Scientists used to believe adult brains did not grow any new neurons, but it has emerged that new neurons can sprout in the brains of adult rats, birds and even humans. Understanding the process could be important, for finding ways to treat diseases such as Alzheimer's in which neurons are destroyed.

Most neurons sprouting in adulthood seem to be in the hippocampus, a structure involved in learning and memory. But they rarely survive more than a few weeks. "We thought they were possibly dying because they were deprived of some sort of input," says Elizabeth Gould, a neuroscientist at Princeton. Because of the location, Gould and her colleagues suspect that learning itself might bolster the new neurons' survival, and that only tasks involving the hippocampus would do the trick.

To test this, they injected adult male rats with a substance that labeled newborn neurons so that they could be tracked. Later, they gave some of the rats standard tasks. One involved using visual and spatial cues, such as posters on a wall, to learn to find a platform hidden under murky water. In another, the rats learnt to associate a noise with a tiny shock half a second later. Both these tasks use the hippocampus — if this structure is damaged, rats can't do them.

Meanwhile, the researchers gave other rats similar tasks that did not require the hippocampus finding a platform that was easily visible in water, for instance. Other members of the control group simply paddled in a tub of water or listened to noises.

The team reported in *Nature Neuroscience* that the animals given the tasks that activate the hippocampus kept twice as many of their new neurons alive as the others. "Learning opportunities increase the number of neurons," says Gould.

But Fred Gage and his colleagues at the Salk Institute for Biological Studies in La Jolla, California, dispute this. In the same issue of *Nature Neuroscience*, they reported that similar water maze experiments on mice did not help new neurons survive.

Gould thinks the difference arose because the groups labeled new neurons at different times. She gave the animals tasks two weeks after the neurons were labeled. When the new cells would normally be dying, she thinks the Salk group put their mice to work too early for new neurons to benefit. "By the time the cells were degenerating, the animals were not learning anything," she says.

6. Not until recently did scientists find out that _____.
   A. new neurons could grow in adult brains
   B. neurons could be man-made in the laboratory
   C. neurons were destroyed in Alzheimer's disease
   D. humans could produce new neurons as animals

7. Gould's notion was that the short-lived neurons _____.
    A. did survive longer than expected
    B. would die much sooner than expected
    C. could actually better learning and memory
    D. could be kept alive by stimulating the hippocampus
8. Which of the following can clearly tell the two groups of rats from each other in the test?
    A. The water used.
    B. The noises played.
    C. The neurons newly born.
    D. The hippocampus involved.
9. Gould theorizes that the Salk group's failure to report the same results was due to _____.
    A. the timing of labeling new neurons
    B. the frequency of stimulation
    C. the wrongly labeled neurons
    D. the types of learning tasks
10. Which of the following can be the best title for the passage?
    A. Use It or Lose It.
    B. Learn to Survive.
    C. To Be or Not to Be.
    D. Stay Mentally Healthy.

Passage Three

Here's yet another reason to lose weight. Heavier people are more likely to be killed or seriously injured in car accidents than lighter people.

That could mean car designers will have to build in new safety features to compensate for the extra hazards facing overweight passengers. In the US, car manufacturers have already had to redesign air bags so they inflate to lower pressures making them less of a danger to smaller women and children. But no one yet knows what it is that puts overweight passengers at extra risk.

A study carried out in Seattle, Washington, looked at more than 26,000 people who had been involved in car crashes, and found that heavier people were at far more risk. People weighing between 100 and 119 kilograms are almost two-and-a-half times as likely to die in a crash as people weighing less than 60 kilograms.

And importantly: the same trend held up when the researchers looked at body mass index (BMI) — a measure that takes height as well as weight into account. Someone 1.8 meters tall weighing 126 kilograms would have a BMI of 39, but so would a person 1.5 meters tall weighing 88 kilograms. People are said to be obese if their BMI is 30 or over.

The study found that people with a BMI of 35 to 39 are over twice as likely to die in a crash compared with people with BMIs of about 20. It's not just total weight, but obesity that's dangerous.

While they do not yet know why this is the case, the evidence is worth pursuing, says Charles Mock, a surgeon and epidemiologist at the Harborview Injury Prevention and Research Center in Seattle, who led the research team. He thinks one answer may be for safety authorities to use heavier crash-test dummies when certifying cars as safe to drive.

Crash tests normally use dummies that represent standard-sized males weighing about 78 kilograms. Recently, smaller crash-test dummies have also been used to represent children inside crashing cars. But larger and heavier dummies aren't used, the US National Highway Traffic Safety Administration in Washington, D.C. told *New Scientist*.

The reasons for the higher injury and death rates are far from clear. Mock speculates that car interiors might not be suitably designed for heavy people. Or obese people, with health problems such as high blood pressure or diabetes, could be finding it tougher to recover from injury.

11. When they redesigned air bags to hold less pressure, the American car manufacturers
    _____.
    A. found it hard to set standards without the definition of obesity
    B. incidentally brought about extra risks to obese passengers
    C. based their job on the information of car accidents
    D. actually neglected smaller women and children
12. When they categorized the obese people, the researchers _____.
    A. showed a preference for BMI in measurements
    B. achieved almost the same results as previously
    C. found the units of kilogram more applicable than BMI
    D. were shocked to know the number of obese people killed in car crashes
13. To address the problem, Mock _____.
    A. suggested that the safety authorities use heavier crash-test dummies
    B. cried for the standardization of crash-test dummies
    C. reduced the weights of crash-test dummies
    D. encouraged obese people to lose weight
14. While exploring the reason for the higher injury and death rates, Mock would most probably say that _____.
    A. cars can be made safer to avoid crashes
    B. it is wise for obese people not to drive drunk

C. it is not just total weight, but obesity itself that is dangerous

D. the main reason behind the problem is drinkers of heavy weight

15. Which of the following questions is closely related to the passage?

A. Are air bags really necessary to be built in cars?

B. Are cars certified as safe to drive?

C. Are crash-test dummies too thin?

D. Are car accidents preventable?

Passage One

 本文话题

麻醉状态下人们仍有记忆。

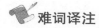 难词译注

anesthetic [ˌænis'θetik] *n.*	麻醉剂
anesthesia [ˌænis'θiːziə] *n.*	麻醉
skeptic ['skeptik] *n.*	怀疑者
bispectral analysis	双谱分析
frontal lobe	大脑额叶

难句译注

But failure by other researchers to confirm such findings has led skeptics to speculate that the patients who remembered these events might briefly have regained consciousness in the course of operations.

【分析】主句的主语为 failure, by other researchers...such findings 作为定语修饰 failure；主句谓语为 has led；不定式 to speculate 后面接一个宾语从句。宾语从句的主语为 the patients，谓语动词结构为 might briefly have regained，宾语从句主语 the patients 由定语从句 who remembered these events 修饰。

【译文】然而其他研究者没能证实上述结果，这导致怀疑者推测，回忆起这些事情的病人在手术过程中可能暂时恢复了意识。

答案及解析

1. 【问题】科学家们已经发现深度麻醉_____。

    A. 可能影响听力   B. 不能阻碍医生的言语

    C. 可造成记忆的严重损伤   D. 可保留有意识或潜意识的记忆

【答案】D

【解析】此题考点为细节定位题，原文有效信息是第二段第一句。

2. 【问题】新研究中，双谱分析有助于科学家_____。

    A．在手术过程中获取脑波变化的平均测量数据

    B．决定病人是否保持有意识的或潜意识的记忆

    C．把测量数据和记录与手术中的语言发音联系起来

    D．确保手术中的麻醉程度

【答案】B

【解析】根据题干中的关键词"bispectral analysis"定位到文章的第三段。本段第一句中出现该技术，并且同位结构解释说明这一技术的作用，即测量手术大脑额叶脑波形式的时时刻刻的变化。本段最后一句提到在这项研究前，研究者们仅对整个手术进行平均测量。A 项错在这一作用不是双谱分析的作用；C 项没提到；D 项错在 assure。

3. 【问题】为了测试病人，科学家们_____。

    A．准备了两套词汇

    B．使用 96 个耳机

    C．使整个试验持续 3 分钟

    D．手术中仅念出 16 个单词的前 3 个字母

【答案】B

【解析】此题可通过定位选项中的数字进行判断。第五段第二句提到使用不同的单词表，但没有提到两套，故 A 项排除；第四段第二句话提到 16 个单词，每个单词重复 3 分钟，因而可判断选项 C 错误；第五段第一句话提到手术后测试病人，每个单词仅展示前 3 个字母，因而 D 项错误。B 项信息在第四段，整个研究的受试者为 96 人，每个病人都戴上耳机，所以 B 项为答案。

4. 【问题】新研究的结果表明病人可能_____。

    A．在手术中恢复意识

    B．会在术后区分词汇

    C．回忆起手术中听到的内容

    D．在手术中对深度麻醉反应过激

【答案】C

【解析】此题为细节定位题，原文第一段开门见山地提到新研究的结果。

5. 【问题】从研究结果中我们可以推断出什么？

    A．手术误操作如何避免。

    B．为什么外科大夫多小心都不为过。

    C．为什么外科大夫应该在手术中保持沉默。

    D．术后病人如何能保持潜意识的记忆。

【答案】C

【解析】此题为推断题。文章最后一段提到研究结果可能意味着手术医务人员应该更加

谨慎，手术中他们交谈的内容可能影响到病人，病人术后可能回忆起手术中听到的内容，因而外科大夫应该在手术中保持沉默，以免影响到病人。故答案为C。

Passage Two

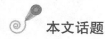 本文话题

成人大脑中也可以产生新的神经元，这一新发现为阿尔茨海默症的治疗提供了新的方法。

难词译注

hippocampus [ˌhipəˈkæmpəs] *n.*　　　　　　海马状突起（脑组织）
bolster [ˈbəulstə] *v.*　　　　　　　　　　　支持，支撑
murky [ˈməːki] *a.*　　　　　　　　　　　　朦胧的

答案及解析

6. 【问题】直到最近科学家才发现_____。
　　　A．成人大脑可以生长出新的神经元
　　　B．在实验室中神经元可以人为制造
　　　C．阿尔茨海默症患者的神经元受损
　　　D．人类同动物一样可以生长出新神经元
　【答案】A
　【解析】此题为细节定位题，文章第一段直接说明新研究的研究结果。

7. 【问题】Gould 的观点是：短命的神经元_____。
　　　A．比预期存活的时间更长　　　　　B．比预期死亡得更快
　　　C．实际上更有助于学习和记忆力　　D．通过刺激海马状突起而存活
　【答案】D
　【解析】此题根据人名定位到文章的第二段最后一句话。第二段的第一句提到海马状突起涉及学习和记忆力。而最后一句提到学习本身有助于新神经元的存活。因而答案为D。

8. 【问题】下列哪一个可以清楚地分清试验中的两组老鼠？
　　　A．使用的水。　　　　　　　　　　B．播放的声音。
　　　C．新生的神经元。　　　　　　　　D．海马状突起。
　【答案】D
　【解析】此题为细节定位题，由原文中的第四段第一句话可以得出答案。

9. 【问题】Gould 认为 Salk 小组没能得出相同的结果是因为_____。
　　　A．标记新神经元的时间　　　　　　B．刺激的频率

C．误标的神经元   D．学习任务的类型

【答案】A

【解析】此题为细节定位题，参考最后一段的第一句话。

10.【问题】下列哪一项是文章最好的标题？

A．使用它，或失去它。   B．学会生存。

C．生存还是毁灭。   D．保持精神健康。

【答案】A

【解析】此题为主旨题。通过第二段可知，学习（learning）可以促使新的神经元生长，而缺乏输入（input）则会使其死亡（dying），故 A 为正确的题目。

Passage Three

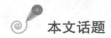 本文话题

本文讨论体重较大者可能在车祸中更危险。

答案及解析

11.【问题】当重新设计安全气囊以承受较少压力的时候，美国汽车制造商 _____。

A．发现若没有肥胖的定义则很难制定标准

B．意外地给肥胖乘客带来了额外的危险

C．根据车祸的相关信息进行工作

D．实际上忽略了娇小女性和儿童

【答案】B

【解析】此题考点为细节信息定位。文章第二段第二句话提到美国汽车制造商重新设计气囊，因为他们减少气囊的压力，从而降低娇小女性和儿童面临的危险。因而 D 项错误。最后一句话转折结构揭示这样的做法可能给超重乘客带来更多的危险，答案为 B 项。

12.【问题】当对肥胖人群进行分类时，研究者们 _____。

A．对 BMI 测量情有独钟

B．几乎得出和先前一样的结果

C．发现公斤单位比 BMI 更实用

D．震惊地获知车祸中肥胖人致死的人数

【答案】B

【解析】此题解题关键在文章第四段第一句话。这句话的意思是：当研究者们看 BMI 测量值时，得出同样的结论。这句话中的 hold up 的含义是"证明属实，经得起检验"。因而答案为 B。

13.【问题】为了解决这个问题，Mock ___。

A．建议安全权威部门使用更重的碰撞测试假人

B．迫切呼吁碰撞测试假人的标准化

C．减少碰撞测试假人的重量

D．鼓励肥胖者减肥

【答案】A

【解析】此题为细节信息定位题，根据人名定位到文章第六段。本段最后一句提到，他认为问题答案可能就在于要检验汽车行驶安全时，权威部门应该使用更重的碰撞测试假人。

14．【问题】当探究重伤和致死率的原因时，Mock 最可能的观点是 _____。

A．汽车要更安全，以避免车祸

B．肥胖者最好不要饮酒驾车

C．不仅是总重量的问题，而是肥胖本身很危险

D．问题背后的主要原因是饮酒者的过重体重

【答案】C

【解析】此题为推断题。文章最后一段提到 Mock 推断汽车内部设计不太适合体重较大的人，或者有高血压、糖尿病等疾病的肥胖者很难从事故受伤中康复。因此我们可以推断 Mock 的观点在于肥胖本身可能是该问题的原因。

15．【问题】下面哪一个问题与文章紧密联系？

A．车内确实有必要安装气囊吗？   B．汽车真的能保证安全驾驶了吗？

C．碰撞测试假人重量不够？   D．车祸可以避免吗？

【答案】C

【解析】此题参考文章主旨：文章第一段。并且可以参考第 13 题。

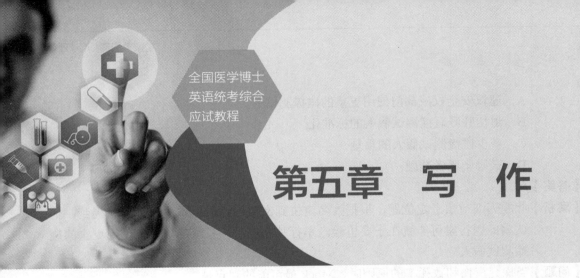

第五章 写 作

一、考试大纲的要求

按 2019 年最新大纲要求，书面表达测试考生使用英语书面表达自己思想的能力。此部分共计 20 分，考试时间约为 50 分钟。测试题型共有以下两种：

1. 文章摘要。要求考生阅读一篇 600~800 字中文文章，然后用英文写出一篇约 200 词的文章摘要。所概括的内容应简洁、全面、准确。在行文上，要求文字通顺，基本符合英语表达习惯，无重大语法错误。近几年文章摘要为主要测试题型，而且中文文章的篇幅也在逐年递增，平均字数约为 1200 字左右。

2. 翻译与写作。这种测试题型包括两个部分，即段落翻译和段落写作。翻译要求忠实原文；段落写作要求切题且意思连贯。在行文上，要求与摘要写作相同。

从近几年的真题来看，一直使用的测试题型就是摘要写作，因而考生应该在此测试题型上多加练习，掌握摘要写作的要领。对于段落翻译和段落写作在平时备考其他测试题型时可以作为基本功，加以训练。

2022 年的全国统考史无前例地选取了翻译的形式来命题，我们将在"命题作文和翻译"这个部分详细讲解。

二、摘要写作基本流程

在备考阶段，考生一定要注意：摘要写作绝对不是将千字中文文章翻译成英文文章。摘要写作依然是写作，因而摘要写作要注意以下基本写作流程：

第一步：浏览中文篇章。

第二步：在中文篇章中画出各段主题句及关键的细节内容。

第三步：根据各段主题句及关键内容组织英文摘要的各主要部分及内容。

第四步：根据中文摘要的内容写相应的英文摘要。

第五步：检查有无拼写、语法、用词等错误，查看有无逻辑关系不明确、语句不通顺等。

例题解析

No.1

珍爱生命从护心开始

生命第一杀手

这些年来，随着我国经济的发展，在人们解决了温饱之后，伴随而来的是与吸烟、缺乏运动、紧张和过度饮食等不良生活方式相关的慢性疾病，尤其是心血管疾病、肿瘤等已经成为危害健康、危及生命的第一杀手。

近年来，"猝死"事件在各地屡有发生。压力过大，劳累过度，使得不少中青年人长期处于亚健康状态，积重难返而猝死。在众多猝死事件中，多数是由心肌梗死引起的。而半数以上的心肌梗死是没有先兆的，突然起病，致死或致残；在心肌梗死的发病早期死亡者中，半数都死在到达医院之前。

在很多人的印象里，高血压、冠心病、心肌梗死好像是中老年人的"专利"，其实不然，现在每天医院急诊室、监护室里都能看到一些非常年轻的心肌梗死患者，而且越来越多。

无知者"无畏"

多数并不是死于无钱，而是死于无知，即缺乏预防意识，缺乏对健康的忧患意识，这在"白骨精"（白领、骨干、精英）中尤为突出。他们白天忙于工作，晚上忙于应酬，很少有人把自己的健康放在心上。

值得注意的是，不健康生活方式所致的心血管病多是"隐形杀手"，平时无明显症状，但在不知不觉或无先兆的情况下，以突然发病的形式瞬间结束人们的生命。相当多的病人第一次发病或第一次有临床表现就是心肌梗死，甚至猝死进而结束生命。

令人担忧的是，现在很多"白骨精"们根本意识不到自己是心血管疾病的高危人群，甚至幻想患病以后再亡羊补牢。实际上，在长期的超负荷"压迫"下，他们一旦发病就会一发不可收拾，第一次就往往可能猝死，所以一定不能心存侥幸。

管住嘴　迈开腿

血脂的异常和胆固醇升高、吸烟、糖尿病、高血压、中心型肥胖、日常生活缺乏运动、饮食缺乏蔬菜水果，都已经被证明是心血管疾病的重要危险因素，既然我们已经知道心血管疾病是一个多种危险因子的疾病，那么应首先从预防危险因素上做起，而不是等到患了高血压再去吃降压药物，得了高血脂再去降血脂。

心血管疾病是可防、可控、可救的。吸烟是万恶之源，不只是危害心血管，也是引起呼吸系统和多种癌症的"罪犯"。吸烟害己更害人，吸烟不是"嗜好"，而是疾病。肥胖和血脂异常也可以明显增加高血压、心肌梗死等的危险。

心血管防治要注重"治未病"，对每一个人来说，要有一个健康的身体，首先要不吸烟，"管住嘴"，特别要从青少年抓起，引导青少年从小养成健康文明的生活习惯，告别吸烟，告别垃圾食品。

> "迈开腿"，除了爬山、游泳等运动以外，要把路走起来。如果大家能坚持每天快步走一万步的话，持之以恒，定将受益匪浅。饭吃八成饱，日行万步路，为最有效的减肥方法。
>
> （1024 字）

↗ 写作解析

1. 分析中文原文

本文一共十三段，而且文章各部分均有副标题，这就对于考生来说很容易抓住文章的主要要点。在阅读中文原文后，我们可以确定每一段的段落大意，并在原文画出相应的关键细节内容。关键细节内容请见原文画线部分。各段的段落大意简要如下：

第一段：副标题1：生命第一杀手。

第二段：不良生活方式相关的慢性病，尤其是心血管疾病和肿瘤成为第一杀手。

第三段："猝死"屡有发生，多数是由心肌梗死引起的，事先没征兆，突然起病。

第四段：现在有越来越多的年轻心肌梗死患者。

第五段：副标题2：无知者"无畏"。

第六段：多数人死于无知，既缺乏预防和忧患意识，"白骨精"尤为突出。

第七段：不健康生活方式所致的心血管疾病是"隐形杀手"。

第八段：很多"白骨精"意识不到自己是高危人群。

第九段：副标题3：管住嘴，迈开腿。

第十段：心血管疾病的高危因素，从预防危险因素做起。

第十一段：吸烟是万恶之源。

第十二段："管住嘴"。

第十三段："迈开腿"。

在确定每段的段落大意后，我们可以很清楚地看到：文章共三个要点，就是三个副标题，因而英文摘要最好是符合副标题，由三个段落组成。根据各个副标题下的具体细节，可以整合内容，形成英文摘要的中文提纲，但要注意段落和句句间的逻辑关系连接。

2. 摘要的中文大纲

第一部分（第1～4段）：生命第一杀手。近些年来，与不良生活方式相关的慢性病，尤其是心血管疾病和肿瘤成为危害健康的第一杀手。压力过大、劳累过度使得不少中青年人长期处于亚健康状态，"猝死"事件屡有发生。心肌梗死趋于年轻化，而且大多没有先兆。

第二部分（第5～8段）：无知者"无畏"。多数人死于无知，即缺乏预防和对健康的忧患意识，这在"白骨精"中尤为突出。值得注意的是，不健康生活方式所致的心血管疾病多是"隐形杀手"，即平时无明显症状，在不知不觉中残害人们的健康。但令人担忧的是，很多"白骨精"们根本意识不到自己是高危人群，心存侥幸。

第三部分（第 9～13 段）：管住嘴，迈开腿。血脂异常、胆固醇升高、吸烟、糖尿病、高血压、中心性肥胖、日常生活缺乏运动、饮食缺乏蔬菜水果、紧张都是心血管疾病的重要危险因素，故应从预防危险因素做起。"管住嘴"首先要不吸烟，吸烟是万恶之源，其次要注意饮食，尤其要从青少年抓起。"迈开腿"是指除了爬山、游泳等之外，坚持每天快步走。

3. 供参考的表达式

第一杀手	top killer
不良生活方式	unhealthy lifestyle
慢性病	chronic diseases
心血管疾病	cardiovascular diseases
肿瘤	tumor
压力过大	excess stress
劳累过度	overwork; overloaded work
中青年人	young and middle-aged individuals
亚健康状态	sub-health
猝死	sudden death
心肌梗死	myocardial infarction
趋于年轻化	younger trend
先兆	sign
死于无知	die of ignorance
意识	consciousness
"白骨精"（白领，骨干，精英）	white-collars; backbones; elite
隐形杀手	invisible killer
高危人群	high-risk group; high-risk population
心存侥幸	count on luck
"管住嘴"	control the diet
"迈开腿"	start a workout or exercise
血脂异常	abnormal blood lipid
胆固醇升高	the increasing cholesterol
糖尿病	diabetes
高血压	high blood pressure; hypertension
中心性肥胖	central obesity

4. 参考范文

Love Your Life, Care Your Heart

In recent years, some chronic diseases related to unhealthy lifestyles, particularly cardiovascular diseases and tumors have been becoming the top killer. Excess stress and overwork contribute to sub-health among many young and middle-aged individuals, which causes high occurrence of sudden deaths without any signs, even frequently happening among young people.

It is believed that most people die of ignorance, that is, lack of prevention and health consciousness. Unfortunately those white-collar workers and elites, counting on luck, don't realize at all that they are high-risk groups. It is worth noting that the cardiovascular diseases induced by unhealthy lifestyles are invisible killers, which have no any obvious symptoms.

Controlling your diet and enjoying workouts are the optimal solutions. It is accepted that abnormal blood lipid, smoking, diabetes, hypertension, inactive life, lack of vegetables and fruits as well as stress are the high risks of cardiovascular diseases; thus, prevention of those risks comes first. First of all, please quit smoking, in combination with diet control, which should be required among young people. Besides, apart from climbing and swimming, walking at fast pace can be beneficial.

（182 words）

No.2

 2009 年真题

水果是否可吃可不吃

水果含有人体必需而又不能自身合成的矿物质，具有强抗氧化作用、防止细胞衰老的维生素以及可以明显降低血液中胆固醇浓度的可溶性纤维等，对人体健康十分有益。但中国人特别是男性，经常吃水果的比例很低。20 世纪 80 年代我在美国分析了美国 100 万人十年追踪研究的资料，发现不吃或很少吃水果的人群，肺癌死亡率为吃水果人群的 1.75 倍。而且从 45 岁到 74 岁的每个 5 岁年龄组均表现出类似的结果，说明这种因果关系非常可靠。美国有句谚语叫："一天一个苹果，不用看医生。"说明他们很早就总结出了水果对疾病的预防作用。世界卫生组织近年来提出了"天天五蔬果"的口号。其含义是，为保障健康，最好每天吃够五种蔬菜和五种水果。近年来美国哈佛大学的一些研究表明，多进食水果和蔬菜还可降低中风和冠心病的发病危险。

那么，到底水果中的什么成分起到了这样的作用？是不是维生素？服用市售维生素制剂是否可起到相同作用？我又进一步分析了肺癌死亡与服用维生素制剂的关系。结果发现，经常服用维生素并不能起到类似的保护作用。再专门分析重度吸烟者肺癌死亡率与进食水果和服用维生素制剂的关系。发现水果仍然起到保护作用，而维生素却没有。该分析研究的结论是人工合成的维生素不能替代水果对肺癌死亡的预防作用。后来的一些研究也得出了同样的结论。对此，营养免疫学家的解释是：天然植物中的维生素并不是单独起作用，而是与其他维生素和营养素相互联合一起工作。一种维生素补充的过多或不足，均会影响和削弱其他营养素或维生素的作用。

由于化学合成的维生素是与其他维生素和营养素分离的，复方的各成分间的比例也与天然的不尽相同，所以他们不能产生与天然物质中所含的维生素一样的功效。有些国外的专家把这种现象戏称为"人造的不如神造的"。另外，蔬菜水果中还可能含有些尚未被人类认识的生理活性物质。目前，天然食物的抗氧化作用已成为一个重要的研究领域，各国营养学家正在进行研究开发。研究已证实，有些蔬菜水果具有强抗氧化作用，如大蒜、胡萝卜、柿子、柑橘、猕猴桃等能提高体内超氧化物歧化酶（SOD）的活性，发挥延缓衰老的作用。

综上所述，在日常生活中，水果应作为每日膳食的重要组成部分，绝不是可有可无的东西。对一般人群来说，维生素制剂绝不能也不应当代替日常对水果、蔬菜的进食。另外，过多地服用维生素制剂还可能引致一些副作用，有些甚至非常严重。如服用过量维生素 D 会导致软组织钙化，对肾脏和心血管系统造成损伤；长期服用维生素 E 易引起血栓等。在病态情况下，由于体内某些维生素的大量消耗或吸收合成转化不良，打破了其正常平衡，则必须适当补给，如，发热、手术、患心肌梗死等疾病时需补充维生素 C；肝肾功能不良时需补充维生素 D 等。但这些均需在医生的指导下使用。

（1110 字）

↗ 写作解析

1. **分析中文原文**

本文一共三段，主要讲述水果对健康的好处，以及维生素制剂对人健康的影响。关键细节内容请见原文画线部分。各段的段落大意简要如下：

第一段：水果中的矿物质、维生素和可溶性纤维对人体健康有益。

第二段：维生素制剂不能替代天然维生素。

第三段：水果是每日膳食必需品，以及维生素制剂的副作用。

在确定每段的段落大意后，我们可以根据选取各段主要具体细节作为论据支持三个段落的主旨。文章中的具体重要细节参见原文中的画线部分。

2. **摘要的中文大纲**

第一部分（第1段）：水果含有人体必需而又不能自身合成的矿物质，具有强抗氧化作用、防止细胞衰老的维生素以及可以明显降低血液中胆固醇浓度的可溶性纤维等，对人体健康十分有益。但中国人特别是男性，经常吃水果的比例很低。一项研究表明，不吃或很少吃水果的人群，肺癌死亡率为吃水果人群的 1.75 倍。世界卫生组织近年来提出了"天天五蔬果"的口号。其含义是，为保障健康，最好每天吃够五种蔬菜和五种水果。美国哈佛大学的一些研究也表明，多进食水果和蔬菜还可降低中风和冠心病的发病危险。

第二部分（第 2 段）：服用市售维生素制剂不能起到水果所起到的作用。一项有关肺癌死亡和维生素制剂的研究发现：人工合成的维生素不能替代水果对肺癌的预防作用。天然植物中的维生素是与其他维生素和营养素共同工作的。但化学合成的维生素是与其他维生素和营养素分离的。另外，蔬菜水果中还可能含有些尚未被人类认识的生理活性物质。研究已证实，有些蔬菜水果具有强抗氧化作用，如大蒜、胡萝卜、柿子、柑橘、猕猴桃等能提高体内超氧化物歧化酶（SOD）的活性，发挥延缓衰老的作用。

第三部分（第3段）：因而在日常生活中，水果应作为每日膳食的重要组成部分。对一般人群来说，维生素制剂不能替代蔬果的进食，过多服用维生素制剂会引起一些副作用。在病态情况下，必须适当补给维生素，但须在医生指导下使用。

3.　供参考的表达式

必需	indispensable
合成	synthesize
矿物质	mineral
抗氧化作用	antioxidant effects
可溶性纤维	soluble fibers
死亡率	death rate
中风	stroke
冠心病	coronary heart disease
发病危险	risk factors for developing a disease
市售	over-the-counter
营养素	nutrient
生理活性物质	physiologically active substance
柿子	persimmon
猕猴桃	kiwi fruit
大蒜	garlic
延缓衰老	delay aging process
膳食	diet
替代	substitute
副作用	side effect

4.　参考范文

Fruits, rich in the minerals that human bodies need but cannot be synthesized by themselves, anti-aging vitamins as well as soluble fibers which considerably decrease cholesterol in the blood, are beneficial to human's health. However, Chinese, particularly males, eat less fruits. It is indicated by a research that people eating less or no fruit have higher risks of lung cancer. WHO has also advocated that consumption of five kinds of vegetable and fruits can improve human health. Another study also suggests that the increasing vegetable and fruit consumption can lower the risks of stroke and coronary heart disease.

Over-the-counter vitamin supplement cannot play the role that fruit does, such as prevention of lung cancer. It is believed that natural vitamins work together with other vitamins and nutrients while synthetic vitamins are separated from other vitamins and nutrients. In addition, research has verified that some vegetable and fruit such as garlic, carrot, orange and kiwifruit have antioxidant effects which can help delay aging.

Therefore, fruit should be the significant component in daily diet. For ordinary people, vitamin supplements can't substitute natural vegetable and fruit, and excess intake of supplements can cause side effect. As patients, they should consume vitamin supplements with the help of physicians' instructions.

（204 words）

No.3

 2010 年真题

新兴学科：药物心理学

药物作用于人体的病变部位，而病人的心理作用会或多或少地影响药物的作用。为了使药物治疗达到最佳疗效，人们必须研究药物心理学，讲究服药心理。

现代医药学认为：药物大多能产生两种效应。药物通过其药理作用来达到治病的目的，此为药物的生理作用。药物还可通过其非生理作用，在病人的心理上产生良好的感觉，加速疾病的康复，此为药物的心理效应。药物的心理效应可促使药物取得更好的疗效，为治疗奠定良好的基础。

药物的心理效应是指由医生的威信，病人对药物的信任感，接受药物治疗的体验、评价，治疗时外界的暗示及药物的广告效应等共同作用而产生的综合效应。药物心理学正是建立在药物心理效应基础之上的一门新兴边缘学科。众所周知，用同样的药物，由专家、名医开出的则效果会更好，这就是药物心理学最简单而明显的例子。

有人做了一个形象的比喻：药物是治疗疾病的"种子"，而心理状态是种子赖以生长、开花和结果的"土壤"。药物的药理作用是药物治疗疾病的基础，而药物的心理效应则在疾病治疗过程中起着十分微妙的作用。特别是在治疗心因性疾病和心理精神疾病中，良好的心态显得更为重要。

与服药心理关系最密切的是药物的信誉。原因为：虔诚的信念和愉快的心情能影响人体的生理机能，增加肾上腺皮质激素的分泌；而适量的肾上腺素能耐受200～400倍致死量的细菌内毒素。药物的良好信誉，能树立人对药物治病救人的鉴定信念。

为什么不良心态会降低药物的生理效应呢？人体是一个复杂的有机整体，不良心态会影响内分泌、心脑血管系统等的功能，从而减弱人体的抗病能力，体内细菌就乘机繁衍滋生，药效当然就降低了。积极的服药心理，可激活内分泌和潜在的免疫功能，药物在免疫器官分泌抗体增多时，能发挥最佳疗效。

药物心理学对人体的作用，在某些人中表现尤为明显：特别是有神经质、意志薄弱、心理缺陷和易受暗示的人。药物心理学揭示了安慰剂止痛和心理安慰的奥秘：安慰剂可通过心理暗示作用刺激大脑产生内源性脑啡肽，其结构类似天然吗啡，作用于疼痛部位，从而减轻疼痛。

许多人有以自觉症状为主的慢性病。许多慢性病有明显的自觉症状，如恶心呕吐、头晕目眩、失眠多梦、食欲不振、腹胀和隐痛等，这些症状与心理和精神状态密切相关。而药物的心理作用正是通过心理暗示来调整人的心态，在不知不觉中治愈或缓解了原有的慢性病。

医护人员的语言、举止和行为对病人的用药心理影响很大。目前世界各国对癌症、类风湿性疾病和自身免疫疾病等尚无特效药。但医生绝不可对患者说："此病为绝症，无药可治。"如对症适时选用安慰剂，有时会收到真正特效药所没有的神奇作用，至少可解除病人精神上的痛苦，在心灵上得到安慰和鼓励，从而增强战胜疾病的信心。

药物心理学的重要组成部分是暗示疗法和安慰剂。安慰剂通过心理暗示作用而影响病人的心理状态，进而影响机体的生理功能，从而起到积极的治疗作用。现代医学证明：药物心理效应不但具有心理上的安慰作用，而且还有改变器官功能活动和躯体症状的多种作用，故可用于治疗某类躯体疾病及多种心理疾病。

（1228 字）

↗ 写作解析

1. 分析中文原文

本文段落较多，内容较复杂，不利于考生快速确定文章中的主要要点。这就要求考生研读每一个段落并抓住段落主旨，然后根据段落主旨确定摘要写作的要点。各段段落大意简要如下：

第一段：病人心理作用影响药物疗效，有必要研究药物心理学。

第二段：药物产生两种效应：生理作用和心理效应。

第三段：药物心理效应的定义。

第四段：药物和心理状态的关系：形象比喻。

第五段：药物信誉。

第六段：服药心理对药效的影响。

第七段：药物心理学对人体的作用。

第八段：心理暗示有效缓解自觉症状。

第九段：医护人员的语言、举止和行为对病人的用药心理影响很大。

第十段：药物心理学的重要组成部分是暗示疗法和安慰剂。

根据这些段落主旨考生可以提炼或总结概括摘要的要点，不难看出这篇文章的要点如下：药物产生的两个效应、药物心理学定义及重要性、药物心理效应对人体的作用、药物心理学的重要组成部分。具体相关细节参见文章画线部分。

2. 摘要的中文大纲

第一部分（第 1~3 段）：药物作用于人体的病变部位，而病人的心理作用会或多或少地影响药物的作用。现代医药学认为：药物能产生两种效应：生理作用即通过药理作用治病，和心理效应，它可促使药物取得更好的疗效。药物心理效应是指医生的威信，病人对药物的信任感，接受药物治疗的体验、评价和治疗时外界的暗示及药物的广告效应等共同作用而产生的综合效应。

第二部分（第 4~6 段）：在治病过程中，药物的心理效应起到十分微妙的作用。服药心理关系最密切的是药物的信誉。药物的良好信誉，能树立人对药物治病救人的坚定信念。不良心态会影响内分泌、心脑血管系统等功能，从而减弱人体的抗病能力。相反，积极的服药心理可激活内分泌和潜在的免疫功能，使药物发挥最佳疗效。

第三部分（第 7~10 段）：药物心理学的重要组成部分是暗示疗法和安慰剂。安慰剂通过心理暗示作用而影响病人的心理状态，进而影响机体的生理功能，从而起到积极的治疗作用。医护人员的语言、举止和行为对病人的用药心理影响很大。对于那些有神经质、意志薄弱、心理缺陷和易受暗示的人，或是有自觉症状的慢性病人，安慰剂可通过心理暗示作用于疼痛部位，从而减轻疼痛，缓解症状。

3. 供参考的表达式

药物心理学	pharmacopsychology
病变部位	the site of pathological changes
药理作用	pharmacological effect
威信	prestige
信任感	sense of trust
心理暗示	psychological implication
综合	comprehensive
药物信誉	credibility of medicine
内分泌	endocrine
心脑血管系统	cardiovascular and cerebrovascular system
抗病能力	resistance to diseases
免疫功能	immune function
疗效	efficacy
安慰剂	placebo
生理功能	physiological function
神经质	neurotic
意志薄弱	weak will
心理缺陷	mental defects
自觉症状	self-sense symptom

4. 参考范文

Medicine imposes effects on the body's disease and patients' psychology can more or less affect the result of medicine. Medicine can produce two effects: physiological effect and psychological effect. The former one means diseases can be cured by pharmacological effects, while the latter one can promote the medicine more effectively. Psychological effect of medicine refers to the comprehensive effects including physicians' prestige, patients' trust on medicine and their experiences of treatments and their evaluation.

In the process of treatment, psychological effect of medicine performs the delicate roles. The credibility of medicine is closely related to patients' psychology. Unhealthy mental attitude would affect endocrine and cardiovascular and cerebrovascular functions, which will lower body's resistance to diseases. On the contrary, positive attitude can activate potential immune functions and increase the efficacy.

The two important components of pharmacopsychology are implication and placebo. Placebo will influence patients' mental state and body's physiological functions through psychological implication, and then enhance the effectiveness of drugs. In this case, medical staff's words and behavior will greatly influence patients' medication attitude. For those people with weak will or mental defects or those with self-sense symptoms, placebo can impose effects on the pains through mental hints, which will relieve pains and symptoms.

（202 words）

No.4

 2021 年真题

"健康中国"的三层含义

《健康中国 2030 规划纲要》的颁布是我国健康现代化建设的一个里程碑。它实现了两个政策突破：首先，把健康中国建设上升为国家战略。其次，确认了健康优先战略，就是"把人民健康放在优先发展的战略地位"，加快推进健康中国建设。

落实规划纲要，首先要科学理解"健康中国"的三层含义。从健康事业角度看，"健康中国"是一个发展目标，是指人民健康、长寿水平达到世界先进水平的中国；从人民生活角度看，"健康中国"是一种生活方式，是人人拥有健康理念和健康生活，家家享有健康服务和健康保障的生活方式；从国家发展角度看，"健康中国"是一种发展模式，是把人民健康放在优先发展的战略地位，把健康融入所有政策，努力实现全方位、全周期保障人民健康的国家发展模式。

"健康中国"建设是一个大战略，必然面临诸多新挑战。从实施规划纲要的角度来看，卫生和计划生育领域的管理部门要进一步强化职能转变。《规划纲要》提出了健康优先发展战略方面的很多要求，现有的机制、手段、措施是远远跟不上的。要加快把卫生、计生系统从行业管理的职能定位向社会治理、公共事务管理上转变。

如何促使《规划纲要》更好地落地？首先要确立以人为本、以健康为中心的服务理念，比如在实施健康儿童计划方面，可以考虑整合现有分散的、以机构为中心的服务体系，在妇女结婚时就为其将来的孩子设立健康档案；其次是要着力加强系统整合，包括加强医疗和预防、卫生服务体系上下联动等方面的系统整合。

《规划纲要》中提出，要建立完善针对不同人群、不同环境、不同身体状况的运动处方库。运动处方是体育科学的最高点。如果每个人都能从医生或体育科学工作者手里拿到一张绿色的运动处方，就能够让个人的健康发展达到有计划、有目的的程度。目前落实这一内容难度很大，只有体育和医学的高度结合，才能促使其真正落地。

↗ 写作解析

1. 分析中文原文

画出中心大意、主题句和核心信息。本文行文结构为总分结构，也可以看作"提出问题—解决问题"的类型，具有明确的段落标志和主题词语。本文主题是以《规划纲要》为依托，阐述"健康中国"的三层含义，以及如何落实《规划纲要》中的目标。

2. 摘要的中文大纲

第一段：《健康中国 2030 规划纲要》的重要意义。

第二段："健康中国"的三层含义。

第三段："健康中国"战略实施过程中的挑战。

第四段：如何落实《规划纲要》？

　　　　第一，确立正确理念。

　　　　第二，加强系统整合。

　　　　第三，建立运动处方库，落实个人健康，结合体育和医学。

3. 表达方式参考

《健康中国 2030 规划纲要》	*the Plan for Healthy China 2030*
健康事业	the issue of health
人民生活	people's living standards
生活方式	lifestyle
运动处方	exercise therapy

4. 参考范文

How to Understand and Implement *Healthy China 2030*

The blueprint of *Healthy China 2030* is a milestone. It confirms the construction of Healthy China as a national strategy, which puts people's health in the priority position.

Scientific understanding is a necessary prerequisite to implement *Health China 2030*.

It is a goal of overall development from the issue of health, a lifestyle to maintain correct concepts, adequate service and protection, as well as a model of development to coordinate health into all the policies.

It also confronts big challenges, which demands the health and family planning administration to carry out institutional reform and innovation.

How should we promote the implementation of the blueprint? First, we must establish a people-oriented and health-centered service concept, paying attention to the health of key groups such as women, children, seniors, migrants and low-income groups. Secondly, we must focus on strengthening the system integration, including strengthening the system integration of medical treatment and prevention, and the linkage between the upper and lower levels of the health service system. Last but not least, it proposes to establish and improve a library of exercise therapy for different groups of people. Only a high degree of integration of sports and medicine can promote its real implementation.

No.5 **2019 年真题**

我国食品安全的现状、问题及对策

民以食为天，食以安为先。进入 21 世纪以来，我国食品安全事件多发、频发，不仅对产业发展造成影响，也给人民的身体健康和安全带来威胁，成为社会关注的重大民生问题。随着经济发展和人民生活水平的提高，我国民众的生活方式在悄然发生转变，由吃到饱、吃到好奔向要吃出健康。那么，舌尖上的美食究竟是否安全呢？

具体而言，我国食品安全水平是不断提高的。2009 年至 2013 年，我国蔬菜、水果、畜禽、水产品质量安全合格率分别在 96%、95%、99% 和 94% 以上，总体保持较高水平。2009 年至 2012 年，我国加工食品监督抽查合格率从 91.1% 上升至 95.6%，质量安全水平逐年提高。这些都与我们国家《食品安全法》的颁布和实施有着密切关系，也与社会各方面的努力分不开。

尽管我们在食品安全方面取得了很大成就，但食品安全治理仍然任重道远。我国凸显四类主要食品安全风险。第一，病原微生物污染是造成食品中毒死亡的主要原因，因此，防控病原微生物的污染是食品安全的刚性需求；第二，农兽药滥用是当前食品安全源头污染的主要来源，我国农兽药的使用仍然处于无序状态；第三，重金属、真菌毒素等污染物对粮食和食品安全构成长远隐患；第四，非法添加（addition）和掺假（adulteration）仍是我国现阶段突出的食品安全问题。

对于食品安全的治理要实施"两步走"的战略。第一步，通过完善法律法规、标准和监管体系，强化过程控制和风险分析等技术支撑，优化产销环境，强化企业主体责任，建立诚信体系和契约机制。第二步，通过产地环境的进一步治理，高效种植、养殖业得到健康发展，到 2030 年，产地环境污染治理初见成效，食源性（foodborne）疾病实现主动预防和控制，食品营养失衡引发的慢性非传染病高发态势得到遏制。

↗ 写作解析

1. **分析中文原文**

   画出中心大意、主题句和核心信息。本文为提出问题——分析问题——解决问题的结构: 首先提出食品安全问题仍然严重,紧接着分析四类食品问题,最后提出"两步走"的解决战略方案。

2. **摘要的中文大纲**

   第一段:食品安全问题仍是国计民生问题,食品健康现状如何?

   第二段:随着法规健全和全社会的共同努力,食品质量安全水平逐年提高。

   第三段:虽然取得了巨大成就,食品安全问题仍然任重道远,四类主要问题仍然凸显。

   第四段:"两步走"的治理方案。

3. **表达方式参考**

食品安全	food safety
民生问题	livelihood issues
治理	harness
病原微生物污染	pathogenic microorganism contamination
农兽药滥用	abuse of agricultural and veterinary drugs
重金属、真菌毒素	heavy metals, mycotoxins
长远隐患	long term hidden danger
主体责任	subject responsibility
诚信体系	integrity system
契约机制	contract mechanism

4. **参考范文**

The Current Situation, Problems and Countermeasures of Food Safety in China

Food safety is always the most important livelihood issue of concern in our society. With the economic development and the improvement of people's living standards, people are not satisfied with being filled with food. What they are more concerned is: is our food really safe in China?

According to some statistics, due to the promulgation and implementation of the Food Safety Law of our country, China's food safety level continues to increase. It is surely inseparable from the efforts of all sectors of society.

However, despite our great achievements, food safety governance still has a long way to go. There are four highlighted food safety risks including the problem of pathogenic microbial contamination, the abuse of agricultural and veterinary drugs, the disorderly use of heavy metals or mycotoxins and last but not least, illegal addition and adulteration.

To address the problems above, a "two-step" strategy should be implemented. In the first step, technical support such as process control and risk analysis will be strengthened through the improvement of laws, regulations, standards and regulatory systems. In the second stage, the efficient planting and breeding industry will be through the further management of production environment.

No.6

 2018 年真题

未来医学发展趋势

根据现代医学的发展轨迹和社会的发展趋势，未来 20 年或 30 年，医学将发生很大的变化。

一、医学的任务将从以防病治病为主逐步转向以维护和增强健康、提高人的生命质量为主。在未来寻求医学服务的，不再仅仅是患者，还会有相当数量的正常人；询医问诊的人，也不仅仅是因为躯体的缺欠或某个系统有病患的患者，相当多的人是为得到生活指导和心理咨询而求医；医生开出的不会全是去药房取药的处方，还有如何提高生活质量的处方。医学的对象将从以患者为主的模式逐步转变成面向整个人群的模式。因此，整个社会卫生资源的配置将重点分为两极，即社区医学服务与医学中心。有相当数量的医生是从事社区服务的全科医生，而比全科医生多得多的，从某种意义上来说，更直接、更有效、更节省资源的是社区护理队伍。社区护理队伍包括家庭病床服务、老年公寓服务以及社区围产与婴幼儿服务等。

二、信息学、生物信息学将改变医学工作的方式。长期以来精心保存的厚厚的病历，将被一张可以记载一个人一生的病情变化、诊疗经过，甚至全部影像资料的卡片代替。病历，不再只是在某医院、某时期的病情档案的记录，而是其一生的健康与疾病变化的记载。预计在不久的将来，作为医学咨询或医疗、预防等辅助手段，电子医疗和网上医院一定会走向社会，走入市场。但必须强调的是：无论科学怎样发达，诊断或治疗手段如何先进，电子医疗、远程会诊都不能代替最基本的医生与患者面对面直接的诊疗。各种先进的医疗手段都很重要，但最重要的还是医生的基本功，而医生使用计算机的能力只是医生的基本功之一。

三、医学工作的范围将从"出生到死亡"扩展为"生前到死后"。既往，人们认为"人从生到死，总离不开医生"。如今，在人还未出生的时候（胎生期），医生就可以对某种疾病做出正确的诊断，并可进行外科治疗，从而矫正畸形、修复缺损，待手术完毕，再把胎儿还纳子宫，使胎儿正常发育，待其成熟后娩出。此时不仅畸形或缺损得以矫正，而且连瘢痕都没有，这就是所谓的胎儿外科。当今的医院儿科还只是从新生儿开始，在不久的将来，在妇产科和儿科之间，将出现一个新兴的交叉学科——胎儿学科。现在，脑死亡者是个宝贵的卫生资源，在医学领域不仅具有可供利用、造福世人的价值，更具有研究的价值，如：器官保存，组织与细胞的保存与增值，都是新的研究课题和有发展前途的医学新领域。

↗ 写作解析

1. 分析中文原文

画出中心大意、主题句与核心信息。本文是明显的总分结构，且有明晰的并列段落的标志词语。主题为未来医学的发展趋势，并从医学任务、医学工作的方式以及医学工作的范围来进行阐述。

2. 摘要的中文大纲

第一段：在未来，医学会发生很大的变化。

第二段：医学任务将从防病治病转向维护健康，对象从病人转向正常人，社区护理队伍将更加壮大。

第三段：医学工作的方式将更多地受到信息学、生物信息学等技术的影响。

第四段：医学工作的范围将从"出生到死亡"扩展为"生前到死后"，更多的新兴学科会在未来兴起，扩展医学新领域。

3. 表达方式参考

防病治病	disease prevention and treatment
以患者为主的模式	patient-oriented model
卫生资源	health resource
社区医学服务和医学中心	community medical service and medical service
信息学	informology
生物信息学	bioinformatics
电子医疗	e-medical treatment
网上医院	online hospital

4. 参考范文

Future Medical Development Trend

According to the development track of modern medicine and the development trend of society, medicine will undergo great changes in the next 20 or 30 years.

First, the medical task will be gradually shifted from disease prevention and treatment to maintaining and enhancing health and improving people's quality of life. To follow this trend, the allocation of the entire social health resources will be divided into two poles, namely the Community Medical Service and Medical Center.

Second, information science and bioinformatics will change the way medical work is done. It is expected that in the near future, e-health and online hospitals will surely go to the society and enter the market, on the solitary basic skills and the ability of doctors to conduct face-to-face treatment for patients as the most important guarantee.

Third, the scope of medical work will expand from "born to death" to "after birth to death". In the near future, there will be emerging interdisciplinary disciplines, which, in the medical field, not only have the value of being available for the benefit of the world, but also have research value. Those topics such as organ preservation, tissue and cell preservation and value-adding are new research topics with a promising future.

No.7　2017 年真题

环境污染与肺癌

　　近几十年来，许多国家的流行病学调查资料都表明，不少传染病的发病率和死亡率在不断下降，而癌症的发病率和死亡率却在不断上升。大量的调查研究表明，癌症等疾病的发病率的上升与环境污染有关。由于环境污染对人体的作用一般具有剂量小、作用时间长等特点，所以容易被人们所忽视。往往病发之日，尚不知谁是元凶。

　　环境污染就像邪恶的阴影，悄悄吞噬着人体的健康。肺及呼吸道是一个开放器官，与外界直接接触，外界很多致癌因素都可以导致肺癌。环境污染就是导致肺癌的一个重要原因。环境污染中最为重要的就是大气污染。大气污染的许多学者惊奇地发现，近 50 年来，随着工业和经济的发展，人们生活水平的提高，肺癌的发病率也显著提高，特别是世界经济发达地区的患者成倍地增加。例如，美国的病人在50 年中，男性增加了 18 倍，女性增加了 6 倍。每 4 名癌症死亡病例中，就有 1 名是肺癌患者；每 100 名死亡病人中。有 5 名死于肺癌。就我国情况看，也有明显增加的趋势。从全国恶性肿瘤排列顺序来看，肺癌占第 5 位；每 100 名癌症病人中，大约有 8 名是患的肺癌。

　　肺癌是最常见的恶性肿瘤之一，据 WHO 统计，每年全球估计有 120 万以上新发肺癌病例，死亡约 110 万人，平均每隔 30 秒就有人死于肺癌。近年来，我国肺癌发病率及死亡率亦不断上升。国内外流行病学研究报告指出，大气污染易诱发肺癌而使死亡率增高。

　　在公认的大气污染物中，颗粒物对健康的危害最大，可增加患肺癌的危险。随着交通的发展、机动车辆的增加、环境的日益破坏，PM2.5 污染越来越严重。研究发现，大气中 PM2.5 在总悬浮颗粒物中的比率逐年增加，沉积在下呼吸道的 96%的颗粒物是 PM2.5。对肺癌死亡率进行分析表明市区大气总悬浮颗粒物与肺癌死亡率增高有一定的相关性。这在世界上许多国家都被证实。美国癌症协会收集的 16年资料，涉及 50 万名美国人的死亡原因数据，发现空气中的 PM2.5 与总死亡率和肺癌死亡相关。在日本进行的 PM2.5 与疾病关系研究也发现，PM2.5 水平与女性肺癌呈正相关。

写作解析

1. 分析中文原文

本文共有四段。第一段开门见山点明文章主旨：癌症等疾病的发病率的上升与环境污染有关。第二段主要讲环境污染与肺癌的直接关系。第三段讲肺癌在全球范围内的严重情况。第四段着重讲大气中颗粒物对健康的影响。

2. 摘要的中文大纲

写作的中文提纲大致如下：

第一段：大量的调查研究表明，癌症等疾病的发病率的上升与环境污染有关。

第二段：环境污染是导致肺癌的一个重要原因。环境污染中最为重要的就是大气污染。近50年来，随着工业和经济的发展，人们生活水平的提高，肺癌的发病率也显著提高，特别是世界经济发达地区的患者成倍地增加。大气污染易诱发肺癌而使死亡率增高。

第三段：大气污染物中的颗粒物对健康的危害最大，可增加患肺癌的危险。对肺癌死亡率进行分析表明市区大气总悬浮颗粒物与肺癌死亡率增高有一定的相关性。

3. 参考的表达

流行病学	epidemiology
传染病	infectious disease
发病率	incidence rate
死亡率	mortality rate
环境污染	environmental pollution
大气污染	air pollution
肺癌	lung cancer
恶性肿瘤	malignant tumor
公认的	widely accepted
悬浮	suspension，suspend
颗粒物	particulate
相关性	relevance
正相关	positive relevance

4. 参考范文

Environmental Pollution and Lung Cancer

According to some epidemiological data, a number of malignant tumors have been caused by the deteriorated environmental conditions, and their incidence rate and mortality rate are increasing.

Environmental pollution is one of the essential factors leading to lung cancer. From some statistics, in recently 50 years, with the industrial and economic development as well as the improvement of people's living standard, the incidence of lung cancer is increasing significantly, especially in the advanced areas where lung cancer patients are doubled. Air pollution leads to higher mortality of lung cancer.

PM2.5 may be the crucial factor in air pollution. According to a new research from the USA, the pm2.5 are abundant in the fog and haze because of overusing cars and destroying of air condition could increase the morbidity of lung cancer. Another research says that the total particle suspending has been found in respiratory system, and there is a positive relevance between the pm2.5 and lung cancer. The above analysis has been approved by scientists in Japan. We have to make efforts to improve the air condition. Not only will it reduce the risk to the lethal disease, but it also can give us a better environment and living quality. The way to the destination, however, is not easy and smooth.

No.8

 2016 年真题

全科医生培养及发展思路

随着医疗卫生事业的不断发展，人们对社区卫生服务的要求也越来越高。目前我国社区卫生服务发展还不平衡。高素质的全科医生（general practitioner）缺乏成为滞后社区卫生发展的主要原因。规范全科医生培养，大力发展全科医生培训工作势在必行。全科医生在社区卫生服务中的功能包括治疗、保健、预防、护理、健康调查、咨询及健康教育等。虽然我国全科医学（general family medicine）已经得到了普及和发展，但其教育与培训还存在一些问题。本文就全科医生的培养和今后的发展作一浅析。

全科医生需具备的基本素质

全科医生需要较全面的知识。某些严重疾病的早期症状可能比较轻微，与一些常见病、多发病表现并无太大区别。这就要求全科医生从众多的疾病中筛选可能的情况，因此要求全科医生临床学科知识面要广。社区卫生工作中，一名合格的全科医生，也应是一名出色的社会工作者。全科医生服务的对象是社区内的居民，而且有可能需要长期面对，因此要求全科医生要有良好的人际关系、协调能力和高度的工作热情，并与患者建立一种亲密而长期的友情，成为病人家庭的良师益友，要具有良好的职业道德。

目前全科医生存在的问题

全科医生工作热情不高。一方面与专业医生相比，收入与社会地位存在差距；另一方面工作环境较艰苦，医疗设备落后，导致全科医生的工作热情和人员稳定性不高。合格的全科医生人员不多。由于全科医学专业在我国发展历史较短，很多医学院校近年刚开设全科医学的专业。全科医生实际工作能力与居民的要求还有距离，同时社区工作也是在逐渐摸索、完善过程中，因此社区卫生服务的工作开展仍不太理想。

解决的方法与思考

　　制定全科医学相关领域的政策和规划、社区卫生服务发展策略和相关人力资源政策，特别是推动全科医学毕业生致力于社区群众服务的激励机制等，促使全科医疗得到健康持续的发展。以全科医生岗位培训为重点，低年资的全科医生要进行专科轮转，至少3年，掌握专科学校的基本理论和基本技能；高年资的全科医生可通过远程教育，参加各省、市中心培训机构组织的临床技能培训，逐步提高技术水平。各省、市可以根据实际需要，增加一些社区工作急需的培训内容。对部分基础较好的医生进行重点培养，然后由这些合格的全科医生再去培养更多的全科医生，促进全科医生的全面提高，进而提高防治社区常见疾病解决社区健康问题的能力，达到全科医生的岗位要求。

↗ 写作解析

1. 分析中文原文

　　本文共有4段，话题突出，并有小标题，这对于考生梳理中文内容、提炼文章结构大有益处。本文话题围绕社区卫生服务中全科医生的培养以及发展思路展开，第一段为背景介绍，谈到社区卫生服务的主要功能、重要性以及全科医学、全科医生教育培养存在不足。第二段主要介绍全科医生的基本素质：知识全面、高度的工作热情以及良好的协调沟通能力。第三段阐述目前全科医生存在的问题及原因。第四段阐述解决方法与思考，既有政策调整又有岗位培训重点及方法。

2. 摘要的中文大纲

　　通过提炼、总结画线部分的内容，写作的中文提纲大致如下：

　　第一段：随着医疗卫生事业的不断发展，社区卫生服务日益重要，其主要功能包括医疗、保健、预防、护理、健康调查、咨询及健康教育等。然而我国全科医学教育培训还存在一些问题，缺乏高素质的全科医生，这些都制约着社区卫生服务的发展。因而规范全科医生培养、大力发展全科医生培训的工作势在必行。

　　第二段：谈到基本素质，全科医生首先需要知识全面。一些严重疾病的早期症状可能较为轻微，与一些常见多发疾病并无太大区别，这就要求全科医生能筛选出可能的情况。其次，作为社会工作者，全科医生需要与社区内居民长期接触，因而饱满的工作热情以及良好的协调沟通能力很必要。

　　第三段：然而，目前全科医生还存在诸多问题。收入与社会地位相对较低，工作环境艰苦，医疗设备较为落后，这导致全科医生工作热情不高。全科医学专业开展时间不长，全科医生实际能力还很欠缺。

　　第四段：为了使全科医疗健康持续发展，首先相关政策、规划的制定以及激励机制很必要。其次全科医学教育应以岗位培训为重点，低年资全科医生要进行至少3年的专科轮转，以掌握基本理论及技能；高年资全科医生可通过多种渠道（例如远程教育或培训班）进一步提高技术水平。对于部分基础较好的医生进行重点培养，再由他们培养更多的全科医生。

3. 供参考的表达

全科医生	general practitioner
全科医学	general family medicine
社区卫生服务	community health service
保健	healthcare
护理	nursing
健康调查	health survey
咨询	consultation
规范（培养）	standardized training
势在必行	imperative
知识全面	well-rounded
（工作）热情	enthusiasm
协调沟通能力	communication and coordination skills
激励机制	incentive mechanism
岗位培训	on-the-job training
低年资的	junior
高年资的	senior
专科轮转	rotation and training
远程教育	distance education

4. 参考范文

With the continuous development of health care, community health services are increasingly significant, which mainly include health care, sickness prevention, health survey, consultation and health education and so on. However, imperfect general practice education and lack of high-qualified general practitioners inevitably restrict the development of community health services. Thus, standardized training and vigorous devotion to general practice education are very imperative.

When it comes to basic qualities of general practitioners, well-rounded knowledge comes first. Some severe diseases tend to be characterized with mild symptoms which are similar with some common disorders. Therefore, general practitioners are required to identify possible cases. Moreover, as social workers, general practitioners are bound to constantly contact people in the community, and hence, enthusiasm in work as well as good communication and cooperation skills is crucial.

Unfortunately many problems arise currently. Unsatisfactory income, lower social status and tough working conditions lead to less devotion to the work. Besides, it has not been long since the major of general family medicine was established. General practitioners have not been equipped with adequate practical skills.

In order to enhance the sustainable development of community health care, firstly, related policies, projects and incentive mechanism are indispensable. Secondly, general practice education should put emphasis on on-the-job training. On the one hand, junior general practitioners are required to take rotation and training for three years at least, so as to master basic theories and skills. On the other hand, senior general practitioners could improve their skills through distance education or training programs. Some potential talents may be chosen as the very group to be trained, in the hope that they can further cultivate more qualified general practitioners.

No.9

2015 年真题

什么是健康

人的健康包括身体健康和心理健康两个方面。一个人的身体和心理都健康才称得上真正的健康。联合国世界卫生组织对健康下的定义是：健康的人不但没有身体疾患，而且有完整的生理、心理状态和社会适应能力。

日前在我们国家，无论在健康人与病人中或者在医务人员中，大都在不同程度上忽略了心理健康。这对提高人的健康水平与提高医疗效果都产生消极的影响。例如在现实生活中，人们往往重视营养，而忽视饮食时的心理因素作用。人们注意身体的锻炼，而不重视心理的锻炼。甚至不知道什么是心理健康以及如何锻炼。在临床实践中，有些医务人员在病因上，重视病毒、感染等因素，忽视疾病的心理因素的作用；在诊断上重视物理诊断等，忽视心理诊断；在治疗上重视药物治疗，忽视心理治疗。其实，身体健康与心理健康是同等重要的。二者是相互联系、相互制约的。身心两方面健康是相辅相成的。

随着 21 世纪的到来，人们更加专注自身的健康。追求长寿、健康生活已成为一种时尚。但是，如何才能健康，怎样才能长寿？健康与长寿的大敌又是什么呢？众多医学保健专家指出，介于疾病与健康之间的"第三状态"是人类健康与长寿的大敌。所谓第三状态，指人们经常感到自己身体难受不适的状态。主要表现为时常感觉身体很累，很疲倦，很想好好睡上一觉。此外，经常出现懒言、少气、食欲欠佳、对什么都不感兴趣，无精打采等症状，也就是人们常说的亚健康状态（sub-health condition）。如果说健康是人的第一状态，疾病是人的第二状态，那么亚健康则为人的第三状态。

有关调查表明，随着经济的高速发展，竞争日趋激烈，生活节奏逐渐加快，亚健康人群的增多已成为一种不可回避的现实。该人群以中年人居多，职业涉及很广。一般来讲，越是有成就，收入越高，亚健康状态的出现频率越高，如经理、秘书、管理人员等都是亚健康状态的高发职业。此外，记者、律师、医生、自由职业者出现亚健康状态的比例也比较高。

　　目前很"时髦"的"疲劳综合征"（exhaustion syndrome）就是亚健康状态的典型代表。疲劳综合不仅在发达国家有相当高的发病率，在发展中国家也不少见。这类疾病表面看来对人体并无多大妨碍，仅仅表现为生理功能低下，但其潜伏的危险性却不容忽视，因为疲劳综合征往往就是某些慢性病的先兆。比如大家所熟悉的高血压、心脑血管疾病、肿瘤等，很多都继发于疲劳综合征。

　　对于亚健康状态，目前国内、国外尚无特效治疗方法，而学会自我调节，对于缓解、纠正人体的亚健康状态非常重要。这里提醒您注意以下几点：一是学会以轻松的心态对待学习、工作和生活，尽量不要故意给自己加压；二是要吃好。所谓吃好，不是指大吃大喝、大鱼大肉，而是指根据自己的实际情况选择饮食；三是一定要睡好，早睡早起。睡上一个好觉，精力、体力就容易恢复。

（1098 个字）

➚ 写作解析

1.　分析中文原文

　　本文主题为亚健康，文章共分 6 段，各段的信息有重合，因而需要考生根据文章的主线重新整理细节信息，使得摘要的内容和结构清晰明了。本文的主线为：健康包括身体健康和心理健康，二者相辅相成，但在我国人们往往忽略心理健康。健康有三种状态，其中第三种状态亚健康是人们健康和长寿的大敌。亚健康的典型代表就是疲劳综合征，然后叙述其表现及危害，最后针对亚健康状态提出建议。

2.　摘要的中文大纲

　　通过提炼、总结画线部分的内容，写作的中文提纲大致如下：

　　第一段：人的健康包括身体健康和心理健康两个方面。按照世卫组织的定义，健康的人不但没有身体疾患，而且有完整的生理、心理状态和社会适应能力。然而在我国，无论在健康人与病人中或者在医务人员中，大都在不同程度上忽略心理健康。人们注意锻炼身体，而不重视心理锻炼。在临床实践中，有些医务工作者也忽略了致病的心理因素以及心理治疗。其实，身体健康与心理健康是同等重要的。二者是相互联系、相互制约的。

　　第二段：人们专注自身的健康，追求长寿，而正如众多医学保健专家指出的，介于疾病与健康之间的"第三状态"是人类健康与长寿的大敌。所谓第三状态也就是人们常说的亚健康状态，目前很"时髦"的"疲劳综合征"（exhaustion syndrome）就是亚健康状态的典型代表，其主要表现为时常感觉身体很疲倦。此外，经常出现懒言、少气、食欲欠佳、对什么都不感兴趣、无精打采等症状。有调查表明,亚健康人群以中年人居多,职业涉及很广,从管理人员、记者到医生。疲劳综合征潜伏的危险性不容忽视,因为疲劳综合征往往就是某些慢性病的先兆,比如高血压、心脑血管疾病、肿瘤等。

第三段:对于亚健康状态,虽然尚无特效治疗方法,但自我调节很重要。一是学会以轻松的心态对待学习、工作和生活,尽量不要故意给自己加压;二是要根据自己的实际情况选择饮食;三是一定要睡好,早睡早起。

3. 供参考的表达式

社会适应能力	social adaptability
心理锻炼	mental exercise
相互联系、制约	interrelated and mutually restricted
介于疾病和健康之间 / 亚健康	subhealth
疲劳综合征	exhaustion syndrome
食欲不佳	poor appetite
无精打采	listlessness
潜伏的危险性	potential risks
慢性病	chronic diseases
高血压	hypertension
心脑血管疾病	cardiovascular and cerebrovascular diseases
肿瘤	tumor
调节情绪	regulate mood
放松心态	relax

4. 参考范文

Health includes people's physical and mental health. WHO defines it as a state of complete physical, mental, and social well-being and not merely the absence of disease or infirmity. People, healthy or not, along with medical staff ignore the mental health to some extent. People tend to attach importance to physical exercise regardless of mental exercise. In clinical practice, some medical staff pay less attention to mental factors and psychological treatments. In fact, physical and mental health is equally significant, which are interrelated and mutually restricted.

People care about their own health and pursue longevity, however the "third state", being subhealthy, serves as the barrier to people's health. Exhaustion syndrome is the typical representative of such a state, which is characterized by fatigue, listlessness and poor appetite. It is reported that subhealthy people are mainly the middle-aged in a variety of professions ranging from administrators to doctors. Potential risks of exhaustion syndrome should not be ignored, which tend to trigger some chronic diseases, such as hypertension, cardiovascular and cerebrovascular diseases and even cancers.

Although there have not been effective treatments towards subhealth, self-regulation would work. First we should be positive towards our study, work and life and try not to impose much pressure on ourselves. Additionally, we'd better choose proper diet and have a sound sleep. Keeping early hours is recommended.

（222 words）

三、评卷人掌握的评分原则

1. 摘要或短文写作的评分原则

总体评分法（global scoring）：通过"内容 + 语言"确定考生作文的基本分数段，再酌情加减分数。

2. 摘要或短文写作的评分标准

20~17 分	文章切题，体裁正确，文笔流畅，完全没有或仅有个别语法或用词错误
16~13 分	文章基本切题，体裁基本符合要求，文笔较流畅，但有数处一般性语法和用词错误
12~9 分	文章大体切题，体裁大体符合要求，文章虽不很流畅但能令人理解其意思，有数处重大语法或用词错误
8~5 分	词数达不到要求，文章尚能切题，体裁不符合要求，句子结构较单调和松散，有多处重大语法和用词错误，但文章尚能表达一些意思
4~1 分	仅写出若干句子符合题意，语法用词和拼写错误较多，表现缺乏写作能力
0 分	仅写几个与题意无关的句子，或虽写几句而错误比比皆是，或根本一句未写，表现无写作能力

3. 解释评分标准

- 词数：要求 200 左右，即左右浮动 20，不可词数太少过于明显（词数偏少体现写作能力不强）。
- 切题：要点要全，否则扣分；不可增加个人看法（摘要）。
- 文笔流畅：体现在用词恰当，句句相扣，段段相扣。
- 错误：重大错误是指句法结构或主谓结构相关的错误，如语序、时态语态等；词性错误、用词错误；拼写错误个别不作扣分主要依据，但多次出现错误就要扣分了。

四、近十年医博摘要写作汇总

年份	中文标题	英文标题
2012	电脑、网络与健康	Computer, Internet and Health
2013	健康处方帮你走出"第三状态"	Health Prescription Gets You Out of the Third State
2014	学会呼吸能长寿	Learn to Breathe, Get Longevity
2015	什么是健康	What is Health?

（续）

年份	中文标题	英文标题
2016	全科医生培养及发展思路	Ideas of Training and Cultivating General Practitioners
2017	环境污染与肺癌	Environment Pollution and Lung Cancer
2018	未来医学发展趋势	Future Medical Development Trend
2019	我国食品安全的现状、问题及对策	The Current Situation, Problems and Countermeasures of Food Safety in China
2020	抗生素的滥用	The Abuse of Antibiotics
2021	健康中国的三层含义	Three Meanings of Healthy China

从近十年的写作命题中可看出，中文文章有以下特点：

1. 无论是宏观层面的环境问题，还是微观层面的饮食习惯，中文题材都是与大健康有关的。因此在进行话题和背景知识准备的时候，最后落脚处均可以落到群体或是个体的健康问题。

2. 从结构上看，中文段落结构清晰。小标题时有时无。每一段内部有主题，有论点，有论据。在备考时需要准确辨识论点和论据，才好在英文摘要的写作中做到详略得当。

五、写作中存在的问题及对策

针对历年考生在医学博士英语统考中写作测试部分出现的错误分析，我们将考生常出现的问题归纳如下，希望考生能引起重视：

1. 不是写摘要，而是将中文文章翻译为英文；
2. 错误较多，如拼写、搭配等；
3. 中式英文现象严重；
4. 语法错误频繁出现；
5. 文章结构不紧凑，凌乱不堪；
6. 常用词汇积累不够，导致文章关键词无法体现；
7. 试图使用长难句，但语句结构混乱；
8. 字迹潦草，辨认不清。

针对以上罗列的问题，希望考生在备考阶段在如下方面多加训练和积累：

1. 平时要注意中文篇章大意的凝练，这是医学博士考试摘要写作的第一道坎，每年很多考生不是栽在英文上，而是栽在母语中文上，所以考生如果这个步骤还有较大问题，分不清主次，不能提炼出文章的关键信息，就一定要多下功夫。

2. 一定要用笔纸实际进行写作，切忌用在电脑上完成写作。众所周知，电脑有语法和拼写纠错功能，这样使得考生自己不能意识到错误的存在，而是依赖电脑的提醒。

3. 鉴于医学博士英语统考的作文部分测试题材以大众医学科普知识和社会医学问题，例如健康与生活方式类、常见病类以及医疗体制，考生在备考阶段应加强医学相关文章的阅读以及表达式的积累，以免考试时有想法，但没有相应的表达式支持，最终导致自己随意创造。在练习阶段，写作不是一个根据个人喜好创作的过程，一定要注意模仿别人的写作结构、表达式等，必要的积累必不可少！待自己的"语料库"相当丰满的时候，才能够做到把自己的想法流畅地表达出来，故希望考生更多地关注积累、使用、替换：即积累新的，使用新的，替换旧的！积累的途径可以是阅读的任何英文文章。

4. 在平时写作中，针对文章出现的错误要引起重视，及时查漏补缺，认真改正。

5. 在平时写作训练中，要按照写作流程进行构思和写作，养成良好的写作习惯。

6. 考生要熟悉基本的英文写作结构模式，以利于文章结构一目了然。一般说来，各段的主题句（topic sentence）放在段落之首，用以概括段落大意，使得全段其他文字都围绕它展开。而各段的主题句正是文章结构框架的重要体现，它们要围绕文章的中心思想展开。

7. 写作时间分配建议

1）5~10分钟：认真阅读中文原文，大致把握文章的内容。

2）5分钟：对中文文章进行提炼，划出各段主题句以及关键的细节内容。

3）5~10分钟：根据在各段划出的主题句和关键细节内容，组织英文摘要的各主要部分及内容，符合英文的写作结构，即：

- 文章的中心思想（main idea）
- 每段的主题句（topic sentence）
- 每段的扩展句（support sentences）
- 结论句（conclusion）

4）20分钟：根据确定的英文摘要的大纲写摘要。

5）5分钟：检查要点是否齐全、语法有无错误、意思表达是否清楚、拼写有无错误等。

六、写作常用词语和句子

1. 开头句型

1）As far as...is concerned 就……而言

2）It goes without saying that... 不言而喻

3）It can be said with certainty that... 可以很肯定地说

4）As the proverb says 正如谚语所说

5）It has to be noticed that... 必须注意的是

6）It's generally recognized that... 人们普遍认识到

7）It's likely that 很可能

8）It's hardly too much to say that... 几乎不用说太多的是

9）What calls for special attention is that 需要特别关注的是

10）There's no denying the fact that... 无可否认的是

11）Nothing is more important than the fact that... 没有什么比这个事实更重要

12）What's far more important is that... 更为重要的是

2. 衔接句型

1） A case in point is… 举个恰当的例子

2） As is often the case… ……是常有的事

3） As stated in the previous paragraph 如前段所述

4） But the problem is not so simple. Therefore… 然而问题并非如此简单，所以……

5） But it's a pity that… 但是遗憾的是……

6） For all that…In spite of the fact that… 是因为……尽管事实是……

7） Further, we hold opinion that… 更进一步，我们的观点是……

8） However , the difficulty lies in… 然而，困难在于……

9） Similarly, we should pay attention to… 同样，我们应该注意……

10） not (that) …but (that) … 不是……，而是……

11） In view of the present situation 鉴于目前形势

12） As has been mentioned above… 正如前述

13） In this respect, we many as well (say) 从这个角度上，我们可以说

14） However, we have to look at the other side of the coin, that is… 然而，我们还得看到事物的另一方面，即……

15） equally important 同样重要的是

3. 结尾句型

1） I will conclude by saying… 总结说来

2） Therefore, we have the reason to believe that… 因而，我们有理由相信……

3） All things considered 总而言之

4） It may be safely said that… 可以放心地说

5） Therefore, in my opinion, it's more advisable… 因而，按照我的观点，……更明智

6） It can be concluded from the discussion that… 从中我们可以得出这样的结论……

7） From my point of view, it would be better if… 在我看来……也许更好

8） in the long run 从长远来看

9） consequently; in conclusion; in short; in summary 结果；总结说来；简而言之

10） It's high time that strict measures were taken to stop… 该是采取严格措施制止……的时候了

11） Taking all these into account, we… 考虑到所有这些，我们……

4. 常见病医学词汇

癌症	cancer
肺癌	lung cancer
肝癌	liver cancer
宫颈癌	cervical cancer

皮肤癌	skin cancer
乳腺癌	breast cancer
胃癌	stomach cancer
心血管疾病	cardiovascular diseases
心脏病发作	heart attack
冠心病	coronary disease
骨质疏松症	osteoporosis
关节炎	arthritis
皮肤病	skin diseases
带状疱疹	zoster
疹子	rash
湿疹	eczema
痘	pox
荨麻疹	hives
静脉曲张	varix
天花	variola
中风	stroke
肺结核	tuberculosis
溃疡	ulcer
气管炎	tracheitis
扁桃体炎	tonsillitis
糖尿病	diabetes
糖尿病人	diabetic
狂犬病	rabies
高血压	hypertension; high blood pressure
低血压	hypotension
肝炎	hepatitis
肥胖症	obesity
血管的	vascular
肿瘤	tumor
血栓	thrombus
脑梗死	cerebral infarction
急性的	acute
慢性的	chronic
胰岛素	insulin
脂肪肝	fatty liver

5. 常见症状英语词汇

发痒的	itchy
超重	overweight
症状	symptom
呕吐	vomit; bring up
眩晕的	dizzy (n. dizziness)
消化不良	indigestion
体重下降	lose weight
反胃	nausea
失眠症	insomnia
紊乱	disorder
气短	short breath
倦怠	listless
抗生素	antibiotics
胆固醇	cholesterol
流鼻涕	runny noses
嗓子痛	sore throats
头疼	headache
昏昏欲睡	drowsy
心不在焉	absent-minded

6. 常用治疗英语词汇及其他

疫苗	vaccine
移植器官	transplant organs
疗法	therapy
物理治疗	physiotherapy
化疗	chemotherapy
临床的	clinical
流行病学	epidemiology
诊断	diagnosis (v. diagnose)
副作用	side effect
缩短寿命	shorten lifespan
夺人生命	claim
蛋白质	protein
止痛药	painkiller
维生素	vitamin
发病	incidence

七、写作专项练习与解析

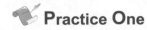 **Practice One**

大健康时代的新思维

人类已进入老龄化社会，拥有长寿的同时也面临着慢性病的威胁。不同于外来病原体引发的传染病，慢性病是机体内部出现问题而导致的，病因复杂多变。更麻烦的是，慢性病表现出明显的个体差异，甚至个体内的异质性。因此，不能简单地停留在"看病"，而是要"看人"。慢性病的发生需要时间，通常是从健康状态逐渐演化成为疾病状态。因此，要利用发病之前的"窗口期"，将抗击疾病的"关口前移"，早期监测和早期干预，实行对生命全周期的健康管理和维护。在卫生领域里，从"疾病"到"健康"。

中国当前进入了一个"大健康"时代。2016年，中国政府召开了第一次全国卫生与健康大会，并在会上提出了建设健康中国的目标——为人民群众提供全生命周期的卫生与健康服务。要注意到"全生命周期"这个词的提出，即维护人民健康的任务不再像过去那样，把医疗卫生服务的重点放在疾病的诊断和治疗方面。这种新观点在国家发布的《健康中国2030规划纲要》里表述地更为清楚："加快转变健康领域发展方式，全方位、全周期维护和保障人民健康"，"实现从胎儿到生命终点的全程健康服务和健康保障"。这个转变的关键点就是要将抗击疾病的"关口前移"，实行"健康优先"。这一点充分反映在《健康中国2030规划纲要》提出的第一个原则："把健康摆在优先发展的战略地位，立足国情，将促进健康的理念融入公共政策制定实施的全过程，加快形成有利于健康的生活方式、生态环境和经济社会发展模式，实现健康与经济社会良性协调发展"。

慢性病的形成是一个由健康状态逐渐向疾病状态转换的过程，在出现临床症状之前，会先出现亚健康状态或前疾病状态等各种过渡态。显然，这样一个发病前的亚健康"窗口期"给人们提供了抗击慢性病的重要机会。人们不应像过去那样，等到疾病出现了才去诊断和治疗。中医有一个经典的说法，叫"上医治未病"，就是说高明的医生在疾病发生之前就已经察觉，就要进行干预了。这个传统观点与今天提出的要把抗击疾病的关口前移的理念非常一致。

抗击慢性病的关口前移，不仅从防治疾病的角度来说是"上策"，而且从社会经济的角度来看，也同样是"上策"。大部分慢性病一旦进入临床阶段，常常就是难以治愈，需要终身服药；更麻烦的是，这些慢性病的预后往往很差，其发展期或并发症危害大，疾病后期的致死致残率高。因此，慢性病的治疗往往"性价比"很低，投入多，获益少。而"关口前移"的策略则能够明显提升抗击慢性病的"性价比"。一个流行的观点是，政府和社会在慢性病预防方面投入一块钱，相当于在治疗方面投入六块钱。

从个体的角度来看，也可以得到同样的结论。不妨把享受生活视为"产出"，把健康的维护作为"投入"，进行一下"投入产出比"分析：当我们身体处于健康状态的时候，维护健康的投入不多，并可以尽情地享受生活，所以"投入产出比"非常理想；一旦得了慢性病，例如糖尿病，维护健康的投入就明显增加了，要去看病吃药，而生活上也有了各种限制，比如饮食要有所控制，"投入产出比"明显变差；如果疾病继续发展，例如糖尿病并发症出现，更多的费用投入到治疗中，生活质量变得更差，如糖尿病眼病会导致失明；这时在个体健康方面的"投入产出比"就可想而知该有多糟。所以，不论是对国家与社会，还是对家庭和个人来说，把抗击慢性病的"战场"移至医院之外，都是一个更为经济合理的选择。

到了 21 世纪，人类进入了一个全新的"大健康时代"。对人类健康的主要威胁已经从传染病转变为慢性病，"关口前移"和"健康优先"是抗击慢性病更为合理、更为经济的策略。因此，在这样一个全新的健康医学时代，关键词应该改为"健康"。围绕着"健康"，我们需要发展出能够对机体病理变化进行早期监测的新技术，发展出能够维护健康和预防疾病的早期干预方法，建立起对个体全生命周期进行健康管理的社区系统，创造出能够支撑全社会以及个体对健康维护费用需求的健康保障系统。

↗ 写作解析

1. 分析中文原文

本文的中心思想是：随着老龄化社会的到来，人类进入全新的"大健康时代"，卫生领域也应从"疾病"转向"健康"。每段的大意如下：

第一段：人类进入老龄化社会，面临慢性病的威胁，应该全方位转变防治思维。

第二段：中国进入"大健康"时代，健康领域发展方式转变的关键点在于从"治病"到"健康"。

第三段：慢性病的治疗思想。

第四、五段：抗击慢性病的关口前移，对社会经济也是有利的。

第六段：总结，大健康时代的新观念。

2. 摘要的中文大纲

第一段：人类已进入老龄化社会，拥有长寿的同时也面临着慢性病的威胁。治疗慢性病，不仅要看病，更要看人，将抗击疾病的"关口前移"，在卫生领域里，从"疾病"转移到"健康"。

第二段：中国当前进入了一个"大健康"时代，要注意到"全生命周期"这个词的提出，即维护人民健康的任务不再像过去那样，把医疗卫生服务的重点放在疾病的诊断和治疗方面。这个转变的关键点就是要将抗击疾病的"关口前移"，实行"健康优先"。慢性病的形成是一个由健康状态逐渐向疾病状态转换的过程。中医有一个经典的说法，叫"上医治未病"，就是说高明的医生在疾病发生之前就已经察觉，就要进行干预了。这个传统观点与今天提出要把抗击疾病的关口前移的理念非常一致。

第三段：抗击慢性病的关口前移，不仅从防治疾病的角度来说是"上策"，而且从社会经济的角度来看，也同样是"上策"。从个体的角度来看，也可以得到同样的结论。

第四段：在这样一个全新的健康医学时代，关键词应该改为"健康"。围绕着"健康"，我们需要发展出能够对机体病理变化进行早期监测的新技术，发展出能够维护健康和预防疾病的早期干预方法，建立起对个体全生命周期进行健康管理的社区系统，创造出能够支撑全社会以及个体对健康维护费用需求的健康保障系统。

3. **供参考的表达方式**

老龄化社会	aging society
长寿	longevity
慢性病	chronic disease
生命全周期	full life circle
防治疾病	disease prevention and treatment
大健康时代	era of big health

4. **参考范文**

New Thinking in the Era of Big Health

Human beings have entered an aging society. Chronic diseases come along with longevity. To deal with the new situation, the key point in the health field is from "disease" to "health".

The formation of chronic diseases is a process of transition from a healthy state to a disease state. The critical point is to fight against diseases before they occur. Therefore it is important to note that in the new era of Big Health, the task of health care is no longer the diagnosis and treatment of diseases but the "health priority" strategy.

To deal with chronic diseases at the early stage is a "top policy" not only from the perspective of disease prevention and treatment, but also in the light of socio-economic way. It is a more economical and reasonable choice to move the "battlefield" outside the hospital, for the country and society, and for families and individuals.

To conclude, the focus is "health". Around this call, we need to develop new technologies that can detect early pathological changes in the body, develop early intervention methods that can maintain health and prevent diseases, and establish a community system that manages the health of individuals throughout their life cycle. A health protection system that supports the entire society and the individual's need for health maintenance should be accomplished.

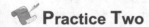 **Practice Two**

关于流感

流行性感冒（以下简称流感）是由流感病毒引起的一种急性呼吸道传染病，在世界范围内引起爆发和流行。

流感起病急，虽然大多为自限性，但部分因出现肺炎等并发症可发展至重症流感，少数重症病例病情进展快，可因急性呼吸窘迫综合征（ARDS）和／或多脏器衰竭而死亡。重症流感主要发生在老年人、年幼儿童、孕产妇或有慢性基础疾病者等高危人群，亦可发生在一般人群。

流感患者和隐性感染者是流感的主要传染源。从潜伏期末到急性期都有传染性。受感染动物也可成为传染源，人感染来源动物的流感病例在近距离密切接触可发生有限传播。流感主要通过打喷嚏和咳嗽等飞沫传播，也可经口腔、鼻腔、眼睛等黏膜直接或间接接触传播。接触被病毒污染的物品也可引起感染。人感染禽流感主要是通过直接接触受感染的动物或受污染的环境而获得。人群普遍易感。

医生建议，如有症状应及时就医，先进行诊断，鉴别普通感冒、其他类型上呼吸道感染或下呼吸道感染，根据临床特征可做出初步判断，病原学检查可资确诊，对临床诊断病例和确诊病例应尽早隔离治疗、中西医对症治疗。

尽管流感来势凶猛，但也并非不可预防。一般来讲，预防手段分为以下几种：

（一）疫苗接种

接种流感疫苗是预防流感最有效的手段，可以显著降低接种者罹患流感和发生严重并发症的风险。推荐老年人、儿童、孕妇、慢性病患者和医务人员等流感高危人群，应该每年优先接种流感疫苗。

（二）药物预防

药物预防不能代替疫苗接种，只能作为没有接种疫苗或接种疫苗后尚未获得免疫能力的重症流感高危人群的紧急临时预防措施。可使用奥司他韦、扎那米韦等。

（三）一般预防措施

保持良好的个人卫生习惯是预防流感等呼吸道传染病的重要手段，主要措施包括：增强体质和免疫力；勤洗手；保持环境清洁和通风；尽量减少到人群密集场所活动，避免接触呼吸道感染患者；保持良好的呼吸道卫生习惯，咳嗽或打喷嚏时，用纸巾或毛巾等遮住口鼻，咳嗽或打喷嚏后洗手，尽量避免触摸眼睛、鼻或口；出现呼吸道感染症状后应居家休息，及早就医。

↗ 写作解析

1. **分析中文原文**

本文的中心思想是，随着流感高峰期的到来，人们应该培养良好的卫生习惯，随时观察症状，随时就医，尽早防治。每段的大意如下：

第一、二段：流感的起因及常见发病人群。

第三段：流感的主要传染源。

第四段至文末：如何预防流感。

2. **摘要的中文大纲**

第一段：流行性感冒（以下简称流感）是由流感病毒引起的一种急性呼吸道传染病，在世界范围内引起爆发和流行。

第二段：重症流感主要发生在老年人、年幼儿童、孕产妇或有慢性基础疾病者等高危人群，亦可发生在一般人群。

第三段：流感患者和隐性感染者是流感的主要传染源。

第四段：医生建议，如有症状应及时就医，预防手段有疫苗接种和药物预防。另外保持良好的个人卫生习惯是预防流感等呼吸道传染病的重要手段。

3. 供参考的表达方式

流感	flu/influenza
病毒	virus
爆发	break out/outbreak
流行	epidemic
并发症	complications
症状	symptom
疫苗接种	vaccination
药物预防	drug prevention
一般预防措施	common prevention
通风	ventilation

4. 参考范文

Influenza is an acute respiratory disease caused by the flu virus, causing outbreak and epidemic in the world.

Some flu may develop to severe cases due to complications, a few of which could progress rapidly. Almost all the people have the possibility to be attacked by severe flu through high-risk groups account for higher potential.

Flu patients and latent infections are the major source of infection, as well as the infected animals can also become the source. Flu mainly spreads not only through sneezing and cough droplets, but also by the oral cavity, nasal cavity, eyes and other mucosal contact, and exposure to contaminated items can also cause infection. Human infection with bird flu is mainly through direct contact with infected animals or contaminated environment. People are generally susceptible.

Doctors suggest that if symptoms show up, you should seek timely medical treatment and diagnosis. Isolation and symptomatic treatment should be done to the clinical diagnosis and confirmed cases without any delay.

Although the flu is fierce, it is not always unpredictable. Vaccination and drug prevention are main preventive measures. Maintaining good personal hygiene is an important means, for example, enhancing physical fitness and immunity; washing hands frequently; keeping the environment clean and well ventilated and so on.

Practice Three

一说心脏病这个话题就有点沉重，据世界心脏联盟预计，2025 年前，在全世界范围内，25 岁以上的成年人中，每 3 人就有 1 人将罹患心血管疾病。心血管疾病的死亡率远远高于包括癌症、艾滋病在内的其他疾病，堪称威胁人类健康的"第一杀手"。在中国，每年大约有 260 万人死于心脑血管疾病。在专家看来，目前预防心脏病意识提高的主要集中在老年人，在过去 15 年里，中国 35 岁至 44 岁年龄组患冠心病的人数增长了 150%，心脏病发病正在年轻化，发病风险最高的是 40 岁至 50 岁的人群。9 月 28 日是世界心脏日，而高血压、糖尿病、肥胖都已成为引发心脏病的潜伏杀手。今年世界心脏病日活动主题也因此命名为 "了解您的危险因素"，目的是敦促人们了解威胁自己心脏健康的危险因素。

许多医学专家指出，要想拥有健康的心脏，必须了解并远离形成心血管疾病的危险因素。目前得到公认的冠心病危险因素包括两方面。一是依据现有的医疗水平认为不能控制的，如年龄和遗传因素。二是目前医疗手段可以控制的，如吸烟、肥胖、高血压、血脂异常、高血糖等。胡吃乱喝、不运动是导致慢性非传染性疾病患病率上升的主要原因。这其中，城市居民禽肉类及油脂消费过多，谷类食物消费偏低。除此以外，现代人的不健康生活方式也是威胁人们健康的杀手之一，如吸烟酗酒、经常熬夜、不合理营养、长期不运动、紧张压抑等。"总有人会说工作太忙、应酬太多、竞争太激烈，导致自己不能有健康的生活方式，但我说，健康是一颗空心玻璃球，一旦掉下去就会粉碎；工作只是一个皮球，掉下去后还能再弹起来。"中华医学会会长、中国工程院院士钟南山在接受记者采访时说。钟南山强调，快节奏、高强度的工作，抽烟、酗酒、经常熬夜吃夜宵、饮食不合理、长期不运动等不健康的生活方式，使越来越多的都市人处于亚健康的灰色地带，"都市人患病 70% 是不合理的生活方式所致"。

那么，我们应该如何预防心血管疾病呢？我们首先要从健康的生活方式做起。①合理安排饮食，避免肥胖和超重。每天进食的总热量不能过高，一般要求的 60 岁以上老年人，男性 2000~2500 千卡，女性 1700~2100 千卡；70 岁以上老年人，男性 1800~2000 千卡，女性 1600~1800 千卡；80 岁以上老年人，男性 1600 千卡，女性为 1400 千卡。应选择低脂肪、低胆固醇、富含维生素的食物，限制含糖食物的摄入。应以蔬菜类、粗粮、水果为主，可常食富含钙、钾、碘、铬、钴的食物，因它具有降血压、保护心脏，减少冠心病发病率的良好作用，如牛奶、虾皮、黄豆、核桃、蒜苗、鲜雪里蕻等。所食油类应尽量用花生油、棉籽油、豆油、菜籽油、玉米油等植物性油类。②保持血压正常，若出现高血压，应积极采取措施，包括药物及非药物措施，使血压降至正常范围。③参加一定量的体育锻炼，促进机体新陈代谢，消耗过多的脂肪，防止肥胖，又可增强心血管系统的调节功能，防止冠心病的发生与发作，如慢跑、散步、练气功、游泳等。④戒烟。香烟中含有大量有害物质随烟雾被吸入肺内，进而进入血液中，通过作用于心脏、血管、神经系统，从而导致动脉硬化及冠心病的发生。⑤生活起居要有规律，保证充足睡眠，保持心情愉快，避免情绪激动。

保护心脏不分早晚、不分年龄大小，改善生活方式和饮食习惯越早越有益。为拥有健康的心脏，应从现在做起。

（1295 字）

↗ 写作解析

1. 分析中文原文

本文的中心思想是远离危险因素，拥有健康的心脏。而且文章结构清晰，易于考生提炼完成英文摘要的提纲。每段的大意如下：

第一段：心血管疾病已成为人类健康头号杀手，今年世界心脏病日活动主题目的是敦促人们了解威胁心脏健康的因素。

第二段：威胁心脏健康的因素。

第三段：如何预防心血管疾病。

第四段：总结。

2. **摘要的中文大纲**

第一部分（第1段）：据估计，2025年前，在全世界范围内，25岁以上的成年人中，每3人就有1人将罹患心血管疾病。心血管疾病的死亡率远远高于包括癌症、艾滋病在内的其他疾病，堪称威胁人类健康的"第一杀手"。在中国，每年大约有260万人死于心脑血管疾病。9月28日是世界心脏日，而高血压、糖尿病、肥胖都已成为引发心脏病的潜伏杀手。

第二部分（第2段）：目前得到公认的冠心病危险因素包括两方面。一是依据现有的医疗水平认为不能控制的，如年龄和遗传因素。二是目前医疗手段可以控制的，如吸烟、肥胖、高血压、血脂异常、高血糖等。胡吃乱喝、不运动是导致慢性非传染性疾病患病率上升的主要原因。除此以外，现代人的不健康生活方式也是威胁人们健康的杀手之一，如吸烟酗酒、经常熬夜、不合理营养、长期不运动、紧张压抑等，这些会使越来越多的人处于亚健康的灰色地带。

第三部分（第3~4段）：为了预防心血管疾病，我们首先要从健康的生活方式做起。①合理安排饮食，避免肥胖和超重。②保持血压正常。③参加一定量的体育锻炼，促进机体新陈代谢，如慢跑、散步、练气功、游泳等。④戒烟。⑤生活起居要有规律，保证充足睡眠，保持心情愉快，避免情绪激动。

3. **供参考的表达式**

心血管疾病	cardiovascular disease
死亡率	mortality
肥胖	obesity
潜伏杀手	invisible killer
遗传因素	hereditary factors
血脂异常	dyslipidemia
高血糖	high blood glucose
不合理营养	unbalanced diet
长期不运动	inactive; sedentary
压抑	depression
新陈代谢	metabolism
充足睡眠	adequate sleep
愉快心情	cheerful mood

4. **参考范文**

It is estimated that one in three adults aged above 25 will have developed cardiovascular diseases by the end of 2025. Thus cardiovascular mortality is much higher than the mortality of other diseases including cancers and AIDS. Up to now, heart diseases have become the top killer, claiming 2.6 million deaths annually in China.

In terms of risks of heart diseases, it is acknowledged that there are two aspects: one aspect contains some uncontrollable factors, such as age and hereditary factors; the other aspect involves some controllable risks, for instance smoking, obesity and high blood pressure. In addition, unhealthy lifestyle is another potential risk: unbalanced diet, lack of physical exercise, pressure and depression, which result in sub-health.

In order to prevent heart disease, we had better start with healthy lifestyle. Firstly, have a well balanced diet and avoid obesity and overweight. In order to control the total amount of calories we take in, low-fat, low-cholesterol and high-fiber food are recommended, such as vegetables, fruit and cereals. Secondly, regular and moderate physical exercise, such as jogging, swimming, can promote metabolism, prevent overweight and lower the incidence of heart attack. Thirdly, stop smoking. Last but not least, healthy living habits are equally significant. Adequate sleep and cheerful mood are beneficial too.

（212 words）

 Practice Four

很多人不重视早餐，常常是随便凑合一下或者干脆不吃。其实早餐对保障人体健康、维持体能、提高学习和工作效率有着至关重要的作用。不仅如此，专家还认为，应该根据人的不同年龄和体质状况，科学合理地搭配早膳，以满足人体健康的需要。

幼儿的早餐 幼儿正值生长发育的旺盛时期，应当注重补充丰富的蛋白质和钙(calcium)，尽量少吃含糖较高的食物，以免引起龋齿（ decayed tooth ）和肥胖。如果在条件许可的情况下，幼儿的早餐通常以适量的牛奶、鸡蛋和面包为佳。当然，也可以用果汁或粥来代替牛奶，或者用饼干、馒头代替面包。

青少年的早餐 青少年时期身体发育较快，是肌肉和骨骼生长的重要时期，需要足够的钙、维生素 C、维生素 A 等营养成分，尤其是要保证充足的热量供应。青少年比较合理的早餐是一杯牛奶、适量的新鲜水果或蔬菜、100 克干点（面包、馒头、大饼或饼干等含碳水化合物（ carbohydrate ）较高的食品）。所含的热量要充分满足青少年脑力活动与体力活动的需要。

中年人的早餐 人到中年，肩挑工作、家务两副重担，身心的负荷相当重，加上中年时期组织器官的功能和生理功能日渐减退，其体力和精力都不如青少年。为了减缓中年人衰退的过程，推迟"老年期"的到来，除了要保持乐观的思想情绪和进行必要的体育锻炼之外，合理地搭配膳食也非常重要。中年人的饮食，既要含有丰富的蛋白质、维生素、钙、磷（ phosphorus ）等，还应保证低热量、低脂肪并适当地控制碳水化合物的摄入量。中年人较理想的早餐是：鸡蛋、豆浆或粥、干点（馒头、大饼、饼干和面包均可）和适量的蔬菜。

老年人的早餐 老年人的新陈代谢（ metabolism ）已经明显衰退，但必需的营养成分不能减少，尤其是要保证钙的供应，以防止老年人的骨质疏松（ osteoporosis ）。老年人的早餐除了供应牛奶和豆浆以外，还可多吃粥、面条、肉松和花生酱等既容易消化、又含有丰富营养的食物。除此之外，老年人的早餐应注意少吃油炸类食品。因为这类食物脂肪含量高，胃肠一般难以承受，容易出现消化不良，并易诱发胆、胰疾患，或使这类疾病复发、加重。多次使用的油里往往含有较多的致癌物质，如果常吃油炸的食品，可增加患癌症的危险。老年人还要少吃甜食，因为多余的糖在体内转化为脂肪，容易引起无机盐缺乏。动物内脏类如肝、肾、脑等胆固醇（cholesterol）含量甚高，老年人如经常食用，会使血中胆固醇增高，从而容易引发冠心病、肝病、动脉硬化、高血压等心脑血管疾病，或使原有的疾病加重。

（953 字）

↗ 写作解析

1. 分析中文原文

本文因为有副标题，故文章结构清晰，要点明确。各段大意如下：

第一段：早餐很重要。

第二段：幼儿的早餐。

第三段：青少年的早餐。

第四段：中年人的早餐。

第五段：老年人的早餐。

2. 摘要的中文大纲

第一部分（第 1 段）：很多人不重视早餐，甚至不吃早餐。其实早餐对保障人体健康、维持体能、提高学习和工作效率有着至关重要的作用。不仅如此，专家还认为，应该根据人的不同年龄和体质状况，科学合理地搭配早膳，以满足人体健康的需要。

第二部分（第 2 段）：幼儿的早餐 幼儿处于生长快速阶段，应当注重补充丰富的蛋白质和钙（calcium），尽量少吃含糖较高的食物，以免引起龋齿（decayed tooth）和肥胖。幼儿的早餐通常以适量的牛奶、鸡蛋和面包为佳。当然，也可以用果汁或粥来代替牛奶，或者用饼干、馒头代替面包。

第三部分（第 3 段）：青少年的早餐 青少年时期身体发育较快，是肌肉和骨骼生长的重要时期，需要足够的钙、维生素 C、维生素 A 等营养成分，尤其是要保证充足的热量供应。青少年比较合理的早餐是一杯牛奶、适量的新鲜水果或蔬菜、100 克干点（面包、馒头、大饼或饼干等含碳水化合物（carbohydrate）较高的食品）。

第四部分（第 4 段）：中年人的早餐 为了减缓中年人衰退的过程，中年人的饮食，既要含有丰富的蛋白质、维生素、钙、磷（phosphorus）等．还应保证低热量、低脂肪并适当地控制碳水化合物的摄入量。中年人较理想的早餐是：鸡蛋、豆浆或粥、干点（馒头、大饼、饼干和面包均可）和适量的蔬菜。

第五部分（第 5 段）：老年人的早餐 老年人的新陈代谢（metabolism）已经明显衰退，但必需的营养成分不能减少，尤其是要保证钙的供应，以防止老年人的骨质疏松（osteoporosis）。老年人的早餐除了供应牛奶和豆浆以外，还可多吃粥、面条、肉松和花生酱等既容易消化、又含有丰富营养的食物。除此之外，老年人的早餐应注意少吃油炸类食品。因为这类食物脂肪含量高，肠胃一般难以承受，容易出现消化不良。老年人还要少吃甜食，动物内脏类如肝、肾、脑等。

3. **供参考的表达式**

不吃早餐	skip breakfast
补充	supplement
蛋白质	protein
钙	calcium
青少年	adolescent
碳水化合物	carbohydrate
粥	porridge
消化	digest

4. **参考范文**

Many people tend not to attach importance to breakfast, and even skip breakfast. Actually breakfast plays vital roles in people's health and their efficiency in work and study. Proper breakfast should be based on their physical conditions and age.

Infants are in the stage of rapid growth, so they should consume plenty of protein and calcium and intake less high-sugar food to avoid decayed teeth and obesity. Milk, eggs and bread are optimal food for breakfast.

Adolescence is a critical period for the growth of muscles and bones. Adequate calcium, Vitamin C and Vitamin A are necessarily required. Milk, fresh fruit and vegetable along with food with carbohydrate can meet the requirement of mental and physical activities.

Due to the age, many middle-aged people suffer from decline in organ function and they have less energy than before. In this case, food for breakfast should be high in protein, vitamin, calcium and phosphorus and they should control the intake of carbohydrate properly. It is suggested that they have eggs, soybean milk, porridge together with bread and vegetable for breakfast.

Old people's metabolism has declined greatly but the adequate nutrients should not be reduced, especially the supply of calcium, in order to prevent osteoporosis. In addition to milk, soybean milk or food easily digested are recommended, such as porridge, noodles.

(219 words)

Practice Five

抑郁症是精神疾病中危害人群最大的一种精神疾病。目前有 1.21 亿人患有抑郁症，该病患病人群仍在不断增加。患抑郁症的人通常会感到异常忧伤、觉得人生毫无价值、对原本感兴趣的活动失去兴趣、精力丧失、疲劳无力、消极悲观、烦躁、甚至会产生自杀的念头。身体症状一般表现在：食欲减退、体重减轻和睡眠障碍。食欲减退、体重减轻：多数病人都有食欲不振，胃口差的症状，美味佳肴不再具有诱惑力，病人不思茶饭或食之无味，常伴有体重减轻。

睡眠障碍：典型的睡眠障碍是早醒，比平时早 2~3 小时，醒后不复入睡，陷入悲哀气氛中。

那么什么样的人容易患上抑郁症呢？ 追求十全十美的人。这类人因为要求自己所做的每一件事都完美无缺，所以把全部精力都放在事物上，从另一个角度而言，即有很强的占有欲、控制欲，在临床上常称这些人具有强迫倾向。过分追求完美的人在某些事情未完成时，就会产生相当强烈的焦虑感，觉得浑身不对劲，所以，不论在任何情况下，他都必须今日事今日毕，一旦碰到什么事没法马上做完时就会紧张万分。倘若跟别人一起做事时，别人不根据他的标准来做的话，他也会觉得如坐针毡。这类人往往更易患焦虑障碍。具有自卑倾向的人。这类人常常会有强烈的不安全感，有些人深信自己的容貌、身体特征、口才、表情、学业成绩、体能状况处处不如人，由于坚信不疑以致这种观念根深蒂固，每当与别人在一起时，这种想法就蜂拥而出，使其无法放松来与别人交谈和交往，总觉得自己处处不如人。有些人在感觉到别人投过来的视线时，脸上的肌肉就会马上僵硬起来，嘴巴张不开，甚至连喉咙也会发生阻塞感。过分自卑往往易发展为社交焦虑障碍。过度关心自己的人。这类人会有焦虑倾向。这些人通常以自我为中心，非常关注自己健康的状况。当他发现自己有任何的身体症状时，他会非常紧张而马上采取各种医疗行为。一些轻微的不适，如头痛、颈酸、腹痛等也会引起他们对严重疾病的强烈恐惧，并有可能发展成为严重的焦虑障碍。

针对如何治疗抑郁症，专家提出以下建议：

给自己安排的计划要现实合理。即使你在慢慢恢复，但也不要总把自己的时间安排得满满的。

试着摆脱由抑郁症引起的如失败感等此类的消极想法，这些想法会随着抑郁症的减轻而逐渐消除。

参加一些你喜欢的、能让自己感到愉快的活动。

当你情绪低落的时候，避免去做人生中的重大决定。如果一定要做出决定，最好向可信赖的朋友或家人寻求帮助。

不要喝酒精饮料或服用非医生开具的药物，因为这可能会与抗抑郁类药物发生严重反应，而且可能会使病情加重。

多锻炼身体，每周锻炼四至六次，每次至少 30 分钟。

（1001 字）

➜ 写作解析

1. **分析中文原文**

   本文结构很清楚，属于分析问题—解决问题型的文章，故摘要结构可依据这种结构完成。

   第一段：抑郁症的症状。

   第二段：易患抑郁症的人群。

   第三至九段：如何治疗抑郁症。

2. **摘要的中文大纲**

   第一部分（第 1 段）：抑郁症是精神疾病中危害人群最大的一种精神疾病。目前有 1.21 亿人患有抑郁症，该病患病人群仍在不断增加。患抑郁症的人通常会感到异常忧伤、觉得人生毫无价值、对原本感兴趣的活动失去兴趣、精力丧失、疲劳无力、消极悲观、烦躁、甚至会产生自杀的念头。身体症状一般表现在：食欲减退、体重减轻和睡眠障碍。

第二部分（第 2 段）：一共有三类人容易患上抑郁症。第一类是追求十全十美的人。这类人因为要求自己所做的每一件事都完美无缺，所以把全部精力都放在事物上，从另一个角度而言，即有很强的占有欲、控制欲，在临床上常称这些人具有强迫倾向。一旦碰到什么事没法马上做完时就会紧张万分。第二类就是具有自卑倾向的人。这类人常常会有强烈的不安全感，有些人深信自己的容貌、身体特征、口才、表情、学业成绩、体能状况处处不如人，使其无法放松来与别人交谈和交往。第三类人是过度关心自己的人。这些人通常以自我为中心，非常关注自己健康的状况。当他发现自己有任何的身体症状时，他会非常紧张而马上采取各种医疗行为。

第三部分（第 3~9 段）：针对如何治疗抑郁症，专家提出以下建议：给自己安排的计划要现实合理；试着摆脱由抑郁症引起的如失败感等此类的消极想法；参加一些你喜欢的、能让自己感到愉快的活动；当你情绪低落的时候，避免去做人生中的重大决定。最好向可信赖的朋友或家人寻求帮助；不要喝酒精饮料或服用非医生开具的药物；多锻炼身体。

3. **供参考的表达式**

抑郁	depression
威胁	endanger; threaten
劳累	tiredness; fatigue
悲观	pessimism
烦躁	irritation
食欲不振	poor appetite
消瘦	weight loss
失眠	insomnia
十全十美	perfection
自卑	be inferior to
没安全感	insecurity
以自我为中心	self-centered

4. **参考范文**

Depression is the biggest mental disease which endangers people. At present, there are 121 million people suffering from depression and the number is increasing. Depression can make people feel extremely sad, worthless and lose enjoyment in what they used to be interested before. Besides loss of energy, fatigue, pessimism, irritation, poor appetite, weight loss, and insomnia are typical symptoms.

It is said three kinds of people are liable to depression. People pursuing perfection strictly require everything be perfect. If something is unfinished, they tend to feel very anxious. People who feel inferior to others, have strong insecurity and they are convinced that they are inferior to others in all aspects. People who concern about themselves excessively are very self-centered and they concern about their health. Even a slight headache may arouse their fear.

There are some helpful tips for the treatment of depression. Firstly, set a reasonable schedule for yourself. Don't arrange a tight schedule for yourself. Secondly, try to remove the negative thoughts. Thirdly, try not to make decisions when you are gloomy. If you have to, you may turn to your friends or parents for help. Fourthly, don't drink alcohol or take unprescribed drugs, which may make your mental health worse. Last but not least, take physical exercise as possible as you can.

(217 words)

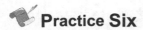 **Practice Six**

失 眠 症

睡眠是每个人的健康需要，也是本应享有的基本权利，但快节奏的生活却"吞噬"着人们越来越多的睡眠时间。在 3 月 21 日"世界睡眠日"之际，世界卫生组织公布的最新数字显示，全球近 1/4 的人受失眠困扰，每年近 8.6 亿人患失眠抑郁障碍。流行病学调查显示，33% 的美国人失眠，欧洲 4%~22% 的人受此影响。美国全国睡眠基金会 3 月最新调查显示，美国人每天平均工作 9 小时 28 分，仅睡 6 小时 40 分。全美约 7000 万人失眠。其中，女性更为严重，2/3 的女性睡不好，近 30% 的女性常吃安眠药。来自法国的数据显示，53% 的人"想在白天躺会儿"，30% 的人出现过睡眠紊乱，而 2006 年，这一比例仅为 19%。澳大利亚睡眠协会的调查则显示，约 6% 的澳大利亚人存在失眠、打鼾等睡眠问题，40% 的人经过一夜睡眠后仍浑身乏力。在日本，每隔 5 年就有一次面向 8 万户家庭 18 万人的睡眠情况调查。结果显示，从 1986 年起，日本人睡眠一直在减少。其中，45~49 岁之间的人睡眠时间最少。统计显示，20%~30% 的中国人患有失眠症，超过 50% 的人有睡眠问题。现代研究证实，有近 90 种疾病与长期失眠相关。有专家表示，虽然当今失眠现象较普遍，但如何正确认识和有效防治失眠，尚未引起人们的高度重视。

上海市中医失眠症医疗协作中心副主任施明提出，中国人目前 50% ~ 55% 的失眠与精神情志因素有关。据有关资料显示，35~55 岁是当今失眠症发病率最高的年龄段，而且失眠有向青年人群蔓延的趋势。失眠人群的职业以经营、管理、财务、文教等脑力劳动人员为主。有专家指出，导致失眠的原因主要有以下几种：1. 疾病：有明确疾病存在的患者，睡眠往往不好。2. 心理因素：如紧张、焦虑、抑郁、兴奋、恐惧、烦闷、忧伤等情绪都会引起失眠。3. 生活习惯：饮用含咖啡因的饮料、抽烟和睡前饮酒，这些都会影响睡眠。晚餐过晚或过饱等不良生活习惯也会造成失眠。4. 生理因素：如老年人与更年期女性的失眠，多数与生理现象有关。5. 环境因素：城市的声光污染、气味、床铺舒适度、室温高低等都会干扰睡眠。6. 生物节律的干扰与紊乱，最常见的是倒时差与倒班。7. 药物：某些慢性病患者，长期服用一些毒副作用较强的药物也会影响正常睡眠。

失眠不仅给患者本人造成很大痛苦，还将给整个社会带来诸如医疗资源消耗增加、事故发生率上升和生产力下降等负面问题。有统计显示，45% 的车祸和失眠有关，55% 的工地事故是人们睡眠不够导致的，约 30% 的高血压和 20% 的心脏病是由不良睡眠引发的。失眠者中患抑郁症的人是睡眠正常人的 3 倍，超过 90% 的焦虑症和抑郁症患者同时伴有失眠。不过如果发生一天或几天睡眠不好的情况，并不算是得了失眠症，一般通过自身调整，睡眠自然就会恢复正常。

针对不同病因，治疗失眠的方法也有所不同。主要方法有：药物治疗、心理治疗、自我调节治疗、器械治疗等。自我调节治疗主要是保持情绪稳定，改变睡前饱食、喝酒、看刺激书刊等影响睡眠的习惯。器械治疗则是指使用有助于健康的床垫、枕头等辅助治疗。除此以外，中医针灸或点按穴位也是治疗失眠比较安全有效的方法。

（1186 字）

↗ 写作解析

1. 分析中文原文

此文主要讨论了导致失眠的原因、失眠的危害以及主要治疗方法。各段中心意思如下：
第一段：失眠问题很普遍。
第二段：失眠的高危人群和原因。
第三段：失眠危害。
第四段：治疗方法。

2. 摘要的中文大纲

第一部分（第 1 段）：失眠问题：当今失眠现象在全世界十分普遍，但如何正确认识和有效防治失眠，尚未引起人们的高度重视。

第二部分（第 2 段）：失眠的高危人群和原因：35～55 岁是当今失眠症发病率最高的年龄段，失眠人群以脑力劳动人员为主。导致失眠的原因主要有以下几种：1. 疾病：有明确疾病存在的患者。2. 心理因素：如紧张、焦虑、抑郁、兴奋、恐惧、烦闷、忧伤等情绪。3. 生活习惯：饮用含咖啡因的饮料、抽烟和睡前饮酒，晚餐过晚或过饱等不良生活习惯。4. 生理因素：如老年人与更年期女性。5. 环境因素：城市的声光污染、气味、床铺舒适度、室温高低等。6. 生物节律的干扰与紊乱，最常见的是倒时差与倒班。7. 药物：长期服用一些毒副作用较强的药物。

第三部分（第 3 段）：失眠的危害：失眠不仅给患者本人造成很大痛苦，还将给整个社会带来诸如医疗资源消耗增加、事故发生率上升和生产力下降等负面问题。

第四部分（第 4 段）：失眠的治疗方法：针对不同病因，治疗失眠的方法也有所不同。主要方法有：药物治疗、心理治疗、自我调节治疗、器械治疗、中医针灸或点按穴位治疗等。

3. 供参考的表达式

失眠	insomnia; sleeplessness; sleep disorder
发病率	incidence
心理因素	psychological factors

生理因素	physiological factors
更年期妇女	female climacteric syndrome patients
生物节律	biological rhythm
时差	jet lag
倒班	shifts
心理治疗	psychotherapy
中医针灸	acupuncture
按穴位	point-pressing

4.　参考范文

Insomnia

Insomnia is becoming a common problem throughout the world now. However, people have neither paid enough attention to the problem nor taken effective measures to cope with it.

The highest incidence of insomnia is found in individuals aged from 35 to 55 and mainly in brainworkers. There are six factors contributing to insomnia. Firstly, people with diseases tend to have such a problem. Secondly, psychological factors such as tension, anxiety, depression and sorrow probably lead to sleep disorder. Thirdly, unhealthy living habits, for instance, drinking alcohol before sleep, late dinner, may affect sleep. Fourthly, insomnia of elderly and female climacteric syndrome patients results from certain physiological factors. Fifthly, insomnia has something to do with environmental factors, for example, pollution, temperature in rooms and comfort degree of bed. Sixthly, people in different shifts or with jet lag can't sleep well. Lastly, medicine with toxic side effects taken by chronic patients is another contribution to insomnia.

Undoubtedly insomnia has many negative effects on patients as well as society. It not only brings great pain to the patients, but also causes many social problems, such as increased medical cost, high accident rates, and reduced production, etc.

Based on various causes, treatments for insomnia can be quite different. Apart from medicine and psychotherapy, self-adjustment and change in living habits may be beneficial to patients. In addition, acupuncture and point-pressing are strongly recommended.

（227 words）

 Practice Seven

喝　水

水是生命之源，人体一切的生命活动都离不开水。对于人体而言，水在身体内不但是"运送"各种营养物质的载体，而且还直接参与人体的新陈代谢，因此，保证充足的摄水量对人体生理功能的正常运转至关重要。但是，很多人对喝水的理解仅仅限于解渴。其实喝水也是一门学问，正确地喝水对维护人的健康非常重要。

喝水多少因人而异

深圳市第二人民医院肾内科主任何永成博士告诉记者，一般而言，人每天喝水的量至少要与体内的水分消耗量相平衡。人体一天所排出的尿量约有 1500 毫升，再加上从粪便、呼吸过程中或是从皮肤所蒸发的水，总共消耗水分大约是 2500 毫升左右，而人体每天能从食物中和体内新陈代谢中补充的水分只有 1000 毫升左右，因此正常人每天至少需要喝 1500 毫升水，大约 8 杯左右。

通常每个人需要喝多少水会根据活动量、环境，甚至天气而有所改变。正常人喝太多水对健康不会有太大影响，只是可能造成排尿量增多，引起生活上的不便。但是对于某些特殊人群，喝水量的多少必须特别注意，比如浮肿病人、心脏功能衰竭病人、肾功能衰竭病人都不宜喝水过多，因为喝水太多会加重心脏和肾脏负担，容易导致病情加剧。而对于中暑、膀胱炎、便秘和皮肤干燥等疾病患者，多喝水则可对缓解病情起到一定效果。此外，人在感冒发烧时也应多喝水，因为体温上升会使水分流失，多喝水能促使身体散热，帮助病人恢复健康。而怀孕期的妇女和运动量比较大的人水分消耗得多，也应多喝水。

温开水是最好的饮料

专家说，从健康的角度来看，白开水是最好的饮料，它不含卡路里，不用消化就能为人体直接吸收利用，一般建议喝 30 摄氏度以下的温开水最好，这样不会过于刺激肠胃道的蠕动，不易造成血管收缩。含糖饮料会减慢肠胃道吸收水分的速度，长期大量地喝含糖饮料，对人体的新陈代谢会产生一定不良影响。何博士告诉记者，像橙汁、可乐等含糖饮料口感虽好，但不宜多喝，每天摄入量应控制在一杯左右，最多不要超过 200 毫升，而对于糖尿病人和比较肥胖的人来说，则最好不要喝这类饮料。

纯净水和矿泉水等桶装水由于饮用方便深受现代人青睐，但是何博士提醒，喝这些水时一定要保证其卫生条件，一桶水最好在一个月内喝完，而且人们不应把纯净水作为主要饮用水。因为水是人体的六大营养素之一，水中含有多种对人体有益的矿物质和微量元素，而纯净水中的这些物质含量大大降低，如果平时人们饮食中的营养结构又不平衡，就很容易导致营养失调。有的人担心自来水硬度太大会不利于身体健康，但何博士介绍说，水的硬度对人体健康基本没有影响，而且现在国内的自来水都符合生活饮用水的标准，饮用煮沸了的自来水是安全的。茶和咖啡具有提神效果，但何博士提醒人们，喝茶宜喝淡茶，并且切忌酗咖啡，咖啡因会影响钙的吸收。

喝水不要大口吞咽

很多人往往在口渴时才想起喝水，而且往往是大口吞咽，这种做法也是不对的。喝水太快太急会无形中把很多空气一起吞咽下去，容易引起打嗝或是腹胀，因此最好先将水含在口中，再缓缓喝下，尤其是肠胃虚弱的人，喝水更应该一口一口慢慢喝。

至于喝水时间，专家则告诉记者，喝水切忌渴了再喝，应在两顿饭期间适量饮水，最好隔 1 小时喝一杯。人们还可以根据自己尿液的颜色来判断是否需要喝水，一般来说，人的尿液为淡黄色，如果颜色太浅，则可能是水喝得过多，如果颜色偏深，则表示需要多补充一些水了。睡前少喝、睡后多喝也是正确饮水的原则，因为睡前喝太多的水，会造成眼皮浮肿，半夜也会老跑厕所，使睡眠质量不高。而经过一个晚上的睡眠，人体流失的水分约有450毫升，早上起来需要及时补充，因此早上起床后空腹喝杯水有益血液循环，也能促进大脑清醒，使这一天的思维清晰敏捷。

（1463 字）

↗ 写作解析

1. 分析中文原文

本文从喝水量、喝什么水、如何喝水、饮水时间四个方面简述喝水的重要性。因为有副标题，故文章结构很清楚，便于确定摘要结构。各段大意如下：

第一段：水的重要性。

第二、三段：一般而言，人每天喝水的量至少要与体内的水分消耗量相平衡。因此正常人每天至少需要喝1500毫升水，大约8杯左右。

第四段：通常每个人需要喝多少水会根据活动量、环境，甚至天气而有所改变。

第五、六段：白开水是最好的饮料，少喝含糖饮料。

第七段：桶装水要注意卫生，喝茶要喝淡茶，切忌酗咖啡。

第八、九段：避免大口吞咽。

第十段：喝水的时间。

2. 摘要中文大纲

第一部分（第1段）：人体一切的生命活动都离不开水。因此，保证充足的摄水量对人体生理功能的正常运转至关重要。但是，很多人对喝水的理解仅仅限于解渴。其实正确地喝水对维护人的健康非常重要。

第二部分（第2~4段）：人每天喝水的量至少要与体内的水分消耗量相平衡。人体一天总共消耗水分大约是2500毫升左右，而人体每天能从食物中和体内新陈代谢中补充的水分只有1000毫升左右，因此正常人每天至少需要喝1500毫升水，大约8杯左右。对于中暑、膀胱炎、便秘和皮肤干燥等疾病患者、感冒发烧患者、孕妇和运动量较大的人应多喝水。但是，对于浮肿病人、心脏功能衰竭病人、肾功能衰竭病人都不宜喝水过多，会加重心脏和肾脏负担。

第三部分（第5~7段）：温开水是最好的饮料。长期大量地喝含糖饮料，对人体的新陈代谢会产生一定不良影响。纯净水和矿泉水等桶装水不应作为主要应用水，容易导致营养失调。喝茶宜喝淡茶，切忌酗咖啡，咖啡因会影响钙的吸收。

第四部分（第8~9段）：口渴时才想起喝水以及大口吞咽，容易引起打嗝或是腹胀，因此最好先将水含在口中，再缓缓喝下。

第五部分（第10段）：喝水应在两顿饭期间适量饮水，最好隔1小时喝一杯。人们还可以根据自己尿液的颜色来判断是否需要喝水，睡前少喝、睡后多喝也是正确饮水的原则。

3. **供参考的表达式**

营养物质	nutrient
新陈代谢	metabolism
生理功能	physiological function
解渴	relieve thirst
浮肿	dropsy
心脏功能衰竭	heart failure
肾功能衰竭	kidney failure
中暑	heat stroke
膀胱炎	cystitis
便秘	constipation
孕妇	pregnant women
纯净水	purified water
矿泉水	mineral water
桶装水	barreled water
提神	refresh oneself
吸收	absorb
打嗝	hiccup
腹胀	abdominal distention
尿液	urine
大口吞咽	gulp; swallow
长期的	long-term; chronic

4. **参考范文**

No living activities of our body can go without water. Therefore, adequate water supply plays a crucial role in maintaining proper physiological functions.

The amount of water we drink each day need to be equivalent to the water we consume. Our body consumes approximately 2,500ml water a day, while it can supplement only about 1,000ml water from food and metabolism. So, a normal person should drink at least 1,500ml water, about 8 glasses. People who suffer from heat stroke, cystitis and constipation, and pregnant women are recommended to drink more, while patients with dropsy, heart failure and kidney failure should not drink too much water.

The best drinking water is warm boiled water. Long-term drinking of beverage with sugar affects the body's metabolism. Purified water and mineral water should not be the main drinks, which might cause malnutrition. Light tea is highly recommended, but drinking too much coffee will affect the absorption of calcium.

Try to avoid gulping, because it tends to cause hiccup and abdominal distention. The correct way is to keep water in the mouth and then wash it down slowly.

全国医学博士英语统考综合应试教程

You should drink moderate water between two meals and drink a glass every one hour. Besides, you can determine whether you need to drink according to your urine color. Furthermore, less water before sleep and more water after sleep is the correct way.

（226 words）

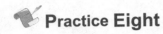 **Practice Eight**

艾滋病和 HIV 的传播

我们自以为熟知如何应付的一种威胁正在迅猛地扩散。在今年 12 月 1 日的世界艾滋病日之际，世界卫生组织发现，全球的艾滋病病毒感染者人数达到了历史最高值：40300000，比 10 年前翻了一倍。4000 多万，这意味着全球每 160 个人当中就有一个艾滋病病毒感染者。

艾滋病（AIDS）不是一个单纯的病，而是一种综合征，叫作获得性免疫缺陷综合征。1981 年在美国首次报道艾滋病病例，后来这个综合征演变成了全球范围的流行病。艾滋病是由人类免疫缺陷病毒（HIV）所引起。这种病毒进入人体后通过杀死或损害人体免疫系统的细胞，逐步损伤机体抵抗感染和某些肿瘤的能力。由于免疫功能的下降，艾滋病人很容易并发一种致命的感染性疾病，叫作条件致病性感染。所谓的条件致病性感染就是，一些病毒或是细菌通常不会导致健康的人感染，但是可以导致艾滋病人患病。

艾滋病的确是一种传染病。但艾滋病本身不会传染，只是 HIV 病毒具有传染性。HIV 传染的最常见的方式是通过与艾滋病患者或者已经感染 HIV 病毒的性伴侣进行无保护措施的性交。在性接触过程中这种病毒可通过阴道、外阴、阴茎、直肠、口腔等进入体内，导致感染。人们也可以通过接触被 HIV 感染的血液导致感染。在献血还没有经过 HIV 感染筛查的年代，HIV 通过输入感染的血液或血液制品进行传播。如今，献血和输血已经有了严格的管理措施，所以输血或血液制品传播 HIV 的危险性已经非常小了。然而，HIV 在吸毒者之间传播还是常见的，他们通常是通过共用注射针头或是被 HIV 感染过的注射器相互之间传染病毒。偶尔也有医务人员被 HIV 污染的针头或其他的医疗器械传染。还有一种传染方式是在感染 HIV 病毒母亲和子女之间进行。感染 HIV 的孕妇可以在怀孕或是分娩期间将病毒传给她们的孩子。尽管如此，艾滋病或 HIV 感染的妇女在得到一定的医学措施护理时，也是可能生下健康的孩子的。如果医务人员为这类孕妇进行适当的治疗和行剖宫产术来分娩婴儿，那么孩子感染 HIV 的概率将降到百分之一。

虽然艾滋病是一种可怕的疾病，但是人们在日常生活中也不必过于害怕，因为 HIV 不会通过一般性接触传染。一般说来，与艾滋病人共用餐具、毛巾、寝具、电话或是坐便等是不会传染这种疾病的。昆虫叮咬一般也不会传播 HIV。

↗ 写作解析

1. **分析中文原文**

   本文一共四段，在阅读中文原文后，我们可以确定每一段的段落大意，并在原文划出相应的关键细节内容。关键细节内容请见原文画线部分。各段的段落大意简要如下：

第一段：艾滋病的威胁迅猛扩散。

第二段：什么是艾滋病。

第三段：HIV 病毒传播的途径。

第四段：在日常生活中不必过于害怕。

2. 摘要中文大纲

第一段：世界卫生组织发现全球艾滋病病毒感染者人数达到历史最高：40300000，这意味着全球每 160 人当中就有一个艾滋病病毒感染者。并且几乎在全球所有国家里，艾滋病病毒感染者数量都在上升。

第二段：艾滋病叫作获得性免疫缺陷综合征。1981 年美国首次报道艾滋病病例，后来该病演变成全球范围流行病。艾滋病是由 HIV 病毒引起，这种病毒进入人体后通过杀死或损害人体免疫系统的细胞，逐步损伤机体抵抗感染和某些肿瘤的能力。实际上艾滋病本身不会传染，但 HIV 病毒具有传染性。

第三段：HIV 病毒传染最常见的方式是通过与艾滋病患者或者已经感染 HIV 病毒的性伴侣进行无保护措施的性交。此外，人们也可以通过接触被 HIV 感染的血液导致感染。HIV 病毒在吸毒者之间通常是通过共用注射针头或是被 HIV 感染过的注射器相互之间传染病毒。偶尔也有医务人员被 HIV 污染的针头或其他的医疗器械传染。最后，HIV 病毒可以在母婴之间传播。

第四段：虽然艾滋病是一种可怕的疾病，但人们在日常生活中不必过于害怕，HIV 病毒不会通过一般性接触感染，如共用餐具、毛巾、寝具、电话；昆虫叮咬也不会传播 HIV。

3. 供参考的表达式

全球范围流行病	worldwide epidemic disease
抗感染	infectious resistance
感染的血液	infected blood
孕妇可以将病毒传染给孩子	mothers can infect their babies with virus

4. 参考范文

WHO has found patients with HIV have reached the peak: 40,300,000, which means there is one with HIV among 160 people around the world.

AIDS (Acquired Immune Deficiency Syndrome) was first reported in the United States in 1981 and has become a major worldwide epidemic disease. AIDS is caused by HIV virus, which destroys the body's ability to fight infections and certain tumors by killing or damaging cells of the body's immune system. In fact, AIDS is not transmitted, but the virus is.

HIV is spread commonly by having unprotected sex with an infected partner. It is also spread through contact with infected blood. HIV is frequently spread among injection drug users by the sharing of needles or syringes contaminated with infected blood. It is rare, however, for a patient to give HIV to a health care worker by accidental sticks with infected needles or other medical instruments. Women can transmit HIV to their babies during pregnancy or birth.

Although AIDS is a terrible disease, but people don't need to feel scared excessively. HIV is spread neither through casual contact such as the sharing of food utensils, towels and bedding, telephones, etc, nor insects biting.

（196 words）

八、命题作文和翻译简析

根据新大纲要求，写作部分还有两种形式备选：命题写作和翻译。大纲中是这么要求的：

翻译（Translation：汉译英）

将一篇 300 字左右的汉语短文翻译为英语，短文可以是一段，也可以是数段，共计 20 分。考试时间 50 分钟，该题型旨在测试考生汉译英的能力，重点考查考生用英语准确再现汉语原文思想和内容的能力。

答题要求：

（1）译文必须忠实于原文，不能随意发挥。

（2）用词恰当，注意词性的必要转换。

（3）注意使用正确的英语语法。

（4）文字通顺，符合英语表达习惯。

命题写作（Essay Writing）

根据题目要求，写一篇 250 个单词左右的文章。共计 20 分，考试时间 50 分钟。该题型旨在测试考生英语议论文的写作能力，重点考查考生在写作中的思想性、逻辑性以及语言应用能力。

答题要求：

（1）紧扣题目，每段只聚焦一个主题思想。

（2）用词恰当、语法正确。

（3）注意句子之间的逻辑关系。

（4）文字通顺，注意篇章的连贯性和一致性。

这两种题型都不是新题型，考生朋友们想必不陌生。下面就分别简单分析一下：

↗ 命题写作

谋篇布局

（1）主题句（The Topic Sentence）

主题句是段落发展的依据，它主要表明作者的观点态度，或指出作者的写作意图，或对文章的内容进行概括，反映了文章的中心思想。因此，主题句写得是否妥贴是文章写得成功与否的关键。

（2）扩展句（Supporting Details）

在经主题句点出段落的中心思想后，接着就是一系列的扩展句。扩展句对主题句的中心思想或者举例说明，或者详细解释。一般来说，扩展句应该具有如下特点：

1）清晰翔实

因为文章的中心思想是通过扩展句来体现的，所以扩展句应写得清晰、翔实，不可含糊其辞或言之无物。同时，扩展句必须具有较强的说服力，不可只考虑篇幅、凑够字数了事，更不可偏离主题，想到什么写什么。

2）条理清楚

为了便于读者掌握作者的意图，扩展句必须有一定的条理。先说哪句话，后说哪句话应有个安排。也就是说，上句为下句铺平道路，下句是上句的自然延伸，层层阐明问题。就作文而言，每句话的平均长度应控制在 10~15 个词为宜。随着自己写作技巧的进步，句子也可稍长些。另外，还要注意，在一篇文章中，各段的篇幅应该大致相当。

（3）结尾句（The Concluding Sentence）

结尾句就是用精练的语言对文章的内容进行归纳总结。因为文章的内容是说明主题句的，所以结尾句须和主题相呼应，或者说是主题句的再现（Restatement of the Topic Sentence）。同时，结尾句还有引发读者对文章内容进一步认识和肯定的作用，因此，其语气比起主题句来须更加中肯切要。

议论文有论点、论证、论据三大要素。论点可以在开头也可以在结尾；论据可以是事实、数据或道理；论证就是摆事实、讲道理。但说理过程要环环相扣，步步深入。从立论到归题，结构要严谨，论证要周密，例证要广泛、充分、翔实和可信，这样方可以理服人。

例 1

Why Women Live Longer

It is a fact that women live longer than men. That difference was not so obvious a long time ago, because everyone died at an early age. Now, however, the average life span of Chinese people is 75 years old. The reasons for the difference are very complex, and scientists can only understand some of them.（主题段：由事实引入主题——什么使得女性寿命更长？）

Disease is chiefly responsible for the difference in life expectancy. At present, heart disease is the main cause of death for men after 40. Doctors have realized that differences in life style and personal habits between men and women are a factor in heart disease. Over the past few decades, men have had poorer diets, have gotten less exercise and have smoked much more than women. Now studies are also beginning to show that the female sex hormones help to protect women from heart disease. More studies are needed to actually tell scientists how these hormones provide their protection.（扩展段 1：对比方法支持说明女性为何患心脏病的概率低。）

It seems clear then that natural factors help to explain why women live longer than men do. These natural factors also interact with life style and personal habits. Women are more often concerned about their health. They are more cautious than men in eating, drinking and sleeping. They are also more careful than men in maintaining their own health. Few women smoke and drink, even if they smoke and drink, the amount is very limited. It has been recognized that smokers will lose their life by 8 years and those who drink alcohol will lose 4 years. At the same time, women are better at grasping emotions and adapting to the environment than men. （扩展段 2：除了自然因素之外，男女寿命差异的原因还在于非自然因素：饮食、生活习惯、掌控情绪的能力等。）

It can be seen that while exploring the mystery of women's longevity, men should be encouraged to create conditions from external factors, strive to prolong their life and share their old age with women. （总结段：既然已经知道女性比男性长寿的原因，那就呼吁男性也努力长寿起来。）

这篇议论文不仅结构严谨，而且列举了一些数字，使文章更具有说服力。

例 2

My View on TCM Development

Traditional Chinese medicine is a treasure of Chinese civilization and the crystallization of more than 5,000 years of civilization. The "14th Five-Year Plan" and the draft of the 2035 long-term goal outline propose that it is necessary to promote the inheritance and innovation of Chinese medicine, adhere to the equal emphasis on Chinese and Western medicine and complement each other's advantages, and vigorously develop the cause of Chinese medicine. With the guidance and strong support of the country, the great development of Chinese medicine is at the right time. （主题段：中药事业源远流长，需要发扬光大。）

In terms of disease prevention, treatment, and rehabilitation, traditional Chinese medicine has unique advantages. Its holistic view and the concept of syndrome differentiation and treatment provide people with all-round and full-cycle health protection, and become a vehicle for advancing the construction of a healthy China and protecting people's health. The Covid-19 epidemic has brought severe challenges to the public health systems of countries around the world. In the absence of specific medicines in the world, Chinese medicine has allowed patients to receive effective treatment in a short period of time, and has played an important role in the fight against the epidemic. （扩展段 1：中药在疾病治疗和预防上的独特优势。）

The combination of Chinese and Western medicine and the combined use of Chinese and Western medicine are a major feature of epidemic prevention and control in China. It is the vivid practice of traditional Chinese medicine inheritance and innovation. This model is making the ancient Chinese medicine culture full of vitality. （扩展段 2：中国中西医结合的独特模式。）

To promote the high-quality development of Chinese medicine, it is necessary to follow the law of Chinese medicine development, dig out the essence, and establish a service and management model that meets its characteristics. It is necessary to clearly realize that there are still shortcomings in the field of Chinese medicine, whether it is subject construction or the talent team, and it needs to work hard to practice internal skills. At the same time, it is necessary to strengthen research and argumentation, summarize and explore the mechanism of TCM disease prevention and treatment, and earnestly inherit, develop and use the precious wealth left by our ancestors, so that the culture of TCM can be deeply rooted in the land of China.（扩展段 3：如何做。）

例 3

Directions: Read the following information and write an essay of ABOUT 200 WORDS. It is all ARGUMENTATIVE ESSAY AND A TITLE is NEEDED.

According to a new study, 92% of college students would rather do their reading in the old-fashioned way, with pages and not pixels. The finding comes from American University linguistics professor Naomi S. Baron, author of the book *Words Onscreen: The Fate of Reading in a Digital World*. Baron led a team that asked 300 college students in the United States, Slovakia, Japan and Germany how they preferred to read. Physical books were the choice of 92% of the respondents, who selected paper over an array of electronic devices. It's not just college students who'd rather spend their time with a book instead of an e-reader. In 2015, e-book sales dropped in the United States, and it's the same story in the United Kingdom.

【参考范文】

Paper Books' Overwhelming Triumph

In this Digital Age, it is surprising to find out that people still favor physical paper-books over e-books. A new study by American linguistics professor Naomi S. Baron shows that 92% of college students prefer pages to pixels. And the decline in e-book sales in both US and UK stands to confirm the same inclination of readers in general, not just college students.（主题段：提及材料，开门见山。）

The news is a comfort to people like me who once worried about the extinction of paper books someday with the rise of digital empire. "Media is the message," quoted Marshall McLuhan, so obviously there would be a big sea difference in reading experience. Although e-book sounds like a pretty smart idea: economic, efficient and environment-friendly, the physical connection is cut off between the reader and the print, a novel, a poem collection or even a textbook. And the heavy weight of paper books becomes a sweet burden to steady your heart and pin you down.（内容段：以自己为例，表明观点和态度。）

It is always a good sign for the world to innovate, to change, to have more choices and to embrace diversity. It is even better to know that our society still needs old-fashioned, harmless habits like reading a book in paper.（总结段：再次表明态度。）

汉译英

　　虽然摘要写作一直是国家医学考试中心最青睐的方式，因为这确实是最能考查考生理解能力和表达能力、综合语言能力素质的方式，但其难度不会因为时间的推移而降低。在特殊时期，传统的纸笔考试有可能被机考或者远程形式代替时，命题形式会更加灵活，所以，命题组采用新大纲中其他两种题型来命题。比如，2022年全国医学博士英语统考的写作部分就选用了汉译英的题型来命题，对此，我们必须对此引起足够的重视。

　　对大多数考生来说，汉译英的难度显然大于英译汉。一般来说，考生对汉语的理解不会有多大困难，但把汉语转换成标准地道的英语就比较有难度了。英译汉重在对原文的理解，汉译英则是对译文的准确表达，而要实现准确的英语表达，就需要深厚的英语写作基础。短文内容主要涉及医学、社会、文化和科技等领域，所选题材以议论文居多。考题看似不难，但译好却不容易。

1. 短文汉译英的应对策略

　　1）理解原文。做题之前，要做的第一步就是理解原文。理解原文不是说能不能看懂，而是要分析其内容，即下笔之前要对段际之间、句际之间、句子内部之间的逻辑关系进行分析，掌握英语语言体系下的主干成分，感受句子所隐含的时态（进行、完成、过去……）、语态（主动、被动）、语义的褒贬，是否要用虚拟语气等。只有这样才能保证表达准确，避免出现偏差。

　　2）确定句数。汉语句子多用逗号，但英语则需要根据逗号前后的结构来对应表达方式。根据英语句子基本句型和结构的根本原则，确定用多少个符合英语句法规则的句子来承载源语言。这一步是最关键的。这里简单用一个口诀来搭建英语的句法框架：

- 谓动乃为山中虎，一山岂能容两只？
- 谓动之前是主语，后面可是宾和表。
- 时态语态语气来，全由谓动来体现。
- 因此谓动常变形，助动情态放在前。
- 多余动词需处理，并列非谓从句用。
- 并列连词要牢记，三种形式非谓重。
- 从句也能分三种，帽子wh-放在先。
- 定从置于名词后，名从就当名词用。
- 状语从句要单记，八种逻辑分清楚。
- 句子如果不正常，比较倒装常备用。
- 谁和谁比更重要，翻译题中最常见。
- 常见特殊句型者，阅读完形写作共。

　　3）确定语法。译文的表达要符合英语语法。英语语法的一大特点就是以动词为核心，构成五种基本句型。英语中无论句子成分多复杂，句子多长，句式如何变幻，都是从这五大句型扩展而来的。所以不管汉语句子如何复杂，如何难以对付，你首先应考虑英语的基本组句框架。这些框架是英语表达的第一步，也是译文的基础。

4）梳理表达。译文要符合英语表达习惯。在许多情况下，考生的译文从语法上看没问题，但却不符合英语的表达习惯，有时候还会闹出笑话。也就是大多数考生容易犯的错误：中国式英语。所以考生在掌握英语语法规则和词汇知识的基础上，还应当熟悉和了解英汉两种语言的风格、特点、规律及表达习惯上的差异。

2. 具体的翻译策略

不要拿到题目就从第一个词译起。英语的句式（尤其是长句）往往同汉语很不一样，逐字翻译有可能谁也看不懂。正确的做法是先弄清句子的结构，然后结合上下文重新安排汉语的表达顺序。英语有五个基本句型，它们是构成英语句子的基础，再长再复杂的句子也是由这五个基本句型（或它们的变体）按一定的规则构建而成的。还要明白，这些基本句型的公式只表示了句子的主要成分，而实际的句子大都还带有一些修饰语，如定语和状语等。这些修饰语可以是单词、短语或句子，如果是句子，又离不开基本句型。

有了这样的认识，我们可以开始理解句子的意思了。对于较长、结构较复杂的句子，我们先要把它分割成一个个意群（可以是动词不定式短语、分词短语、动名词短语、介词短语、形容词短语、名词短语或各种从句等），然后确定意群和意群间的联系。这里我们还应记住两点：①英语的每个成分，甚至每个词，在句中都有它应有的位置，不能游离于句子之外；②某个单词如果属于某个意群，就不能随意把它移到别的意群里去翻译。

3. 真题分析

No.1

 2023 年回忆版真题

原文：

随着新一轮科技革命的发展，以人工智能、大数据分析、5G 为代表的信息化技术赋能万物。科技变革为各领域研究跨越式发展提供了更高效的技术工具，由此引发精准医学、转化医学、数字医学、分子医学、再生医学等新的医学理念和研究范式的兴起。

当前，跨学科、跨领域的科技竞争日益白热化。医学院校要及时跟上形势，为健康中国建设和教育强国建设提供强大的人才支撑。这是新时代赋予医学教育创新发展的重要课题，也是我国医学教育的使命和责任。

面向未来科技和医学发展的新趋势和新需求，医学教育面临着新机遇和新挑战。在新医科背景下，需加快医学教育改革，创新医学人才培养模式，培养复合型医学人才，以精准对接国家发展新战略，为推进健康中国建设、保障人民健康提供强有力的人才保障。

下面我们先确定句数，再确定语法、梳理表达。

① 随着新一轮科技革命的发展，以人工智能、大数据分析、5G 为代表的信息化技术赋能万物。

解析过程：

伴随状语：随着……

主语：信息化技术 + 以 …… 为代表的（名扩结构）

谓语：赋能

宾语：万物

这是一个简单句，考查重点是核心名词的抓取以及后置定语的处理。"随着"是一个标准的表示伴随状语的标志词：With a new round development of scientific revolution。主语为名词 + 名扩结构：information technology represented by artificial intelligence, big data analysis and 5G。"赋能"可翻译为 empower，gives the power 等。整个句子连接起来就是：With a new round development of scientific revolution, information technology represented by artificial intelligence, big data analysis and 5G empowers everything.

②科技变革为各领域研究跨越式发展提供了更高效的技术工具，由此引发精准医学、转化医学、数字医学、分子医学、再生医学等新的医学理念和研究范式的兴起。

解析过程：

句间逻辑关系：两个分句，因果关系（由此）

主语：科技变革

谓语：【为各领域研究跨越式发展】提供了

宾语：（更高效的）技术工具

结果状语：引发 + 医学理念和研究范式（精准医学、转化医学、数字医学、分子医学、再生医学等）的兴起

两个小分句，原本是两套主谓结构。连接两套以上主谓结构的方式有四种：拆成独立小分句、并列结构、从句、非谓语动词。两个小分句间有逻辑关系词"由此"，一般更多地使用非谓语动词。我们来试一试：Scientific and technological changes have provided more efficient technical tools for the leapfrog development of research in various fields, thus triggering the rise of new medical concepts and research paradigms such as precision medicine, translational medicine, digital medicine, molecular medicine, regenerative medicine, etc.

③当前，跨学科、跨领域的科技竞争日益白热化。

解析过程：

状语：当前

主语：科技竞争 + 跨学科、跨领域的（前置定语、名扩结构均可）

谓语：日益白热化

这个句子没有明确的谓语动词，需要在翻译时补充：Currently, interdisciplinary technological competition is becoming increasingly intense.

④医学院校要及时跟上形势，为健康中国建设和教育强国建设提供强大的人才支撑。

解析过程：

主语：医学院校

谓语：跟上形式……提供人才支撑

状语：及时……为健康中国建设和教育强国建设

这个句子可以理解为两个并列谓语动词，我们暂且尝试用并列连词来处理：Medical colleges should keep up with the situation timely and provide strong talent support for the construction of a healthy China and an educational powerhouse.

⑤这是新时代赋予医学教育创新发展的重要课题，也是我国医学教育的使命和责任。

解析过程：

主语：这

谓语：是

表语：重要课题……使命和责任

这明显是个头轻脚重的句子，使用的结构为带有并列连词的结构：This is an important task entrusted to the innovative development of medical education in the new era, as well as its mission and responsibility.

⑥面向未来科技和医学发展的新趋势、新需求，医学教育面临着新机遇和新挑战。

解析过程：

状语：面向未来……

主语：医学教育

谓语：面临着

宾语：新机遇和新挑战

这是个简单句：Facing the new trends and demands of future technology and medical development, medical education is facing new opportunities and challenges.

⑦在新医科背景下，需加快医学教育改革，创新医学人才培养模式，培养复合型医学人才，以精准对接国家发展新战略，为推进健康中国建设、保障人民健康提供强有力的人才保障。

解析过程：

状语：在新医科背景下

主语：缺失

谓语：加快……创新……培养……

宾语：医学教育改革……医学人才培养模式……复合型医学人才

状语：对接新战略，提供……人才保障

这是个很长的句子，句子结构难在两点：无主句的处理以及目的状语的处理。无主句可以尝试使用被动语态或者添加主语（特殊句型），目的状语可以理解为嵌套式，即发展新战略与提供人才保障为同等关系。当然也可理解为并列关系，即两个目的：对接战略、提供人才保障。这句话可以翻译为：In the context of the new medical science, it is necessary to accelerate the reform of medical education, innovate the training mode of medical talents, cultivate composite medical talents, to accurately align with the new national development strategy, and provide strong talent protection for promoting the construction of a healthy China and ensuring the health of people.

综上，我们将每一句的翻译合并到一起，将顺句间和句内的逻辑关系，修改不贴切的词，简化前后重复的地方，再做最后的修正：

With the upcoming latest technological revolution, information technology represented by artificial intelligence, big data analysis, and 5G empowers everything. Scientific and technological changes have provided more efficient technical tools for the huge improvement of research in various fields, triggering the rise of new medical concepts and research paradigms such as precision medicine, translational medicine, digital medicine, molecular medicine, regenerative medicine, etc.

Currently, interdisciplinary technological competition is becoming increasingly intense. Medical colleges should keep up with the situation timely and provide strong talent support for the construction of a healthy China and an educational powerhouse. This is an important task entrusted to the innovative development of medical education in the new era, and it is also the mission and responsibility of Chinese medical education.

Facing the new trends and demands of future technology and medical development, medical education is facing new opportunities and challenges. In the context of the new medical science, it is necessary to accelerate the reform of medical education, innovate the training mode of medical talents, cultivate composite medical talents, which enables us to accurately align with the new national development strategy, and provide strong talent protection for the construction of a healthy China and ensuring the health of people.

No.2

 2022 年真题

原文：

　　互联网的广泛应用正以前所未有的力度和速度改变着人类的工作、生活甚至思维方式。我们在欢呼信息技术带来便利的同时，也深刻体会到潜在危机的存在。近年来，医生个人隐私泄露事件的频繁发生给医生带来了困扰，甚至影响了医生个人的正常生活。因此，研究互联网＋背景下的隐私问题日益重要。

　　在"互联网＋"的时代背景下，大数据的海量挖掘、分析、再利用加速了医生个人隐私的"公开化"，在客观上侵犯了医生个人隐私权益。因此，要加快医生隐私保护相关法律法规的立法工作；完善医生隐私保护的监管体系，健全社会规范，管理部门、企业履行各自的社会责任；加强互联网技术建设，做好防范措施；增强数据控制者和医生的隐私保护意识。保障医生个人隐私权益真正得以实现，还需要各方携手，共同努力。

下面我们先确定句数，再确定语法、梳理表达。

① 互联网的广泛应用正以前所未有的力度和速度改变着人类的工作、生活甚至思维方式。

解析过程：

主语：广泛应用 + 互联网的（名扩结构后置）

谓语：改变着（有"正在……着"，表示进行状态）+ 以前所未有的力度和速度（方式状语）

宾语：人类的工作、生活甚至思维方式。（顿号，表示并列结构）

因此第一句的翻译至少可以平铺直叙如下：The wide application of the Internet is changing our work and life, and even the way of thinking with unprecedented efforts and speed. （语序下一步调整）

② 我们在欢呼信息技术带来便利的同时，也深刻体会到潜在危机的存在。

解析过程：

主语：我们……我们……

谓语：欢呼……体会（深刻：方式状语）

宾语：信息技术带来便利……存在 + 潜在危机（名扩结构后置）

很明显，通过分析我们发现这是两套主谓宾结构，连接两套以上主谓结构的方式有四种：拆成独立小分句、并列结构、从句、非谓语动词。我们选用并列结构来尝试一下：We are cheering for the fact that information brings convenience and we deeply feel the existence of potential risks as well.

③ 近年来，医生个人隐私泄露事件的频繁发生给医生带来了困扰，甚至影响了医生个人的正常生活。

解析过程：

时间状语：近年来

主语：频繁发生 + 医生个人隐私泄露事件（名扩结构：后置定语）

谓语：带来了……影响了……

宾语：困扰 + 给医生（方向）……医生个人的正常生活……

这里有两个谓语动词，仍然用上一句中的四种处理方式之一来处理，我们仍然选择并列：The frequent occurring of doctors' privacy leaking has brought troubles for them, and even disturbed their personal normal lives.

④ 因此，研究互联网 + 背景下的隐私问题日益重要。

解析过程：

句间逻辑关系：因此

主语：研究互联网 + 背景下的隐私问题

谓语：日益重要（缺乏谓语动词：补充系动词）

这里有两个考点：主语为带有动词的词组，名词性成分中含有动词时，处理方式有三种：非谓语动词化、从句、特殊句型。同时该句中没有谓语动词，处理方式有两种：补充谓语动词、特殊句型。既然两个考点都可以用特殊句型，我们就用此方式来翻译（形式主语）：Therefore, it is increasingly important to study the privacy issues with the Internet plus background.

⑤ 在"互联网 +"的时代背景下，大数据的海量挖掘、分析、再利用加速了医生个人隐私的"公开化"，在客观上侵犯了医生个人隐私权益。

解析过程：

条件状语：在"互联网＋"的时代背景下

主语：大数据的海量挖掘、分析、再利用

谓语：加速了

宾语：医生个人隐私的"公开化"

句间逻辑关系：结果——在客观上侵犯了医生个人隐私权益

句间逻辑关系有两种处理方式：带谓语的从句、非谓语化的结构，两种方式都需要加上表示逻辑关系的连词：In the era of Internet plus, massive data mining, analysis and reuse of large data speed up the "publicity" of doctors' personal privacy, thus objectively violating the privacy rights of doctors.

⑥ 因此，要加快医生隐私保护相关法律法规的立法工作；完善医生隐私保护的监管体系，健全社会规范，管理部门、企业履行各自的社会责任；加强互联网技术建设，做好防范措施；增强数据控制者和医生的隐私保护意识。

解析过程：

句间逻辑关系：因此

主语：无主语

谓语：加快

宾语：立法工作 ＋ a. 完善医生隐私保护的监管体系，健全社会规范，管理部门、企业履行各自的社会责任（名扩结构 ＋ 后置定语）＋ b. 加强互联网技术建设 ＋ c. 做好防范措施 ＋ d. 增强隐私数据控制者和医生的隐私保护意识

这是很长的一句话，很明显长的原因是由冒号后的并列结构导致。对于这种情况处理方式有两种：并列结构、另立门户单独成句。本句还有一个考点：无主句的翻译。无主句可以补充主语，或者使用特殊句型：Therefore, we should speed up the legislation related to the protection of doctors' privacy: to improve the supervision system of doctors' privacy protection and social norms, make management departments and enterprises fulfill their social responsibilities, strengthen the construction of Internet technology and take preventive measures and enhance privacy awareness of data controllers and doctors.

⑦ 保障医生个人隐私权益真正得以实现，还需要各方携手，共同努力。

解析过程：

主语：保障医生个人隐私权益真正得以实现

谓语：需要

宾语：各方携手，共同努力

这里的主语部分考点同④，需要非谓语动词化或者特殊句型。同时该句宾语部分用意译的方式更好，表达团结一心即可：To ensure the real realization of doctors' personal privacy rights and interests, all parties need to work together.

综上，我们将每一句的翻译合并到一起，捋顺句间和句内逻辑关系，修改不贴切的词，简化前后重复的地方，再做最后的修正：

The wide application of the Internet is changing the way of our work, life and even thinking with unprecedented strength and speed. While hailing the convenience brought by information technology, we also deeply realize the existence of potential crisis. In recent years, the frequent leakage of doctors' personal privacy has brought trouble to doctors, and even affected their normal life. Therefore, the study of privacy issues in the Internet plus context is becoming increasingly important.

In the era of Internet plus, massive data mining, analysis and reuse of large data make doctors' privacy speedily open, violating the privacy rights of doctors objectively. That's why we should speed up the legislation to protect doctors' privacy. It includes improving the relevant supervision system and social norms, requiring government sectors and enterprises fulfill their social responsibilities, strengthening the construction of Internet technology, taking preventive measures and enhancing data controllers' and doctors' awareness of privacy protection. Coordinated efforts are needed to ensure the real realization of doctors' personal privacy rights and interests.

4. 例题详解

【例句】说到底是年轻人的压力很大，处于创业阶段，需要不时地拼搏，而中年人大功告成，可以卸下担子，逃避风雨，享受一下所谓的宁静淡泊与闲适了。

【参考译文】

The crux of the problem is that young people are under extreme pressure, for being at the start of their career; they have to exert themselves to the utmost. The middle-aged people, however, may relieve themselves of their load and retreat into a quiet, non-ambitious and leisurely life since they have accomplished whatever they have.

【解析】

1）这个句子有两层意思，一层是讲年轻人，另一层是讲中年人，翻译时可以作为断句的依据。

2）第一层意思中"年轻人压力很大"是主要信息，"处于创业阶段，需要不时地拼搏"是说明"压力大"的原因，是次要的，不能用同样结构，可以用状语从句。而其中"处于创业阶段"又是说明为什么"需要不时地拼搏"的，语言结构还要次一等，可以用短语 being at the start of their career。

3）第二层意思中，"大功告成"是后面"卸下担子"和"享受"的原因。同样不能用同一语言结构，被说明的用主句，说明原因的用从句 since they have accomplished whatever they have。

【例1】根据美国科学家发表在 *Proceedings B* 上的研究结果：医院的医务工作人员快速持续地实施控制紧急感染的程序，比如戴面罩、穿工作服、严格洗手等，是在没有疫苗应用的情况下控制感染性疾病唯一而又最重要的措施。

通过建立 SARS 的数学模型，科学家探讨怎样最有效地应对未治疗的感染性疾病在医院里的快速传播。他们发现，花费不多、易于实施的全院接触预防措施是所有疾病控制措施中最有效的一种，甚至可以替代诸如病人隔离设施、检疫、医务工作者的隔离等花费较多的措施。

他们的研究结果对全世界所有国家具有重要的意义，尤其是那些医疗资源有限的国家。由于全球化带来的空前的人口大流动，新的、未治疗的传染病有不断增加的危险，这将对全球的公共卫生系统提出很大的挑战。

【参考译文】

According to the research results published in *Proceedings B* by American scientists: Hospital medical staff implement procedures for controlling emergency infections quickly and continuously, such as wearing face masks, working clothes, and strictly brushing hands, etc., to control infections, which is the only and most important measure for infectious diseases without the application of vaccines.

Scientists have established a mathematical model of SARS to explore how to best deal with the rapid spread of untreated infectious diseases in hospitals. They found that hospital-wide contact preventions that are inexpensive and easy to implement are one of the most effective of all disease control measures, and can even replace those such as expensive patient isolation facilities, quarantine, and medical staff isolation.

The results of their research are of great significance to all countries, especially those with limited medical resources. Due to the unprecedented large-scaled population movements brought about by globalization, new and untreated infectious diseases are causing increasing risks. This will put great challenges on the global public health system.

【解析】

1）"根据"往往用 according to，based on 等表达方式，"比如"可用 such as，including 等。第一段的主句是冒号后的内容。先分析该句的主干：实施控制紧急感染的程序＋是＋措施。翻译时可使用主系表的基本句型。然后再看"的""地""得"等标志词的定语和状语部分，进行对应翻译后放到被修饰词的前后。在表语"是在没有疫苗应用的情况下控制感染性疾病唯一而又最重要的措施"中，"唯一的""最重要的"可直接做前置定语，置于核心词 measure 前，"没有疫苗应用的情况下"是伴随条件，可使用介词结构 without 来表达。

2）"通过建立 SARS 的数学模型，科学家探讨怎样最有效地应对未治疗的感染性疾病在医院里的快速传播"中，"通过"表示方式，可以用 through，with，by 等，此时主干为"科学家＋探讨有效应对快速传播＋through 数学模型"。

3）"他们发现……"句中难点在宾语从句上。"花费不多、易于实施的全院接触预防措施是所有疾病控制措施中最有效的一种，甚至可以替代诸如病人隔离设施、检疫、医务工作者的隔离等花费较多的措施"，该句中主干为"预防措施是最有效的一种"，"花费不多、易于实施的"可作为并列结构在定语从句中体现，"甚至可以替代……"可作为并列谓语处理，因为在语义上和"最有效的一种"是并列的，当然也可使用定语从句来对"最有效的一种"做进一步解释说明。

4）"由于全球化带来的空前的人口大流动，新的、未能治疗的传染病有不断增加的危险，这将对全球的公共卫生系统提出很大的挑战"中，由于"due to""because""because of""thanks to"等表示因果逻辑关系，该句的主干为"这将挑战公共卫生系统，由于……"，原因状语可置于句首，也可放在主句后面。

【例2】医疗上的决策应该基于具体的观察和确切的证据。通常，确切的证据并不存在，或当它确实存在的时候，又没有被采纳。随着我们盯着电脑屏幕的时间越来越长，观察病人的时间越来越少，具体的观察也被渐渐忽略掉了。

尸检始终表明，四分之一的死亡是由医疗意外或并发症造成的。我们越来越多地基于前瞻性的临床判断和大量的数据来做出决断。然而，正如天气一样，即便你有数以亿计的数据支持，对生命进行预测也是不可能的。现如今，海量的数据及其确定性是医学和学术领域里最热门的潮流。我们了解缘由：我们热爱技术。这合乎情理，可以理解。我们拼命地想要理解并划分人的情况，以减少其变异性，从而能合乎逻辑地定量使用资源。但是面对医学上的不确定性，当真正的病人坐在我们面前跟我们要答案的时候，答案很有可能并不存在。临床试验和计算机数据库很少能代表真实具体的临床挑战。所以我们聆听、观察，然后共同做出决定。医学诊断和直觉并不都是合乎逻辑的。

【参考译文】

Decisions on medicine are supposed to rest on concrete observations and hard evidence. Often, hard evidence does not exist or when it does, it isn't adopted. As we stare at computer screens longer and at patients less, concrete observation tends to be missed.

Autopsies have consistently shown that one in four deaths occur from unexpected accidents or complications. We make decisions on the base of foregoing clinical judgement and large amount of data. Like the weather, however, life is impossible to predict even when you have a billion data. Massive data and its certainty are our hottest trend in medicine and academics right now, the reason of which is clear: we love technology. It is rational and understandable. We want desperately to understand and compartmentalize types of human conditions, to minimize its variability, so we can ration our resources logically. But in the face of medical uncertainty, the real patient that sits before us demands an answer where, more likely than not, no real answer exists. Real concrete clinical challenges are rarely represented in a clinical trial or computer database. So we listen. We observe. Then we decide, together. Medical judgment and intuition are not always logic.

【解析】

1）"基于"有多种表达方式：rest on, base on 等；"随着我们盯着电脑屏幕的时间越来越长，观察病人的时间越来越少"中的两个比较级，用对应的 longer and less 来表达。tend to do 的意思是"常常，趋向于"。

2）"四分之一"的表达方式：one fourth，one in four，one out of four。

3）"海量的数据及其确定性是医学和学术领域里最热门的潮流。我们了解缘由：我们热爱技术。"该句是两个简单句，根据句子之间的逻辑关系，用 which 将第二个简单句变成定语从句，使得句子间逻辑关系更紧密。当然，用两个简单句来表达也没有问题。

4）"所以我们聆听、观察，然后共同做出决定。医学诊断和直觉并不都是合乎逻辑的。"这句话在翻译时，保留了简单句的格式，清晰、简单、明确，用句式体现出做决策前的必备条件。将其整合成一个并列句"We listen, observe and decide."也没有问题。

【例 3】如果你认为服用维生素将减少患肺癌的危险性，那么要三思了。研究者在调查了 77721 人之后指出，摄入维生素 E 太多的人，尤其是吸烟者，有一小部分的人有更高的患肺癌的风险。他们跟踪了使用多元维生素、维生素 C 和维生素 E 的情况，研究使用维生素是否能使人免于患上肺癌。然而他们发现没有一种维生素与减少患病的危险性相关。这项研究的被试者被跟踪了四年，521 位患上了肺癌，而绝大多数患者是吸烟者或曾经的吸烟者。在那些患者中，研究者发现，除了有吸烟史、家族史及年龄增长等因素外，少量更高的患癌风险率与过度补充维生素 E 密切相关。研究者说，对于那些每天服用 400 毫克维生素 E 长达 10 年的人来说，患病风险性增加至 28%。

【参考译文】

If you think that taking vitamins will reduce the risk of lung cancer, think twice. After investigating 77,721 people, the researchers pointed out that a small part of people who consume too much vitamin E, especially smokers, have a higher risk of lung cancer. They tracked the use of multivitamins, vitamin C and E, and studied whether the use of vitamins can prevent people from developing lung cancer. However, they found that none of the vitamins was associated with reducing the risk of illness. Participants in this study were followed for four years. 521 had lung cancer, and the vast majority of patients were smokers or former smokers. Among those patients, the researchers found that in addition to smoking history, family history, and age, a small amount of higher cancer risk is closely related to excessive vitamin E supplementation. The researchers said that for those who took 400 mg of vitamin E daily for up to 10 years, the risk of disease increased to 28%.

【解析】

1）三思而行：think twice。

2）"研究者在调查了 77721 人之后指出，摄入维生素 E 太多的人，尤其是吸烟者，有一小部分的人有更高的患肺癌的风险。"先确定该句的主干结构：研究者指出……，再确定宾语从句：一小部分人有更高的患癌风险。接着安排"摄入维生素 E 太多的人"，用定语从句 who consume too much……。最后再完善状语等修饰词组。

3）"这项研究的被试者被跟踪了四年，521 位患上了肺癌，而绝大多数患者是吸烟者或曾经的吸烟者。"翻译该句的时候要注意：如果用简单句处理，该句需要拆分成两个分句，如参考译文所示。如果用复合句处理，则需要使用定语从句来连接：Participants in this study were followed for four years, 521 of whom had lung cancer, and the vast majority were smokers or former smokers.

4）长达：up to；增加至：increase to。如果表达增幅，则用 by 或者 of。

5. 汉译英专项练习

Practice One

世界卫生组织确定了传染病出现的五个阶段：出现前、出现、局部传播、流行和大流行。哈佛大学的医学家提出，最大程度地降低未来暴发疫病的风险，应该关注"检测和遏制新出现的人畜共患病（zoonotic diseases）的威胁"，具体应做到监测病原体、更好地管理野生动物贸易和狩猎，以及减少森林砍伐，尽可能阻止疾病从动物传播到人类，预防未来的流行病。相比之下，检测、治疗和疫苗，虽能减少死亡，但不能阻止病毒传播，且永远无法阻止新病原体出现。

专家说，人类对野生动物的保护应该像对人类自身的保护一样，有一个规范的管理制度，保护环境，维持生态平衡，与动物和平相处，不要改变它们的生活习惯。另外，相关部门应当对野生动物贸易加强病原体监测，规范禽畜养殖、运输、屠宰、贮存、出售等过程的防疫流程。

参考译文：

The World Health Organization has identified five stages of the emergence of infectious diseases: preemergence, emergence, local transmission, epidemic and pandemic. Harvard medical experts proposed that we must aim at "detecting and curbing the emerging threat of zoonotic diseases" to minimize the risk of future outbreaks. We should specifically monitor pathogens, better manage wildlife trade and hunting, reduce deforestation, prevent the spread of diseases from animals to humans as much as possible, and prevent future epidemics. In contrast, although detection, treatment and vaccine can reduce death, they cannot prevent the spread of the virus, and can never prevent the emergence of new pathogens.

Experts said that human beings should protect wild animals as they do to themselves. A standardized management system should be built to protect the environment and maintain ecological balance. It can ensure us to live in peace with animals without changing their living habits. In addition, relevant departments should strengthen pathogen monitoring for wildlife trade and standardize the epidemic prevention process of livestock breeding, transportation, slaughter, storage and sale.

Practice Two

我们的大脑就像一个运转的机器，支配我们的思想和运动，经常使用就会越来越顺畅和灵敏。反之，思考得越少，就会变得越迟钝。怎样锻炼自己的大脑呢？

规划是个不错的办法。先将想做的事情列个清单，尝试在执行过程中不参考笔记，完成后与笔记对照，不仅有益于高效完成工作，还能锻炼大脑。为了更好地实施，在这里提供几个选择。

规划下厨：老人可以尝试将自己安排的菜谱、学做新菜等所有流程写下来，然后不参考笔记自己试着烹饪。完成后再与笔记对照是否相符。

规划出门路径：如果只需步行就可到达，或者是曾经走过的路线，建议不要使用导航软件，而是用大脑去规划从 A 点到 B 点的路径。

　　除此之外，日常使用回想法也可以锻炼大脑。如每晚睡前回忆当天发生的事或者写日记记录。如果觉得困难，刚开始时可以只回想每天吃过的食物，然后循序渐进。

　　参考译文：

　　Our brain, like a running machine, controls our thoughts and movements. It will become more and more sensitive if used often. On the contrary, the less you think, the slower you become. How to exercise your brain?

　　Planning is useful. Make a to-do list. Try not to refer to it in the process of execution. After completion, compare them with your notes, which helps to complete work efficiently when exercising your brain. For better implementation, several options are provided here.

　　Plan cooking: The elderly can learn to cook new dishes. Write down all the processes of their own recipes first and then try to cook without referring to their notes. Check whether it is consistent with the notes after completion.

　　Plan the way out: Within walking distance or by familiar routine, don't use navigation software. Use your memory instead.

　　In addition, recalling can also exercise the brain, such as remembering what happened or keeping a diary before going to bed. If you find it difficult, start with the food you eat every day and then step by step.

Practice Three

　　中国作为一个发展中国家面临着发展经济和保护环境的双重任务。然而，我国人口众多，资源相对不足，经济规模越来越大，经济发展与资源和环境之间的矛盾日益突出。环境污染严重，生态状况恶化、资源耗费巨大、回收率低而导致环境破坏等问题，已成为中国经济可持续发展的瓶颈。

　　从国情出发，中国在全面推进现代化的过程中，已将环境保护作为一项基本国策，将实现经济持续发展作为一项重要战略，同时在全国范围内开展污染防治和生态环境保护，环境恶化的状况基本得到了控制。实践表明，我们协调经济发展和环境保护两者之间的关系的做法是行之有效的。人类发展只有合理地利用自然界，与自然界保持和谐，才能维持和发展人类所创造的文明，才能与自然界共生共荣、协调发展。中国作为国际社会的成员，在努力保护自己环境的同时，还积极参与国际环保事务，促进国际环保合作，并认真履行国际义务。所有这些都充分表明了中国政府和人民保护全球环境的诚意和决心。

　　参考译文：

　　As a developing country, China is faced with the dual tasks of economic development and environmental protection. However, China has a large population, relatively insufficient resources, growing economic scale, and the contradiction between economic development and resources and environment is becoming increasingly prominent. Serious environmental pollution, deterioration of ecological conditions, huge resource consumption and low recovery rate have become the bottleneck of China's sustainable economic development.

Based on China's national conditions, during comprehensively promoting modernization, China has taken environmental protection as a basic national policy and the realization of sustainable economic development as an important strategy. At the same time, China has carried out pollution prevention and ecological environmental protection throughout the country, and the deterioration of the environment has been basically controlled. Practice shows that our practice of coordinating the relationship between economic development and environmental protection is effective. Only by making rational use of nature and maintaining harmony with nature, can human development maintain and develop the civilization created by human beings and coexist with nature for common prosperity and coordinated development. As a member of the international community, while striving to protect its own environment, China has also actively participated in international environmental protection affairs, promoted international environmental protection cooperation, and earnestly fulfilled its international obligations. All these fully demonstrate the sincerity and determination of the Chinese government and people to protect the global environment.

Practice Four

俗话说：情绪有多糟糕，身体就有多糟糕。其实，再如何养生都不如保持一个好心态。

国医大师卢芳曾在采访中谈到，良好的精神状态对人体健康有直接影响。频繁生气或者暴怒，一方面无法解决问题，另一方面也对身体不好。他认为，养生首先要控情绪。人的一生不可能完全顺风顺水，当你遇到困境、挫折的时候，要注意控制自己的情绪，努力以乐观的情绪去面对。

自古以来，我们发现身边的长寿老人都是心态好的、笑口常开的。却很少见谁整天哀怨忧愁可以到期颐之年的。现实研究也证实确实如此。一项刊发在《美国国家科学院院刊》上的针对 7 万多名志愿者长达 30 年的随访发现：乐观的人活到 85 岁及以上的概率更大。

当你情绪不好，再多养生都是徒劳。学会有个好心态，尽量让自己处在轻松、愉悦的生活环境中，这比吃什么都重要！

参考译文：

As the saying goes: your health is as bad as your emotion. In fact, a good mindset is essential to your health.

As Lu Fang said in an interview, who is a master of Chinese medicine, a good mindset has a direct impact on human health. Frequent anger or rage cannot solve the problem; it is even bad for your health. He believes controlling emotions is the key to stay healthy. None will have an extremely easy life. When you encounter difficulties and setbacks, put your emotions into control and try to face them with optimism.

Since ancient times, we have found that the long-lived people around us have a good state of mind and often laugh. It's rare to see someone who can live long full of sorrow. The result has been confirmed by studies. A 30-year follow-up of more than 70,000 volunteers, published in the *Proceedings of the National Academy of Sciences*, found that optimistic people were more likely to live to 85 and over.

When you are in a bad mood, it is no use to talk about health. Learn to have a good attitude and try to put yourself in a relaxed and pleasant living environment, which is more important than what you eat!